The Medical Management of AIDS

Second Edition

MERLE A. SANDE, M.D.

Professor and Vice-Chairman, Department of Medicine,
University of California, San Francisco;
Chief, Medical Service, San Francisco General Hospital,
San Francisco, California

PAUL A. VOLBERDING, M.D.

Associate Professor, Department of Medicine,
University of California, San Francisco;
Director, AIDS Program, San Francisco General Hospital,
San Francisco, California

W.B. SAUNDERS COMPANY
Harcourt Brace Jovanovich, Inc.

Philadelphia, London, Toronto, Montreal, Sydney, Tokyo

W. B. SAUNDERS COMPANY

Harcourt Brace Jovanovich, Inc.

The Curtis Center
Independence Square West
Philadelphia, PA 19106

Library of Congress Cataloging-in-Publication Data

The Medical management of AIDS / edited by Merle A. Sande, Paul A.
   Volberding. —2nd ed.
      p.   cm.
   Includes bibliographical references.
   Includes index.
   ISBN 0-7216-3505-9
   1.   AIDS (Disease)—Treatment.   I.   Sande, Merle A.
II.   Volberding, Paul.
   [DNLM: 1.   Acquired Immunodeficiency Syndrome.   2.   HIV.   WD308
M489]
RC607.A26M43   1990
616.97′92—dc20
DNLM/DLC   90-8584
for Library of Congress   CIP

Listed here is the latest translated edition of this book together with the language of the translation and the publisher.

Spanish—*first edition*—NEISA Cedro 512 06450 Mexico D.F., Mexico

Sponsoring Editor: Martin Wonsiewicz

The Medical Management of AIDS   ISBN 0-7216-3505-9

Last digit is the print number: 9   8   7   6   5   4   3

Dedicated to our devoted staff
of nurses, physicians, administrators, social workers,
and colleagues at San Francisco General Hospital,
who have extended their hands
and opened their hearts to provide compassionate care
for the many AIDS patients of our city

CONTRIBUTORS

DONALD I. ABRAMS, M.D.
Associate Professor of Clinical Medicine,
University of California, San Francisco;
Assistant Director, AIDS Activities Division,
San Francisco General Hospital, San Francisco, California
Hematologic Manifestations of HIV Infection

DONALD ARMSTRONG, M.D.
Professor of Medicine, Cornell University Medical College, Ithaca, New York;
Chief, Infectious Disease Service, and Director,
Microbiology Laboratory, Memorial Sloan-Kettering Cancer Center,
New York, New York
Fungal Infections in AIDS: Histoplasmosis and Coccidioidomycosis

TIMOTHY G. BERGER, M.D.
Assistant Clinical Professor,
University of California, San Francisco;
Chief, Department of Dermatology,
San Francisco General Hospital, San Francisco, California
Dermatologic Care in the AIDS Patient: A 1990 Update

BRUCE BREW, M.B., B.S.
Senior Lecturer in Medicine,
University of New South Wales;
Staff Specialist Neurologist,
St. Vincent's Hospital,
Sydney, Australia
Management of the Neurologic Complications of HIV-1 Infection and AIDS

WILLIAM BUHLES, D.V.M., Ph.D.
Department Head, Department of Immunology and Antiviral Therapy,
Institute of Clinical Medicine,
Division of Syntex, Inc.,
Palo Alto, California
Management of Herpes Virus Infections (CMV, HSV, VZV)

JOHN P. CELLO, M.D.
Professor of Medicine,
University of California, San Francisco;
Chief, Gastroenterology, San Francisco General Hospital,
San Francisco, California
AIDS-Associated Gastrointestinal Disease

RICHARD E. CHAISSON, M.D.
Director, AIDS Services,
Assistant Professor of International Health, and
Assistant Professor of Epidemiology,
Johns Hopkins University School of Hygiene and Public Health,
Baltimore, Maryland
Infections Due to Encapsulated Bacteria, Salmonella, Shigella, *and* Campylobacter

DAVID A. COOPER, B.Sc. (Med), M.D., F.R.A.C.P., F.R.C.P.A.
Associate Professor of Medicine and Director,
National Centre in HIV Epidemiology and Clinical Research,
University of New South Wales;
Senior Staff Specialist in Immunology,
Centre of Immunology, St. Vincent's Hospital,
Sydney, Australia
Primary HIV Infection: Clinical, Immunologic and Serologic Aspects

BRIAN R. DANNEMANN, M.D.
Postdoctoral Fellow, Division of Infectious Diseases,
Stanford University School of Medicine,
Stanford, California
Toxoplasmosis in Patients with AIDS

BASIL DONOVAN, M.B., B.S., Dip. Ven. (Lond.), F.A.C.Ven.
Senior Staff Specialist and Director,
Sydney STD Centre, Sydney Hospital,
Sydney, Australia
Primary HIV Infection: Clinical, Immunologic and Serologic Aspects

W. LAWRENCE DREW, M.D., Ph.D.
Associate Professor, Medicine and Laboratory Medicine,
University of California, San Francisco;
Director, Clinical Microbiology and Infectious Diseases, and
Director, Biskind Pathology Research Laboratory,
Mount Zion Hospital and Medical Center,
San Francisco, California
Management of Herpes Virus Infections (CMV, HSV, VZV)

RONALD J. DWORKIN, M.D.
Fellow, Infectious Diseases,
Mount Zion Hospital and Medical Center,
San Francisco, California
Management of Herpes Virus Infections (CMV, HSV, VZV)

KIM S. ERLICH, M.D.
Infectious Disease Consultant,
Seton Medical Center,
Daly City, California
Management of Herpes Virus Infections (CMV, HSV, VZV)

MARGARET A. FISCHL, M.D.
Professor of Medicine,
University of Miami School of Medicine;
Director, Special Immunology, Jackson Memorial Hospital,
Miami, Florida
Treatment of HIV Infection

JULIE LOUISE GERBERDING, M.D.
Assistant Professor of Medicine, Infectious Diseases,
University of California, San Francisco, School of Medicine;
Physician Specialist and Director, HIV Counseling and Testing Service,
San Francisco General Hospital,
San Francisco, California
Occupational HIV Transmission: Issues for Health Care Providers

PHILIP C. GOODMAN, M.D.
Professor of Clinical Radiology and Medicine,
University of California, San Francisco,
San Francisco, California
The Chest Film in AIDS

DEBORAH GREENSPAN, B.D.S.
Clinical Professor, Department of Stomatology,
School of Dentistry,
University of California, San Francisco;
Clinical Director, Oral AIDS Center,
San Francisco, California
Diagnosis and Management of the Oral Manifestations of HIV Infection and AIDS

JOHN S. GREENSPAN, B.Sc., B.D.S., Ph.D., F.R.C.Path.
Professor and Chairman, Department of Stomatology,
School of Dentistry, and Professor of Pathology,
School of Medicine,
University of California, San Francisco;
Director, Oral AIDS Center,
San Francisco, California
Diagnosis and Management of the Oral Manifestations of HIV Infection and AIDS

MOSES GROSSMAN, M.D.
Professor and Vice Chairman of Pediatrics,
University of California, San Francisco;
Chief, Pediatric Services, San Francisco General Hospital,
San Francisco, California
Special Problems in the Child with AIDS

JULIE HAMBLETON, M.D.
Chief Medical Resident,
San Francisco General Hospital,
University of California, San Francisco,
San Francisco, California
Hematologic Manifestations of HIV Infection

HARRY HOLLANDER, M.D.
Associate Professor of Clinical Medicine,
University of California, San Francisco;
Director and Attending Physician, AIDS Clinic,
San Francisco General Hospital,
San Francisco, California
Care of the Individual with Early HIV Infection: Unanswered Questions, Including the Syphilis Dilemma

PHILIP C. HOPEWELL, M.D.
Professor of Medicine,
University of California, San Francisco;
Chief, Chest Service,
San Francisco General Hospital,
San Francisco, California
Pneumocystis carinii *Pneumonia*

ALLISON IMRIE, B.Sc.
Senior Scientific Officer,
Centre for Immunology, St. Vincent's Hospital,
Sydney, Australia
Primary HIV Infection: Clinical, Immunologic and Serologic Aspects

DENNIS M. ISRAELSKI, M.D.
Assistant Clinical Professor,
Infectious Diseases in Medicine,
Department of Medicine, Stanford University School of Medicine,
Stanford, California;
Medical Director, Palo Alto Veterans Administration Hospital,
AIDS Program, Palo Alto, California;
Medical AIDS Position, San Mateo County General Hospital,
San Mateo, California
Toxoplasmosis in Patients with AIDS

MARK A. JACOBSON, M.D.
Assistant Professor of Medicine in Residence,
University of California, San Francisco;
Attending Physician,
San Francisco General Hospital,
San Francisco, California
Mycobacterial Diseases: Tuberculosis and Mycobacterium avium *Complex*

PAULA JESSON, J.D.
Deputy City Attorney for the City and County of San Francisco,
San Francisco, California
Legal Ramifications of AIDS

LAWRENCE D. KAPLAN, M.D.
Assistant Clinical Professor of Medicine,
University of California, San Francisco;
AIDS/Oncology Program,
San Francisco General Hospital,
San Francisco, California
The Malignancies Associated with AIDS

JAY A. LEVY, M.D.
Professor of Medicine and
Research Associate,
Cancer Research Institute,
University of California, San Francisco, School of Medicine,
San Francisco, California
Features of HIV and the Host Response That Influence Progression to Disease

GRACE MINAMOTO, M.D.
Instructor in Clinical Medicine,
Columbia University, College of Physicians and Surgeons;
Junior Assistant Attending Physician,
St. Luke's–Roosevelt Hospital Center,
New York, New York
Fungal Infections in AIDS: Histoplasmosis and Coccidioidomycosis

LORI A. PANTHER, M.D.
Chief Medical Resident,
San Francisco General Hospital,
San Francisco, California
Cryptococcal Meningitis in AIDS

RONALD PENNY, M.D., D.Sc., F.R.A.C.P., F.R.C.P.A.
Professor of Clinical Immunology,
University of New South Wales;
Director, Centre for Immunology,
St. Vincent's Hospital,
Sydney, Australia
Primary HIV Infection: Clinical, Immunologic and Serologic Aspects

JOHN P. PHAIR, M.D.
Professor of Medicine,
Northwestern University Medical School,
Chicago, Illinois
Natural History of HIV Infection

RICHARD W. PRICE, M.D.
Professor and Head and Clinical Chief,
Department of Neurology,
University of Minnesota Hospital and Clinic,
Minneapolis, Minnesota
Management of the Neurologic Complications of HIV-1 Infection and AIDS

THOMAS C. QUINN, M.D., M.S.
Senior Investigator,
National Institute of Allergy and Infectious Diseases;
Associate Professor of Medicine,
Johns Hopkins University,
Baltimore, Maryland
Global Epidemiology of HIV Infections

JACK S. REMINGTON, M.D.
Professor of Medicine, Division of Infectious Diseases,
Stanford University School of Medicine,
Stanford, California;
Marcus A. Krupp Research Chair and Chairman,
Department of Immunology and Infectious Diseases,
Research Institute,
Palo Alto Medical Foundation,
Palo Alto, California
Toxoplasmosis in Patients with AIDS

MERLE A. SANDE, M.D.
Professor and Vice Chairman,
Department of Medicine,
University of California, San Francisco;
Chief, Medical Service,
San Francisco General Hospital,
San Francisco, California
Cryptococcal Meningitis in AIDS

JOHN D. STANSELL, M.D.
Clinical Instructor of Medicine,
University of California, San Francisco;
Attending Physician, AIDS Consult Service,
San Francisco General Hospital,
San Francisco, California
Cardiac, Endocrine, and Renal Complications of HIV Infection

BRETT TINDALL, B.App.Sc., M.Sc.
Senior Project Scientist,
National Centre in HIV Epidemiology and Clinical Research,
University of New South Wales;
Scientific Officer, Centre for Immunology,
St. Vincent's Hospital,
Sydney, Australia
Primary HIV Infection: Clinical, Immunologic and Serologic Aspects

PAUL A. VOLBERDING, M.D.
Associate Professor of Medicine,
University of California, San Francisco;
Director, AIDS Program,
San Francisco General Hospital,
San Francisco, California
Clinical Care of Patients with AIDS: Developing a System

JAMES R. WINKLER, D.M.D.
Assistant Professor, Periodontology,
University of California, San Francisco,
San Francisco, California
Diagnosis and Management of the Oral Manifestations of HIV Infection and AIDS

CONSTANCE B. WOFSY, M.D.
Professor of Clinical Medicine,
University of California, San Francisco;
Co-Director, AIDS Activities Program,
Assistant Chief, Infectious Diseases Division, and Director,
AIDS Provider Education Experience,
San Francisco General Hospital,
San Francisco, California
Prevention of HIV Transmission

PREFACE

No disease in modern times has had quite the impact on the civilized world as has the acquired immunodeficiency syndrome (AIDS). The disease has rapidly afflicted over 100,000 persons in the United States, and between 1 and 2 million more are believed to be infected with the causative agent, the human immunodeficiency virus (HIV). The scope of the epidemic is even more dramatic in equatorial Africa, where millions of people are already infected. Although the outlook in the near future for curative treatment or effective vaccine is grim, some measure of success in responding to this tragedy has been achieved. The medical and scientific communities have effectively cooperated to quickly accumulate epidemiologic, clinical, and basic science knowledge about this pandemic infection. We have rapidly expanded our knowledge of retrovirology and have turned many of our most creative minds toward unraveling the biology of HIV. Also, we have developed highly efficient mechanisms for treating HIV-infected individuals.

Amid the social and political upheaval precipitated by the AIDS epidemic, a critical problem has silently but steadily emerged: Who is to provide care for the increasing numbers of afflicted individuals? There is a desperate need for physicians, nurses, and other health care workers to provide skilled care for these patients. Although few practitioners have denied their responsibility to provide care, there is a reluctance on the part of some to actively assume a role in caring for these stricken individuals. In some, the reluctance is undoubtedly due to fears of acquiring the infection through patient care activities. For others, inadequate reimbursement schedules for HIV-related problems reduce the economic incentive to devote the large amounts of time and resources required to treat HIV-infected patients. Perhaps most importantly, the newness of AIDS and the rapid evolution of knowledge about the complications of HIV infection have made it difficult for practitioners not directly involved in AIDS research to keep abreast of new developments in the field. It is common for individual physicians, especially those who have limited opportunities for immediate consultation, to feel poorly equipped to handle AIDS patients.

For these reasons, we believe that an important contribution to the medical literature can be made by publishing an up-to-date text that addresses the clinical issues commonly encountered by practitioners who accept the challenges that AIDS provides. In our second edition, we have again compiled contributions from many of the world's leading authorities on AIDS. The biology and epidemiology of HIV infection and approaches to reduce sexual and nosocomial transmission of the virus are reviewed. The initial diagnostic evaluation of HIV-infected patients is outlined, and a summary of the multidisciplinary approach to treating these patients within the community is provided. We have also addressed the controversies related to HIV testing and have discussed some of the legal ramifications that the physician must face when caring for this patient population. Probably the most important and rapidly changing section deals with zidovudine—how and when to use it.

The infectious complications of HIV infection, including diagnosis and treatment of *Pneumocystis carinii* pneumonia and other protozoal, mycobacterial, fungal, and bacterial and viral infections, have been reviewed from a clinical perspective, as have the AIDS-related malignancies, including Kaposi's sarcoma and lymphomas. In this edition we have also included a review of the hematologic, endocrine, renal, and cardiac complications of AIDS. In each chapter an attempt has been made to present information in a practical format that should allow the primary care physician dealing with the disease for the first time to attack the problem in a logical and up-to-date fashion. Discussions on the approach to antiviral treatment for HIV infection and the special problems faced by HIV-infected children have also been included.

We hope that this will provide a useful update and review of contemporary clinical issues relevant to caring for individuals with HIV-related illnesses. We also hope that it will help alleviate some of the apprehensions elicited when patients with HIV infection and its myriad complications are encountered for the first time, so that patients can be approached with confidence and compassion.

We would like to thank The Burroughs Wellcome Company for providing the educational grant that made this publication, and the associated conference, possible. Also, special thanks are extended to Jan Rogerson and her staff for their valued assistance and to our publisher, the W. B. Saunders Company, who again with the second edition has set a record in completing publication 6 months from the time the chapters were completed. This rapid turnaround has allowed us to provide the most up-to-date review possible of the clinical aspects of caring for patients with AIDS.

MERLE A. SANDE, MD

General Guidelines for Initiation of ZDV Therapy in Early HIV Disease

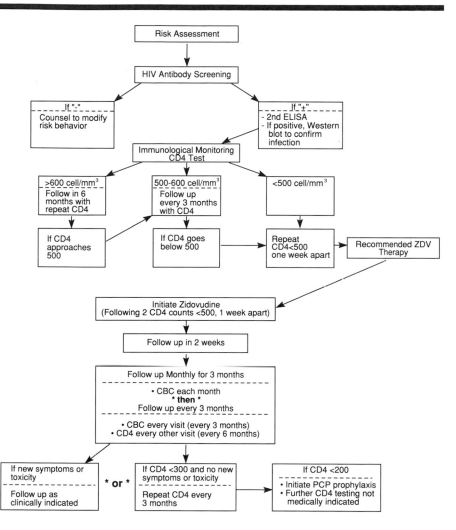

An expert panel convened by the National Institute of Allergy and Infectious Diseases participated in a March 3-4, 1990, State-of-the Art Conference on AZT Therapy for Early HIV Infection. The panel recommended use of low doses (500 mg) of zidovudine for HIV-infected individuals with CD4 cell counts of less than 500/mm³ and published a series of recommendations derived from its deliberations. Because of the importance of these recommendations, we have adapted the following composite algorithm from the panel's algorithms for management of HIV-infected patients.

COLOR PLATE IA. Maculopapular rash on trunk of an individual with acute HIV infection (See page 68.)

COLOR PLATE IB. Hairy leukoplakia on tongue. (See page 138.)

mentioned with fig 11-6

COLOR PLATE IC. Giemsa stain of induced sputum demonstrating cysts and trophozoites of *Pneumocystis carinii.* There is no uptake of stain by cyst wall; therefore, walls appear as clear-to-white circles. Trophozoites appear as dark dots. (×960) (See page 218.)

COLOR PLATE ID. Acid-fast stain of lymph node tissue demonstrating large numbers of red-staining *Mycobacterium avium-intracellulare.* (See page 298.)

COLOR PLATE IE. Severe edema complicating advanced lower extremity cutaneous Kaposi's sarcoma. (See page 342.)

COLOR PLATE IF. Cytomegalovirus-associated retinitis. Note characteristic hemorrhages and exudates. (See page 317.)

COLOR PLATE IG. Widespread cutaneous Kaposi's sarcoma in a Caucasian individual: typical violacious appearance of skin lesions. (See page 342.)

COLOR PLATE IH. Typical appearance of early Kaposi's sarcoma involving the palate. (See page 342.)

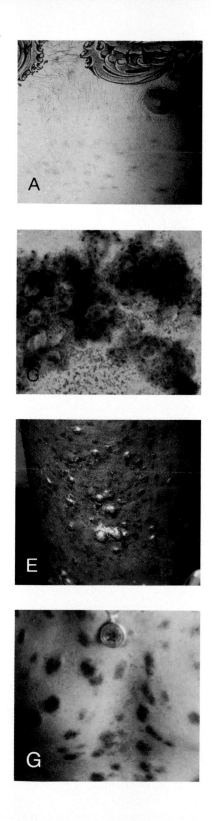
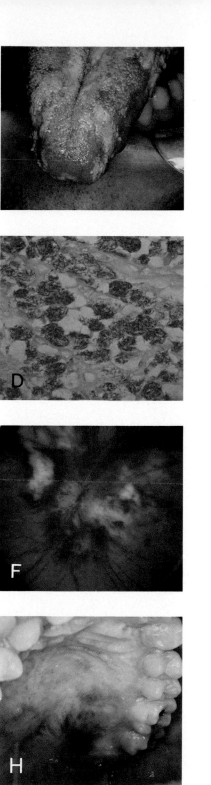

CONTENTS

III SPECIFIC INFECTIONS AND MALIGNANT CONDITIONS

IV SPECIAL ASPECTS OF AIDS

I

THE VIRUS:

Its Transmission and Infection

1

GLOBAL EPIDEMIOLOGY OF HIV INFECTIONS

THOMAS C. QUINN, MD, MS

Since 1981 more than 220,000 cases of acquired immunodeficiency syndrome (AIDS) have been reported from 153 countries. Because of underreporting in many developing countries resulting from the lack of sophisticated diagnostic equipment and health infrastructure required to identify AIDS cases, the World Health Organization (WHO) estimates that more than 500,000 cases of AIDS have occurred worldwide with more than 300,000 deaths during this period.[59,66] Since the recognition of the human immunodeficiency virus type 1 (HIV-1) as the etiologic agent of AIDS in 1984,[3,94] it has become evident that the clinical syndrome of AIDS and its associated deaths represent only a small part of the greater epidemic of HIV-1 infection. Consequently, WHO now estimates from serologic studies that 5 to 10 million people are infected with HIV-1 worldwide, and from this asymptomatic human reservoir of HIV-1 infection continued transmission of HIV-1 to other persons will occur and nearly 1 million cases of AIDS will develop within the next several years.[59,78]

GLOBAL PATTERNS OF SPREAD

Although the immunologic features and pathogenesis of HIV-1 infection appear to be similar throughout the world, geographic variations exist in the epidemiologic patterns and clinical expression of the disease, as well as in the distribution of different human retroviruses such as HIV-1, HIV-2, and human T cell lymphotropic virus (HTLV) infections.[48,83] Epidemiologic studies have consistently demonstrated that HIV-1 has three major modes of transmission: sexual transmission, which may be homosexual, bisexual, or heterosexual; parenteral transmission, including trans-

3

fusion of infected blood products or injection with blood-contaminated needles or syringes; and perinatal transmission.[71,114] The relative frequency of these types of transmission and the rate of HIV-1 introduction and dissemination account for three basic epidemiologic patterns worldwide.[66,77]

The first pattern is observed primarily in developed areas such as Western Europe, Australia, New Zealand, North America, and some urban areas of Latin America. Homosexual or bisexual men and intravenous drug users are the major infected groups. HIV-1 was found first in homosexual men in the mid-1970s, and in some areas more than 50 percent of homosexual men are currently infected.[42] Intravenous drug use accounts for the next largest portion of HIV-1 infection. Heterosexual and perinatal transmission are not a major problem in developed countries, but these modes of trans-mission are increasing, particularly among populations in which HIV-1 infections among intravenous drug users and bisexual men are common, both serving as a bridge for the virus to the heterosexual population.

The second pattern is predominant in Africa and increasing in some areas of Latin America and the Caribbean. Heterosexual transmission is the major mode of transmission in these areas. The virus may have been introduced into these populations in the early or late 1970s, and recent serologic surveys demonstrate that 10 to 20 percent of 20- to 40-year-old persons in some areas are infected.[11,25,47,71,77,83,104,110] Perinatal transmission has also become a major problem in these areas, where 5 to 15 percent of pregnant women are HIV-1 seropositive.[44,112] The ratio of infected males to females is approximately 1:1, and transmission through homosexual activity or intravenous drug use is either absent or at a very low level. Because of the rapid spread of HIV-1 among heterosexuals, these areas tend to have the highest rates of HIV-1 infection among the general pop-ulations that have been surveyed and represent the most difficult areas for control of the epidemic.

The third pattern is evident in Eastern Europe, North Africa, the Middle East, Asia, and most parts of the Pacific, excluding Australia and New Zealand. HIV-1 was probably introduced in these areas during the early to mid-1980s, and only a small number of AIDS cases have been reported. Indigenous homosexual, heterosexual, and intravenous drug use trans-mission have only recently been documented. Although the number of AIDS cases remains small, rapid spread of HIV-1 infection is being doc-umented in some of these countries, particularly among female prostitutes and intravenous drug users.[41,48]

In certain West African countries infection with a second human retro-virus, referred to as HIV-2, has become epidemic.[2,27] High prevalence rates in high-risk individuals, such as hospitalized patients, female prostitutes, and patients in sexually transmitted disease (STD) clinics, suggest that HIV-2 spreads by the same modes of transmission as HIV-1. Systematic surveys for HIV-2 outside West Africa have documented isolated cases in central Africa, North America, and Brazil.[20] During the past 2 years 12 cases of HIV-2 have been diagnosed in North America among patients who have visited or lived in West Africa.[21,22,73,87,98] HIV-2 has been isolated in a Cuban who lived in Angola, and more recently investigators in Brazil have identified several patients with serologic evidence of HIV-2 infection.[31,106]

AIDS SURVEILLANCE

Based on the WHO/Centers for Disease Control (CDC) case definition for AIDS, 222,740 cases of AIDS had been reported from 153 countries as of March 1, 1990 (Fig. 1–1). In the Americas, 147,159 cases or 68 percent of the total have been reported from 44 countries. In the United States alone, 121,645 cases or 85 percent of the cases in the Americas have been reported. For the rest of the Americas, exponential increases in AIDS cases are being reported with 16,458 cases reported in Central and South America and 5547 cases reported from the countries in the Caribbean basin. The Caribbean subregion has reported a number of AIDS cases dispro-

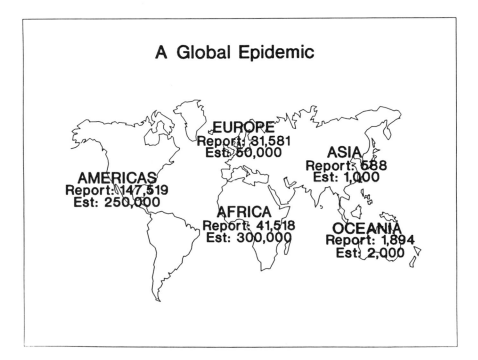

FIGURE 1–1. Worldwide distribution of reported AIDS cases by continent as of March 1, 1990. Because of underreporting in some areas the estimated numbers of cases shown are based on serologic studies and limited surveillance. (Data from World Health Organization.)

portionate to its population base. Excluding the United States, the English-speaking Caribbean countries with only 2 percent of the population and Latin Caribbean countries with 6 percent of the population have reported 10 percent and 21 percent, respectively, of all cases for the Caribbean and Latin America.[83] In contrast to other areas of the Americas, the Caribbean has a male/female ratio of reported AIDS cases of 2.4:1, reflecting an increased number of infected women because of heterosexual transmission of HIV-1.[10] In countries with an increasing number of female AIDS cases in a declining male/female ratio, the proportion of persons with AIDS who are less than 13 years of age also increases proportionately because of perinatal transmission.[45,51] For example, in the Caribbean 11 percent of reported AIDS cases were in children under 5 years of age, reflecting increased mother-to-infant transmission.

In Europe more than 31,000 cases have been reported from 29 countries. The proportions of AIDS cases among high-risk groups are similar in Europe and the United States. Among adults the male/female ratio is 7.4:1, but the sex ratio is closer to 1:1 among intravenous drug users, those having heterosexual contact with other high-risk individuals, and transfusion recipients.[46] In 1988 AIDS cases increased 60.7 percent among homosexuals and bisexuals and 130 percent among intravenous drug users. In some countries such as Italy and Spain more than 60 percent of AIDS cases have occurred among intravenous drug users.

With a late introduction of HIV-1 into Asian and Pacific countries, the number of AIDS cases remains low in those areas, with 1894 cases reported from seven Pacific countries and 588 cases reported from 25 Asian countries. Serologic studies in some of these countries have demonstrated high rates of HIV-1 infection among persons with hemophilia because of importation of factor VIII and IX concentrates from the United States and Europe before the institution of blood screening in 1985. In Southeast Asia the predominant HIV transmission is now among intravenous drug users and their heterosexual partners. In India seroprevalence studies among prostitutes have noted increasing rates of HIV infection, although the number of AIDS cases remains low.[69]

The 41,518 cases reported from 48 African countries is an underestimate of the true number. As documented by serologic studies, HIV infection has spread rapidly, particularly in urban centers of central Africa. Peak infection rates are among women 20 to 39 years of age and men 30 to 49 years of age.[11,25,47,77,104,110] The male/female ratio is 1:1.5, and because of the large number of infected women (up to 10 percent), pediatric cases constitute 15 to 20 percent of the total AIDS cases. Selected seroprevalence studies among diverse urban population groups clearly demonstrate the relatively high frequency of HIV infection among blood donors (up to 20 percent), pregnant women (5 to 10 percent), hospitalized patients (25 to 50 percent), men attending STD clinics (30 to 45 percent), and female prostitutes (40 to 90 percent).[11,25,41,44,47,77,104,110,112] Thus, of all the regions, the countries of central Africa have probably felt the greatest impact of HIV infection and now pose the greatest challenge to control of this epidemic.

CURRENT STATUS OF AIDS IN THE UNITED STATES

Of the 121,645 cases reported in the United States as of Feb. 1, 1990, 119,590 (98.3 percent) occurred among adults and 2055 (1.7 percent) among children less than 13 years of age (Table 1–1). Of the adults, 108,538 (90.8 percent) were men and 11,052 (9.2 percent) were women. Mean age at diagnosis was 37 years. The overall mortality rate was 55 percent at the time of reporting and greater than 90 percent 5 years after diagnosis.[114] AIDS-related deaths disproportionately occurred in persons between 20 and 49 years of age, leading to substantial decreases in life expectancy. Deaths occurring in 1987 among persons with AIDS that were reported to the CDC represented 9 percent of all deaths among persons 25 to 34 years of age and 7 percent of all deaths among persons 35 to 44 years of age. In 1987 AIDS was the seventh leading cause of death before 65 years of age in the United States.[52,72]

The number of AIDS cases was disproportionately high in blacks and Hispanics in the United States, reflecting higher reported rates among black

TABLE 1–1. AIDS CASES BY SEX AND EXPOSURE CATEGORY IN THE UNITED STATES, REPORTED THROUGH JANUARY 1990

	MALES		FEMALES		TOTAL	
TRANSMISSION CATEGORY	No.	%	No.	%	No.	%
Adults/Adolescents						
Homosexual/bisexual	72,153	66	—		72,153	60
Intravenous drug user (IVDU)	19,489	18	5,711	52	25,200	21
Homosexual male/intravenous drug user	8,326	8	—		8,326	7
Hemophilia/coagulation disorder	1,071	1	28	0	1,099	1
Heterosexual contact	2,399	2	3,454	31	5,853	5
Transfusion recipient	1,814	2	1,109	10	2,923	2
Other/undetermined	3,286	3	750	7	4,036	3
Subtotal	108,538	100	11,052	100	119,590	100
Children						
Parent with/at risk for AIDS	846	76	829	89	1,675	82
Hemophilia/coagulation disorder	104	9	4	0	108	5
Transfusion recipient	141	13	76	8	217	11
Undetermined	27	2	28	3	55	3
Subtotal	1,118	100	937	100	2,055	100
TOTAL	109,656	100	11,989	100	121,645	100

From Centers for Disease Control: HIV/AIDS Surveillance Report February 1990, pp. 1-18.

and Hispanic intravenous drug users, their sex partners, and their infants.[52,80] Blacks accounted for 27 percent of the adult cases and 53 percent of the pediatric cases, and Hispanics for 15 percent of the adult cases and 25 percent of pediatric cases. In contrast, blacks and Hispanics account for only 11.6 percent and 6.5 percent, respectively, of the U.S. population. The relative risk of AIDS for blacks and Hispanics is nearly 10 times as high in the northeastern United States as in other regions of the country, partly because of the regional concentration of AIDS transmitted by intravenous drug use. In 1988 the annual incidence of AIDS cases associated with intravenous drug use was 11.5 times higher among blacks and 8.8 times higher among Hispanics than among whites.[56]

Of male patients, 66 percent had a history of homosexual or bisexual activity without intravenous drug use, 18 percent acknowledged intravenous drug use without homosexual or bisexual activity, and 8 percent acknowledged both homosexual activity and intravenous drug use. Another 2 percent had a history of blood transfusion, 1 percent had hemophilia or other coagulation disorders, 2 percent had sex partners at increased risk for HIV-1 or known to be infected with HIV-1, 1 percent were born in countries with predominantly heterosexual transmission of HIV-1, and 3 percent had undetermined means of exposure. This distribution has remained relatively stable except for a decrease in men with a history of homosexual or bisexual activity without intravenous drug use from 70 percent of those reported in 1987 to 63 percent of those reported in 1988. The percentage of men with histories of intravenous drug use and no homosexual or bisexual activity increased from 14 percent in 1987 to 20 percent in 1988. These data suggest that the rate of AIDS among homosexual men is slowing, partly because of adherence to preventive measures such as safe sex guidelines.[42,56,80] In contrast, the incidence of AIDS is continuing to rise among intravenous drug users and their heterosexual partners, groups that need more intensive educational efforts.[24,58,85,89]

The proportion of AIDS patients who are women increased from 8 percent in 1987 to 10 percent in 1988. Mean age at diagnosis was 35.7 years; 51.6 percent were black, 27.9 percent white, 19.5 percent Hispanic, and 0.8 percent other racial groups. As in men, the cumulative incidence of AIDS between 1981 and 1988 was 13.6 times higher among black women and 1.2 times higher among Hispanic women than among white women. Among women with AIDS, 52 percent had a history of intravenous drug use, 31 percent had sex partners at increased risk for or known to be infected with HIV-1, 11 percent had histories of blood transfusion, and 7 percent had undetermined means of exposure. The proportion of women with AIDS who had sex partners at increased risk for HIV-1 rose from 15 percent before 1984 to 26 percent in 1988.[52,67]

Between 1987 and 1988 the number of pediatric cases diagnosed increased 65 percent, reflecting increasing numbers of HIV-1 infections among women who are intravenous drug users or sex partners of users.[52]

Of the 2055 children, 82 percent were born to parents who had or were at risk of AIDS; 11 percent had received infected blood transfusions; and 5 percent were hemophiliacs who had received factor VIII or IX concentrates infected with HIV-1. The remaining 3 percent included patients for whom risk factor information was incomplete. As among adults with AIDS, black and Hispanic children between 1981 and 1988 had a cumulative incidence of AIDS 10 times higher than that of white children.[52]

In the other or undetermined category, one patient was a health care worker who had seroconversion to HIV-1 and development of AIDS after needlestick exposure to blood infected with HIV-1. The undetermined category included 4036 adults and 55 children, of whom 17 percent had died, were lost to follow-up, or refused interview, 72 percent are still under investigation, and 11 percent had an undetermined mode of exposure to HIV-1. Among the last, 103 (39 percent) of 264 persons gave a history of STDs and 63 (35 percent) of 180 men interviewed reported sexual contact with a prostitute. Probably some of these persons represent unreported or unrecognized heterosexual transmission of HIV-1.

MODES OF TRANSMISSION

Sexual Transmission

Serologic surveys and AIDS surveillance suggest that sexual transmission accounts for more than 75 percent of HIV-1 infection worldwide. In developed countries such as the United States, homosexual transmission has been the predominant sexual mode of spread and has been strongly associated with a number of sexual partners and the frequency of receptive anal intercourse.[23,50,57,91,109,113,114] Other practices that lead to rectal trauma, such as receptive "fisting" and douching, appear to increase the risk of infection. Since 1984 more than 50 serologic studies of homosexual and bisexual men in the United States have shown HIV-1 prevalence rates ranging from 10 percent to as high as 70 percent with most between 20 percent and 50 percent.[42,80] Fortunately, recent seroincidence studies of HIV-1 infection among homosexual men have demonstrated a decline in the infection rate in this group, probably because of safer sex practices and a lower frequency of high-risk behaviors.[42,56]

With increasing rates of HIV-1 infection among bisexual men and intravenous drug users, an increasing number of women are being infected with HIV-1 through heterosexual exposure.[67] Among heterosexuals, female prostitutes, patients attending STD clinics, and heterosexual partners of HIV-1-infected persons appear to be at high risk for HIV-1 infection.[26,62] In the United States the proportion of reported cases associated with heterosexual contact increased from 1.1 percent in 1982 to 5 percent in mid-1989. Approximately 70 percent of the index partners for these patients were intravenous drug users, and 18 percent of the index partners for female patients were bisexual men. Interestingly, the male/female ratio of heterosexual contact cases in the United States is 1 : 1.4, similar to the male/female ratio in African countries where heterosexual transmission is the predominant mode of spread.[47,68,77,79] This predominance of women in the heterosexual contact category in the United States is probably due to the larger pool of infected men classified as bisexual or intravenous drug users, but the efficiency of male-to-female versus female-to-male transmission may also be relevant.

The efficiencies of bidirectional transmission have not been well documented, but clearly most heterosexual transmission occurs during vaginal intercourse and receptive anal intercourse also increases the risk of infection in women.[74,90] In one study the relative risk of HIV-1 infection in spouses who engaged in anal intercourse compared with those who had only vaginal sex was 2.3 : 1.[96] Of nine studies of anal intercourse, four found a significantly increased risk of transmission in couples who reported both anal and vaginal intercourse, but the other five studies showed no association with anal intercourse.[79] In several studies investigators have also reported the number of genital-genital exposures for HIV-1 infected persons and their spouses or monogamous sexual partners.[1,18,96,111,115,116] Specifying which sexual exposure resulted in HIV-1 transmission is impossible, but maximum and minimum rates for single exposure can be defined.[74,90] Presumably the lower limit of such transmission is only one exposure that resulted in infection of the susceptible partner, and the upper limit is that all exposures in couples in which both partners are HIV-1 infected involved HIV-1 transmission. The per-contact infectivity for male-to-female transmission of HIV-1 has generally been calculated at less than 0.2 percent, that is, the binomial probability that 15 percent of persons exposed are infected after more than 100 unprotected sexual contacts. However, some persons become infected with HIV-1 after a single or few sexual exposures, whereas others remain uninfected despite hundreds of unprotected sexual contacts. This finding suggests that the likelihood of HIV-1 infection may be substantially affected by intrinsic properties of the HIV-1-infected partner, the virus itself, or the noninfected partner.[74] Variable rates of heterosexual transmission among sex partners of HIV-1-infected individuals have been documented in studies in the United States. Reported rates of infection range from 9 to 20 percent for female partners of infected male hemophiliacs[1,38,64,101]; 26 percent for female sexual partners of bisexual men[53,96]; 19.7 percent and 14.8 percent, respectively, for female and male sexual contacts of transfusion recipients[18]; and 47.8 percent and 50 percent, respectively, for female and male sexual contacts of intravenous drug users.[53,96,115] Even in African studies such as one that examined 250 married couples in which at least one spouse was seropositive, 20 percent were concordantly seropositive and in 80 percent only one partner was infected despite a mean period of 8 years of marriage and unprotected sexual intercourse.[32] This finding is in contrast to another African study of 124 HIV-1 seropositive couples and 150 seronegative couples in which the authors demonstrated that seropositivity in the husbands was significantly associated with sexual contact with prostitutes and a history of STDs within the previous 2 years.[13] Thus, although many couples included in studies of heterosexual HIV-1 transmission have had unprotected sex for prolonged periods, an average of 50 to 60 percent of partners have been infected in most studies. This suggests that, in addition to behavioral factors, biologic factors contribute to the efficiency of HIV-1 transmission.

Some infected individuals may be more efficient transmitters than others, and infectiousness may vary during the course of infection. In a prospective study of the partners of infected hemophiliacs, Goedert et al reported that the best predictor of HIV-1 transmission is the absolute number of T-helper lymphocytes in the hemophiliac.[39,40] Their preliminary data suggest that, as these patients became more immunosuppressed as evidenced by a CD4 + cell count of fewer than 200/ml, and as viral titers increased as evidence of increasing p24 antigenemia, their sex partners were more likely to become infected with duration of infection and frequency of exposures controlled for. This is consistent with the finding that the ability to isolate HIV-1 significantly increases as the number of CD4 + cells declines and the clinical course progresses.[70] These studies in hemophiliac heterosexual partners have been confirmed in other groups. In a study of 77 heterosexual partners (62 women, 15 men) of 72 HIV-1-infected persons (39 African, 38 European), low CD4 + cell concentrations in the index cases were associated with significantly increased risk of HIV-1 infection in their partners.[102] Similarly, in two studies, one in West Germany[117] and one in Miami,[53] of heterosexual partners of HIV-1-infected persons, the likelihood of infection increased with severity of disease, low CD4 + lymphocyte counts, and p24 antigenemia.

Studies in the United States and Africa have also documented a strong association of HIV-1 transmission with a history of STDs, such as genital ulcers, and lack of circumcision.[34,60,76] In one of the first studies of female prostitutes in Africa, HIV-1 infection was strongly associated with a history of genital ulceration and gonorrhea.[65] In a subsequent study of 115 heterosexual men in Nairobi, Kenya, who had genital ulcers when examined in an STD clinic, HIV-1 infection was positively associated with lack of circumcision and a past history of genital ulceration.[63] In a study of 340 men attending that clinic, of whom 11.2 percent were HIV-1 seropositive, HIV-1 infection was independently associated with the presence of genital ulceration and lack of circumcision.[39] Confirmation of this association was sought in a prospective study of HIV-1-seronegative men who attended the clinic and had had recent contact with a female prostitute.[34] In men who were circumcised and had no genital ulcers when examined, the seroconversion rate was 2.5 percent. The seroconversion rate was 13.4 percent in 111 uncircumcised men with genital ulcers, 29 percent in 27 uncircumcised men without genital ulcers, and 52.6 percent in 61 uncircumcised men with genital ulcers. The association of HIV-1 seroconversion with the lack of circumcision could not be related to differences in sexual behavior between the circumcised and uncircumcised men, nor to increased frequency of genital ulcers in the uncircumcised men. A recent ethnographic review of circumcision practices in 409 African ethnic groups demonstrated a direct correlation between lack of circumcision and increased HIV-1 seroprevalence rates in capital cities of Africa ($R = 0.9; p > 0.001$).[76] Balanitis maceration of the skin of the glans penis, trauma to the intact foreskin, or simply the microenvironment of the tissue under the foreskin may possibly allow greater survival and penetration of HIV-1.

Even among patients attending STD clinics in the United States, a strong association between HIV-1 and a history of genital ulcerations caused by syphilis or herpes simplex virus type 2 (HSV-2) has been documented. In combined studies of more than 8000 patients attending STD clinics in Baltimore between 1987 and 1988, 5 percent were HIV-1 seropositive. Of heterosexuals who denied having other traditional risk factors, 2.3 percent were seropositive; in those individuals HIV-1 infection was significantly associated with a history of syphilis, a positive serologic test for syphilis, and serologic evidence of HSV-2.[7,37,84] Although STDs may be covariates of another primary risk factor, a strong association between HIV-1 infection and syphilis and HSV-2 infection has also been documented among homosexual men, even after controlling for sexual behavior such as the number of lifetime sexual partners or receptive anal intercourse.[82,107] In these studies HIV-1 seroconversion was also strongly associated with HSV-2 seroconversion within the year before HIV-1 seroconversion.[82] Consequently, genital ulcers and other STDs may allow penetration of HIV-1 into a susceptible host by causing epithelial disruption or by increasing the person's susceptibility through an increase in the population of CD4+ lymphocytes, target cells for HIV-1 at the site of infection within the genital tract.[6] In a study by Van de Perre et al CD4+ lymphocytes and HIV-1 p17 antigen were demonstrated in genital fluid in nine of 14 seropositive women.[33] The finding that HIV-1 can be isolated from genital ulcers and vaginal fluid is significant, since it implies that HIV-1 transmission can occur at any time and that infected lymphocytes may increase in the genital tract in association with STDs, inflammation of the cervix, and menstruation. Thus the probability that any single episode of genital-genital or anogenital sexual intercourse will result in transmission of HIV-1 may be determined by multiple biologic factors of the infectious person, the virus itself, or the exposed susceptible person.[8,74] Some of these factors are known or suspected, and they may explain the observed differences in the sexual transmission of HIV-1 in different parts of the world, notably Africa, where genitoulcerative disease is more common and strongly influences the epidemiologic pattern of HIV-1.[77,79]

Perinatal Transmission

Perinatal transmission of HIV-1 may occur in utero, perinatally at the time of delivery, or postnatally through breast-feeding. Risk factors associated with perinatal transmission remain unknown, and prospective studies are under way to assess the efficiency and determinants of such transmission. Detection of HIV-1 in fetal tissues and within the placenta supports the hypothesis that infection can occur in utero.[61,100] Similarly, HIV-1 transmission at birth through exposure to infected maternal blood or vaginal secretions seems likely, but it is difficult to differentiate from in utero transmission.[14,28,44,112] A series of case reports of women who were apparently infected with HIV-1 by blood transfusions given during the immediate postpartum period and who subsequently infected their infants also suggests that breast-feeding is a route of HIV-1 transmission.[12,103]

Studies of the rate of perinatal HIV-1 transmission have been complicated by the lack of reliable diagnostic procedures to detect HIV-1 infection in newborn infants. Because infants born to HIV-1-infected mothers have detectable maternally derived antibodies to HIV-1, long-term study of seropositive infants is necessary to detect the loss of maternal antibodies and the development of serologic or virologic markers of infection in the infants. Prospective studies in the United States, Europe, and Africa have suggested a 25 to 40 percent rate of perinatal transmission.[14,28,36,44,112] In one study in Kinshasa, Zaire, where nearly 6 percent of pregnant women are infected, the rate of perinatal transmission after 2 years of follow-up was estimated to be 39 percent.[44] In a French collaborative study at least 27 percent of 117 infants followed to 18 months of age were infected.[28] In the aforementioned Zaire study the rate of perinatal transmission correlated directly with the finding of a CD4+ lymphocytes count of fewer than 200/mm^3 in the mother.[44] In that study perinatal transmission was higher in women of very low socioeconomic status and with symptomatic HIV-1 infection. Infants born to symptomatic HIV-1-seropositive women were also shown to have an increased risk of death within the first year of life. Twenty-one percent of the children born to HIV-1-seropositive mothers died in the first year, compared with 3.8 percent of infants born to seronegative mothers. AIDS developed within the first year in 7.9 percent of the surviving infants born to HIV-1-seropositive mothers. Infants born to HIV-1-seropositive mothers also had a lower mean birth weight and a lower mean gestational age than infants in the seronegative control group. At 1 year the mortality rate of infants born to seropositive mothers was 284:1000 liveborn children compared with 36:1000 in the seronegative group. HIV-1 infection may have already increased the infant mortality rate by as much as 15 percent in Kinshasa.[44]

The contribution of breast-feeding to perinatal transmission of HIV-1 is unclear. HIV-1 has been isolated from breast milk, and postnatal transmission, probably through breast milk, has been reported.[12,15,16,17] In the French collaborative study, five of six breast-fed infants born to seropositive mothers became infected, compared with 25 of 99 children of seropositive mothers who did not breast-feed.[28] This finding plus the anecdotal findings of postnatal transmission in women transfused with HIV-1-infected blood after birth suggests that breast-feeding represents a small incremental risk of mother-to-infant transmission. In the developed world where alternative nutritional support is available, breast-feeding by an HIV-1-infected mother should probably not be recommended. However, in developing countries where safe and effective alternatives for breast-feeding are not available, breast-feeding by the biologic mother should continue to be the feeding method of choice, irrespective of the mother's HIV-1 status.[15,77,81,112]

The recent availability of the polymerase chain reaction (PCR), a new technique that amplifies proviral sequences of HIV-1 within DNA for detection of HIV-1 in infant's lymphocytes, should provide further insight into the incidence of perinatal transmission among infected women.[108] In a recent study by Rogers et al,[81] PCR was positive in five of seven infants in whom AIDS later developed. The test was positive in one of eight newborns in whom nonspecific signs and symptoms suggesting HIV-1 infection later developed, and no proviral sequences were detected in neonatal samples from nine infants who were born to HIV-1-infected women but remained well up to 16 months after birth. Thus PCR was highly specific, producing positive results only in children who later had symptomatic HIV-1 infection, but larger studies are required to determine the overall sensitivity of the test and the efficiency of perinatal transmission.

Parenteral Transmission

Sharing needles or other drug-related paraphernalia results in HIV-1 transmission between intravenous drug users. The incidence of HIV-1 infection is increasing at a faster rate among intravenous drug users than in other high-risk populations, and the intravenous transmission varies markedly by geographic region.[52,89] Data from more than 18,000 drug users tested in more than 90 surveys in the United States have consistently shown high prevalence rates (50 to 60 percent) in the Northeast.[42] Since patients undergoing treatment for drug abuse are believed to represent only 15 percent of the estimated 1.1 million intravenous drug users in the United States, the exact number of habitual or intermittent intravenous drug users infected with HIV-1 is unknown. In a study of selected intravenous drug users in New York City between 1984 and 1987, the seroprevalence rate stabilized between 55 and 60 percent.[58] This relatively stable rate is attributed to new infection, new seronegative persons beginning drug injection, seropositive persons leaving drug injection, and increasing conscious risk reduction. Nonwhite intravenous drug users have a higher rate of HIV-1 infection than white users with histories of similar frequencies of intravenous drug use and needle sharing.[89,92] This difference may reflect a tendency of drug users to share needles with others of their race, which influences further spread of HIV-1 among that racial group.

Parenteral exposure to whole blood, blood components, and blood products has accounted for HIV-1 infection in transfusion recipients and hemophiliacs. Before screening of all blood donors was implemented in 1985,[43] nearly 70 percent of individuals with hemophilia A and 35 percent of those with hemophilia B had already become infected with HIV-1. Although screening for HIV-1 among blood donors is highly effective in preventing HIV-1 transmission, it does not appear to be 100 percent efficient. In a recent study Ward et al[86] demonstrated that HIV-1 infection can result from blood transfusion despite wide-scale screening of donations for HIV-1. They identified 13 patients who were seropositive for HIV-1 and had received blood from seven donors screened as negative for HIV-1 antibody at the time of donation. All of these donors were later found to be infected with HIV-1, suggesting that they had been infected shortly before blood donation and were seronegative at the time of donation. Currently, based on data from more than 17 million U.S. Red Cross blood donations, the estimated odds of contracting HIV-1 infection by this route are 1:153,000 per unit transfused.[75] A patient who receives an average transfusion of 5.4 units has odds of 1:28,000. This risk has been decreasing by more than 30 percent per year. Possibly the risk of undetected infectious units can be further reduced by transfusing fewer units, recruiting more women and fewer men as new donors, and encouraging more frequent donation from donors who have been tested repeatedly. Among 15 million blood donors tested between 1985 and May 1988, the seroprevalence rate for HIV-1 was 0.018 percent in the United States, declining from 0.035 percent in 1985 to 0.01 percent in 1988.[80]

HIV-1 blood screening has not yet been introduced in some developing countries because of economic and technical constraints. However, technologic advances with recombinant antigens have resulted in the development of highly sensitive and specific rapid diagnostic assays.[19,93] It is hoped that these and other inexpensive assays may be used for the immediate implementation of serologic screening for HIV-1 in all areas of the world.

Parenteral exposure to blood has also resulted in a small but definite occupational risk of HIV-1 infection for health care workers. Of the 169 health care workers reported to have AIDS, 28 have incomplete risk factor assessments because of death or refusal to be interviewed, 97 are still being investigated, and 44 have received full investigations that failed to reveal any risk factors.[95] Eighteen health care workers reported exposure to blood or other body fluids from patients during the last 10 years. Only one worker in this category was documented to have seroconversion to HIV-1 and development of AIDS after a needlestick exposure to infected blood. In prospective seroprevalence studies of health care workers worldwide, seroconversion after occupational exposure has been documented in 18, 13 of whom were from the United States.[88] Another six cases of HIV-1 infection are generally considered to be occupation related, although full documentation of seroconversion could not be obtained. The CDC cooperative needlestick seroprevalence study includes 1201 health care workers with documented exposure.[54] Of 860 workers who had needlestick injuries or cuts with other sharp instruments, only three have undergone seroconversion. Thus the risk of virus infection after needlestick transmission is calculated at 0.35 percent (3 : 860).[54] This low but very real risk emphasizes the importance of universal precautions, since other studies have clearly shown increasing rates of HIV-1 infection among patients in whom HIV-1-related risk factors were unknown or unrecognized.[30,105]

Transmission by Other Routes

The AIDS epidemic has been monitored for more than 8 years, and no evidence for casual or household transmission of HIV-1 has been found. In several household studies performed in the United States, Europe, and Africa, the rate of HIV-1 seropositivity did not differ significantly between nonspousal household contacts of AIDS patients and household contacts of uninfected control subjects.[5,38,49,53] Virtually all seropositive children studied have identifiable risk factors for HIV-1 infection, and the low seroprevalence rates among children 5 to 15 years of age and low rates of HIV-1 infection in rural areas in contrast to urban areas in Africa strongly argue against arthropod transmission of HIV-1.[25,47,77] Laboratory studies of insects fed HIV-1-contaminated blood, interrupted, and then allowed to feed on uncontaminated blood failed to show HIV-1 transmission.[35,97]

SUMMARY

During the past decade AIDS has become a global health problem with nearly 200,000 cases reported from 152 countries and an estimated 5 to 10 million people infected with HIV-1. With a mean incubation period of 10 years from time of infection to development of AIDS, the disease will appear in nearly all currently HIV-1-infected individuals within the next decade, and silent HIV-1 transmission will continue among asymptomatic individuals. The major modes of transmission worldwide remain sexual, parenteral, and perinatal, although the proportions of cases within each risk behavior category differ among geographic regions. Serologic studies have demonstrated increasing rates of HIV-1 infection among intravenous drug users and heterosexual contacts of individuals at high risk for HIV-1 infection, but incidence rates have declined among homosexual men. Higher rates of infection and AIDS cases are being documented among minority populations, particularly in the inner cities of the United States. The likelihood of HIV-1 transmission appears to be related to the likelihood of HIV-1 infection with any given population, behavioral factors that increase the risk of contact with infected individuals, a wide variety of biologic factors that determine the infectiousness of the infected individual, and factors that influence the susceptibility of the uninfected individual such as the presence of other sexually transmitted diseases. Prevention and control of HIV-1 infection therefore depend on the recognition of these variables of transmission and educational efforts to prevent infection.

REFERENCES

1. Allain JP: Prevalence of HTLV-III/LAV antibodies in patients with hemophilia and in their sexual partners in France. (Letter.) N Engl J Med 315:517-518, 1986
2. Anderson RM, Medley GF, May RM, et al: A preliminary study of the transmission of dynamics of the human immunodeficiency virus (HIV), the causative agent of AIDS. J Math Appl Med Biol 3:229-263, 1986
3. Barre-Sinoussi F, Chermann JC, Rey F, et al: Isolation of a T-lymphotropic retrovirus from a patient at risk for acquired immunodeficiency syndrome (AIDS). Science 220:868-871, 1983
4. Blanche S, Rouzioux C, Moscato M-LG, et al: A prospective study of infants born to women seropositive for human immunodeficiency virus type 1. N Engl J Med 320:1643-1648, 1989
5. Bongaarts J, Reining P, Way P, et al: The relationship between male circumcision and HIV infection in African populations. AIDS 3:373-377, 1989
6. Brickner PW, Torres RA, Barnes M, et al: Recommendations for control and prevention of human immunodeficiency virus infection in intravenous drug users. Ann Intern Med 110:833-837, 1989
7. Cameron DW, Simonsen JN, D'Costa LJ, et al: Female to male transmission of human immunodeficiency virus type 1: Risk factors for seroconversion in men. Lancet 2:403-407, 1989
8. Cannon RO, Hook EW, Glasser D, et al: Association of herpes simplex virus type 2 with HIV infection in heterosexual patients attending sexually transmitted disease clinics. Presented at the Fourth International Conference on AIDS, Stockholm, Sweden, 1988
9. Carael M, Van de Perre PH, Lepage PH, et al: Human immunodeficiency virus transmission among heterosexual couples in Central Africa. AIDS 2:201-205, 1988
10. Castro KG, Lieb S, Jaffe HW, et al: Transmission of HIV in Belle Glade, Florida: Lessons for other communities in the United States. Science 239:193-197, 1988
11. Centers for Disease Control: AIDS and the human immunodeficiency virus infection in the United States: 1988 update. MMWR 38(suppl):1-38, 1989
12. Centers for Disease Control: AIDS due to HIV-2 infection—New Jersey. MMWR 37:37-39, 1988
13. Centers for Disease Control: Guidelines for prevention of transmission of human immunodeficiency virus and hepatitis B virus to health-care and public safety workers. MMWR 38:S6, 1989
14. Centers for Disease Control: Human immunodeficiency virus infection in the United States: A review of current knowledge. MMWR 36:1-48, 1987
15. Centers for Disease Control: Provisional public health service interagency recommendations for screening donated blood and plasma for antibody to the virus causing acquired immunodeficiency syndrome. MMWR 34:1-5, 1985

16. Centers for Disease Control: Recommendations for prevention of HIV transmission in health care settings. MMWR 36:2S-10S, 1987
17. Centers for Disease Control: Update: Acquired immunodeficiency syndrome associated with intravenous-drug use—United States, 1988. MMWR 38:165-170, 1989
18. Centers for Disease Control: Acquired immunodeficiency syndrome—United States, 1981-1988. MMWR 38:229-236, 1989
19. Centers for Disease Control: Update: Heterosexual transmission of AIDS and HIV infection—U.S. MMWR 38:423-434, 1989
20. Centers for Disease Control: Update: HIV-2 infection—United States. MMWR 38:572-574, 579-580, 1989
21. Centers for Disease Control: Years of potential life lost before age 65—United States, 1987. MMWR 38:27-29, 1989
22. Chamberland ME, Dondero TJ: Heterosexually acquired infection with human immunodeficiency virus (HIV). (Editorial.) Ann Intern Med 107:763-768, 1987
23. Chin J, Mann J: Global surveillance and forecasting of AIDS. Bull WHO 67:1-7, 1989
24. Clavel F: HIV-2, the West African AIDS virus. AIDS 1:135-140, 1987
25. Clavel F, Guetard D, Brun-Vezinet F, et al: Isolation of a new human retrovirus from West African patients with AIDS. Science 233:343-346, 1986
26. Clavel F, Mansinho K, Chamaret S, et al: Human immunodeficiency virus type 2 infection associated with AIDS in West Africa. N Engl J Med 319:1180-1185, 1987
27. Colebunders RL, Kapita B, Nekwei W, et al: Breast-feeding and transmission of HIV. Presented at the Fourth International Conference on AIDS, Stockholm, Sweden, 1988
28. Coombs RW, Collier A, Nikora B, et al: Relationship between recovery of HIV from plasma and stage of disease (Abstract No. WP 5.4). In Abstracts of the Third International Conference on AIDS. Washington, DC, 1987.
29. Coombs RW, Kreiss J, Nikora B, et al: Isolation of HIV from genital ulcers in Nairobi prostitutes (Abstract No. 1244). In Program and abstracts of the 28th Interscience Conference on Antimicrobial Agents and Chemotherapy. Washington DC, American Society for Microbiology, 1988
30. Cortes E, Detels R, Aboulafia D, et al: HIV-1, HIV-2 and HTLV-1 infection in high risk groups in Brazil. N Engl J Med 320:953-958, 1989
31. Cumming PD, Wallace EL, Schorr JB, et al: Exposure to patients to human immunodeficiency virus through the transfusion of blood components that test antibody negative. N Engl J Med 260:510-513, 1988
32. Curran JW, Jaffe HW, Hardy AM, et al: Epidemiology of HIV infection and AIDS in the United States. Science 239:610-616, 1988
33. Darrow WW, Echenberg DF, Jaffe HW, et al: Risk factors for human immunodeficiency virus (HIV) infections in homosexual men. Am J Public Health 77:479, 1987
34. Des-Jarlais DC, Friedman SR, Novick DM, et al: HIV-1 infection among intravenous drug users in Manhattan, New York, 261:1008-1012, 1989
35. Des Jarlais DC, Friedman SR, Stoneburner RL: HIV infection and intravenous drug use: Critical issues in transmission dynamics, infection, outcome and prevention. Rev Infect Dis 10:151-158, 1988
36. Fischl MA, Dickinson GM, Scott GM, et al: Evaluation of heterosexual partners, children, and household contacts of adults with AIDS. JAMA 257:640-644, 1987
37. Friedland GH, Klein RS: Transmission of the human immunodeficiency virus. N Engl J Med 317:1125-1134, 1987
38. Gallo RC, Salahuddin SZ, Popovic M, et al: Frequent detection and isolation of cytopathic retroviruses (HTLV-III) from patients with AIDS and at risk for AIDS. Science 224:500-503, 1984
39. Goedert JJ, Eyster ME, Biggar RJ, et al: Heterosexual transmission of human immunodeficiency virus: Association with severe depletion of T-helper lymphocyte in men with hemophilia AIDS. Rev Hum Retroviruses 3:355-361, 1988
40. Goedert JJ, Eyster ME, Ragni MV, et al: Rate of heterosexual HIV transmission and associated risk with HIV-antigen. Presented at the Fourth International Conference on AIDS, Stockholm, Sweden, 1988
41. Goedert JJ, Sarngadharan MG, Biggar RJ, et al: Determinants of retrovirus (HTLV-

III) antibody and immunodeficiency conditions in homosexual men. Lancet 2:711, 1984

42. Greenblatt RM, Lukehart SA, Plummer FA, et al: Genital ulceration as a risk factor for human immunodeficiency virus infection. AIDS 2:47-50, 1988
43. Guinan ME, Hardy A: Epidemiology of AIDS in women in the United States. JAMA 257:2039-2042, 1987
44. Hearst N, Hulley SB: Preventing the heterosexual spread of AIDS: Are we giving our patients the best advice? JAMA 259:2428-2432, 1988
45. Holmberg SD, Horsburg CR, Ward JW, et al: Biologic factors in the sexual transmission of human immunodeficiency viruses. J Infect Dis 160:116-125, 1989
46. Holmberg SD, Stewart JA, Gerber AR, et al: Prior herpes simplex virus type 2 infection as a risk factor for HIV infection. JAMA 259:1048-1050, 1988
47. Horsburgh CR Jr, Holmberg SD: The global distribution of human immunodeficiency virus type 2 (HIV-2) infection. Transfusion 28:192-195, 1988
48. Jason JM, McDougal JS, Dixon G, et al: HTLV-III/LAV antibody and immune status of household contacts and sexual partners of persons with hemophilia. JAMA 255:212-215, 1986
49. Johnson AM, Laga M: Heterosexual transmission of HIV. AIDS 2:S49-S56, 1988
50. Jovaisas E, Koch MA, Schafer A, et al: LAV/HTLV-III in a 20-week fetus. Lancet 2:1129, 1985
51. Kanki PJ, M'Boup S, Ricard D, et al. Human T-lymphotropic virus type 4 and the human immunodeficiency virus in West Africa. Science 236:827-831, 1987
52. Kelen GD. Human immunodeficiency virus (HIV-1) and the emergency department: Risks and risk protection for health care workers. Ann Emerg Med 19:242-248, 1990
53. Kelen GD, DiGiovanna T, Bisson L, et al: Human immunodeficiency virus infection in emergency patients: Epidemiology, clinical presentations, and risk to health care workers; The Johns Hopkins experience. JAMA 262:516-522, 1989
54. Kingsley LA, Detels R, Kaslow R, et al: Risk factors for seroconversion to human immunodeficiency virus among male homosexuals. Lancet 1:345-349, 1987
55. Kloser PC, Mangia AJ, Leonard J, et al: HIV-2 associated AIDS in the United States: The first case. Arch Intern Med 149:1876-1877, 1989
56. Kreiss JK, Kitchen LW, Prince HE, et al: Antibody to human T-lymphotropic virus type III in wives of hemophiliacs: Evidence for heterosexual transmission. Ann Intern Med 102:623-626, 1985
57. Kreiss JK, Koech D, Plummer FA, et al: AIDS virus infection in Nairobi prostitutes: Spread of the epidemic to East Africa. N Engl J Med 314:414-418, 1986
58. Laga M, Taelman H, Bonneux L, et al: Risk factors for HIV infection in heterosexual partners of HIV infected Africans and Europeans (Abstract No. 4004). In Program and abstracts of the Fourth International Conference on AIDS. Stockholm, Swedish Ministry of Health and Social Affairs, 1988
59. Lapointe N, Michaud J, Pekovic D, et al: Transplacental transmission of HTLV-III virus. N Engl J Med 312:1325, 1985
60. Lepage P, Van de Perre P, Caracel M, et al: Postnatal transmission of HIV from mother to child. Lancet 2:400, 1987
61. Lyons SF, Jupp PJ, Schoub BD: Survival of HIV in the common bedbug. Lancet 2:45, 1986
62. Mann JM, Chin J: AIDS: A global perspective. N Engl J Med 319:302-304, 1988
63. Mann JM, Chin J, Piot P, et al: The international epidemiology of AIDS. Sci Am 10:82-89, 1988
64. Mann JM, Quinn TC, Francis H, et al: Prevalence of HTLV-III/LAV in household contacts of patients with confirmed AIDS and controls in Kinshasa, Zaire. JAMA 256:721-724, 1986
65. Marcus R, et al: Surveillance of health care workers exposed to blood from patients infected with the human immunodeficiency virus. N Engl J Med 319:1118-1123, 1988
66. May RM: HIV infection in heterosexuals. Nature 331:655-656, 1988
67. Melbeye M, Njelesani EK, Bayley A, et al: Evidence for heterosexual transmission and clinical manifestations of human immunodeficiency virus infection and related conditions in Lusaka, Zambia. Lancet 2:1113-1116, 1986

68. Mortimer PP, Cooke EM: HIV infection, breastfeeding, and human milk banking. Lancet 11:452-453, 1988
69. Moss AR, Osmond D, Bacchetti P, et al: Risk factors for AIDS and HIV seropositivity in homosexual men. Am J Epidemiol 125:1035, 1987
70. Narain JP, Hull B, Hospedales CJ, et al: Epidemiology of AIDS and HIV infection in the Caribbean. In AIDS: Profile of an Epidemic. Pan American Health Organization, Sci Pub No 514, 1989, pp 61-72
71. Neumann PW, O'Shaughnessy MV, Lepine D, et al: Laboratory diagnosis of the first cases of HIV-2 infection in Canada. Can Med Assoc J 140:125-128, 1989
72. N'Galy B, Ryder RW: Epidemiology of HIV infection in Africa. J Acquired Immune Deficiency Syndrome 1:551-558, 1988
73. Nzila N, Ryder R, Colebunders R, et al: Married couples in Zaire with discordant HIV serology (Abstract). Presented at the Fourth International Conference on AIDS, Stockholm, Sweden, 1988
74. Office of Technology Assessment, United States Congress: Do Insects Transmit AIDS? Washington, DC: US Government Printing Office, 1987
75. Ou CY, Kwok S, Mitchell SW, et al: DNA amplification for direct detection for HIV-1 DNA of peripheral blood mononuclear cells. Science 239:295-297, 1988
76. Padian N, Marquis L, Francis DP, et al: Male-to-female transmission of human immunodeficiency virus. JAMA 258:788-790, 1987
77. Pape JW, Johnson WD: HIV-1 infection and AIDS in Haiti. In Kaslow RA, Francis DP (eds): The Epidemiology of AIDS. New York, Oxford University Press, 1989, pp 194-221
78. Pepin J, Plummer FA, Brunham RC, et al: The interaction of HIV infection and other sexually transmitted diseases: An opportunity for intervention. AIDS 3:3-9, 1989
79. Peterman T, Curran JW: Sexual transmission of human immunodeficiency virus. JAMA 256:2222-2226, 1986
80. Peterman TA, Stoneburner RL, Allen JR, et al: Risk of HIV transmission from heterosexual adults with transfusion-associated infection. JAMA 259:44-48, 1988
81. Piot P, Kreiss JK, Ndinya-Achola JO, et al: Heterosexual transmission of HIV. AIDS 2:1-10, 1988
82. Piot P, Plummer FS, Mhalu JL, et al: AIDS: An international perspective. Science 239:573-579, 1988
83. Piot P, Plummer FA, Rey MA, et al: Retrospective seroepidemiology of AIDS virus infection in Nairobi populations. J Infect Dis 155:1108-1112, 1987
84. Quinn TC, Cannon RO, Glasser D, et al: The association of syphilis with risk of human immunodeficiency virus infection in patients attending sexually transmitted diseases clinics. Arch Intern Med (in press)
85. Quinn TC, Glasser D, Cannon RO, et al: Human immunodeficiency virus infection among patients attending clinics for sexually transmitted diseases. N Engl J Med 318:197-203, 1988
86. Quinn TC, Kline R, Francis H, et al: Rapid latex agglutination assay using recombinant envelope polypeptide for the detection of antibody to the human immunodeficiency virus. JAMA 260:510-513, 1988
87. Quinn TC, Mann JM, Curran JW, et al: AIDS in Africa: An epidemiologic paradigm. Science 234:955-963, 1986
88. Quinn TC, Zacarias FRK, St John RK: AIDS in the Americas: An emerging public health crisis. N Engl J Med 320:1005-1007, 1989
89. Quinn TC, Zacarias FRK, St John RK: HIV and HTLV-I infections in the Americas: A regional perspective. Medicine 68:189-209, 1989
90. Redfield RR, Markham PD, Salahuddin SZ, et al: Frequent transmission of HTLV-III among spouses of patients with AIDS-related complex and AIDS. JAMA 253:1571-1573, 1985
91. Rogers MF: Breast-feeding and HIV infection. (Letter.) Lancet 11:1278, 1987
92. Rogers MF, Ou CY, Rayfield M, et al: Use of polymerase chain reaction for early detection of the proviral sequence of human immunodeficiency virus in infants born to seropositive mothers. N Engl J Med 320:1649-1654, 1989

93. Ronald AR, Ndinya-Achola JO, Plummer FA, et al: A review of HIV-1 in Africa. Bull NY Acad Med 64:480-490, 1988
94. Ruef C, Dickey P, Schable CA, et al: A second case of the acquired immunodeficiency syndrome due to human immunodeficiency virus type 2 in the United States: The clinical implications. Am J Med 86:709-712, 1989
95. Rwandan HIV Seroprevalence Study Group: Nationwide community-based serological survey of HIV-1 and other human retrovirus infections in a central African country. Lancet 1:941-943, 1989
96. Ryder RW, Hassig SE: The epidemiology of perinatal transmission of HIV. AIDS 2(suppl 1):S83-S89, 1988
97. Ryder RW, Nsa W, Hassig SE, et al: Perinatal transmission of the human immunodeficiency virus types 1 to infants of seropositive women in Zaire. N Engl J Med 320:1637-1642, 1989
98. Ryder RW, Piot P: Epidemiology of HIV-1 infection in Africa. In Piot P, Mann JM, (eds): Bailliere's Clinical Tropical Medicine and Communicable Diseases. London, Bailliere-Tindall, 1988, pp 13-30
99. Schoenbaum EE, Hartel D, Selwyn PA, et al: Risk factors for human immunodeficiency virus infection in intravenous drug users. N Engl J Med 321:874-879, 1989
100. Simoes EA, Babu PG, John TJ, et al: Evidence for HTLV-III infection in prostitutes in Tamil Nadu (India). Indian J Med Res 85:335-338, 1987
101. Simonsen JN, Cameron W, Gakinya MN, et al: Human immunodeficiency virus infection among men with sexually transmitted diseases: Experience from a center in Africa. N Engl J Med 319:274-278, 1988
102. Spielberg F, Kabeya CM, Ryder RW, et al: Field testing and comparative evaluation of rapid, visually read screening assays for antibody to human immunodeficiency virus. Lancet 1:580-583, 1989
103. Sprecher S, Soumenkoff G, Puissant F, et al: Vertical transmission of HIV in a 15-week fetus. Lancet 2:288, 1986
104. Stall RD, Coates TJ, Hoff C: Behavioral risk reduction for HIV infection among gay and bisexual men: A review of results in the United States. J Am Psychol 43:878-885, 1988
105. Stamm WE, Handsfield HH, Rompalo AM, et al: Association of genital ulcer disease with risk of HIV infection in homosexual men. JAMA 260:1429-1433, 1988
106. Stazewski S, Rehmet S, Hofmeister WD, et al: Analysis of transmission rates in heterosexual transmitted HIV infection (Abstract No. 4068). Presented at the Fourth International Conference on AIDS, Stockholm, Sweden, 1988
107. Tanphaichitra D, Armstrong D, Gold J, et al: HIV testing in Bangkok, Thailand. (Letter.) AIDS 2:228, 1988
108. The European Collaborative Study: Mother to child transmission of HIV infection. Lancet 2:1039-1042, 1988
109. Thiry L, Sprecher-Goldberger S, Jockheer T, et al: Isolation of AIDS virus from cell free breast milk of three healthy virus carriers. Lancet 2:891-892, 1985
110. Van de Perre P, De Clercq A, Cogniaux Hectere J, et al: Detection of HIV p17-antigen in lymphocytes but not epithelial cells from cervicovaginal secretions of women seropositive for HIV: Implications for heterosexual transmission of the virus. Genitourin Med 64:30-33, 1988
111. Van Griensven GJD, Tielman RAP, Goudsmit J, et al: Risk factors and prevalence of HIV antibodies in homosexual men in the Netherlands. Am J Epidemiol 125:1048, 1987
112. Veronesi R, Mazzsa CC, Santos-Fereira MO, et al: HIV-2 in Brazil. (Letter.) Lancet 2:405, 1987
113. Ward JW, Holmberg SD, Allen JR, et al: Transmission of human immunodeficiency virus (HIV) by blood transfusion screened as negative for HIV antibody. N Engl J Med 318:473-478, 1988; 321:941-946, 1989
114. Winkelstein W, Lyman DM, Padian N, et al: Sexual practices and risk of infection by the human immunodeficiency virus: The San Francisco Men's Health Study. JAMA 257:321-325, 1987

115. World Health Organization: Acquired immunodeficiency syndrome (AIDS): Global projections of HIV/AIDS. Wkly Epidemiol Rec 64:229-231, 1989
116. World Health Organization: AIDS surveillance update in the WHO European Region. Wkly Epidemiol Rec 64:221-228, 1989
117. Ziegler JB, Cooper DA, Johnson RO, et al: Postnatal transmission of AIDS-associated retrovirus from mother to infant. Lancet 1:896-898, 1985

2

FEATURES OF HIV AND THE HOST RESPONSE THAT INFLUENCE PROGRESSION TO DISEASE

JAY A. LEVY, MD

HIV was initially isolated in 1983 from patients with AIDS and the AIDS-related complex (ARC). The virus was called lymphadenopathy-associated virus (LAV), human T cell lymphotropic virus, type III (HTLV-III), and the AIDS-associated retrovirus (ARV). [4,18,45] An international committee on taxonomy of viruses recommended in 1986 a new term, HIV, to distinguish this virus as a newly recognized human pathogen.[11] In following that recommendation, we at the University of California, San Francisco, have renamed our isolates of HIV type 1, HIV-1$_{Sand Francisco}$ (HIV-1$_{SF}$). The second subtype of HIV, HIV-2, discussed below, is identified in our laboratory with the University of California subscript (HIV-2$_{UC}$). In this chapter we will primarily refer to studies of HIV-1, designated in the text as HIV.

Studies by several groups indicated that HIV was associated with AIDS and the diseases linked to this syndrome.[4,18,45,48,64] Moreover, antibodies to the virus were found in individuals with disease or belonging to one of the groups known to be at risk for AIDS.[18,33,34,66,67] These included homosexual or bisexual men, intravenous drug users, newborn children of seropositive mothers, transfusion and blood product recipients (hemophiliacs), and heterosexual contacts of virus-positive individuals. Moreover, individuals from

My work and that of my colleagues cited in this paper were supported by grants from the American Foundation for AIDS Research, the California State University-Wide Task Force on AIDS, and the National Institutes of Health (grant Nos. ROl-AI-24499 and POl-AI-24206).

TABLE 2–1.   CHARACTERISTICS OF HIV THAT RESEMBLE A LENTIVIRUS

Clinical
  1. Association with a disease with a long incubation period
  2. Involvement of hematopoietic system
  3. Involvement of the central nervous system
  4. Association with immune suppression

Biologic
  1. Cytopathic effect in certain infected cells (for example, T-helper cells) (fusion; multinucleated cells)
  2. Infection of macrophages
  3. Accumulation of unintegrated circular and linear forms of proviral DNA in infected cells
  4. Latent infection in some infected cells
  5. Morphology of virus particle by electron microscopy: cylindric nucleoid

Molecular
  1. Large provirus size (9.7 kb)
  2. Primer binding site, tRNA^{Lys}
  3. Truncated *gag* gene: several processed *gag* proteins
  4. Similar genomic base composition
  5. Polymorphism, particularly in the envelope region
  6. Novel central open reading frame in the viral genome that separates the *pol* and *env* regions
  7. Presence of regulatory and accessory genes

Haiti and Africa had a high prevalence of HIV infection.[38,57,75] The source of infection in Haitians and Africans appeared to be heterosexual activity, but transfusions and reuse of needles could also be factors. These epidemiologic and virologic studies indicated that the major route of HIV infection was by blood and intimate sexual contact. They conclusively demonstrated that HIV was the etiologic agent of this newly recognized human disease.

Studies conducted by several laboratories have now clearly demonstrated that HIV is a member of the lentivirus subfamily of human retroviruses.[47,61] Other subfamilies include the Oncovirinae and the Spumavirinae, characterized by human T cell leukemia virus, type 1, and the human foamy virus, respectively. All these viruses, as retroviruses, code for an enzyme, RNA-dependent DNA polymerase or reverse transcriptase, that permits the viral RNA to be transcribed into a DNA copy (cDNA). In this form it can integrate into the cellular genome and replicate via the proviral DNA (see later discussion). The characteristics the AIDS virus shares with lentiviruses include its long genome (9.7 kilobases [kb]), its highly variable envelope genes (as demonstrated by selective serologic studies), its induction of a slow disease, and its cytopathic properties in cell culture. Moreover, like the animal lentiviruses, it infects the brain (Table 2–1).[23,27,35]

The major HIV proteins have been located in the virion by immunoelectron microscopy.[20] As demonstrated in Figure 2–1, the external envelope protein (gp120) is associated with small protrusions or spikes on the surface of the virion and attached to the viral capsid via the transmembrane

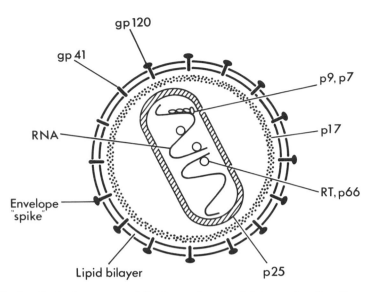

FIGURE 2–1. The basic structure of the human immunodeficiency virus. The diagram shows the location of the major structural proteins of the virion. (From Levy JA: Human immunodeficiency viruses and the pathogenesis of AIDS. JAMA 261:2997, 1989. Copyright 1989, American Medical Association.)

protein, gp41. The *gag* proteins make up the core and the phosphoproteins that are found inside this nucleoid. The major *gag* protein has a molecular weight of 25,000 and is called p25 (or p24); it forms the core shell. The *gag* protein p17 is located outside the core, right below the virion outer membrane (see Fig. 2–1). This location may explain the ability of some sera with antibodies to p17 to neutralize HIV.[65] Part of p17 may protrude through the viral capsid. Finally, reverse transcriptase (RT) is present in the core intimately associated with the two strands of viral RNA, which are exact copies of each other. This diploid state is characteristic of all retroviruses and is important for their replicative cycle (for review, see Levy[40]).

WHAT CELLS ARE INFECTED BY HIV?

The initial studies of the AIDS virus revealed its presence in peripheral blood mononuclear cells (PMCs), particularly T-helper lymphocytes.[4,18,45] Subsequently, HIV was recovered from macrophages and was shown to infect a variety of other human cells, including B lymphocytes, promyelocytes, fibroblasts, and epidermal Langerhans' cells.[47,73,74] The virus has been recovered from lymph nodes, bowel epithelium, and brain (see later discussion).

Integrated viral DNA has been detected in brain tissue,[69] and infectious virus has been isolated from all regions of the brain and cerebrospinal fluid

TABLE 2–2. CELLS SUSCEPTIBLE TO HIV

Hematopoietic	Skin
T lymphocytes	Langerhans' cells
B lymphocytes	Fibroblasts
Macrophages	**Other**
Promyelocytes	Colon carcinoma cells
Brain	Bowel epithelium
Astrocytes	Renal epithelium
Oligodendrocytes	
Capillary endothelium	
Macrophages	

(CSF).[27,46] The detection of infectious virus in CSF does not necessarily correlate with neurologic findings, since individuals with fever or headaches alone have been found to have virus in this body fluid.[29] In situ hybridization studies have demonstrated HIV RNA primarily in brain macrophages but also in capillary endothelial cells and possibly glial cells in the brain, including oligodendrocytes.[39,43,80] Moreover, tissue culture studies have indicated the susceptibility of brain astrocytes to infection by the virus.[9]

HIV has been detected in the renal epithelium[11] as well as in bowel epithelium, particularly in crypt cells and enterochromaffin cells.[55] This observation may explain the malabsorption and chronic diarrhea observed in some infected individuals and the syndrome of "slim disease" first described in Uganda.[68] The enterchromaffin cells have endocrine functions that control motility and digestive functions of the bowel. Thus, when infected, they could be responsible for the diarrhea. All these studies indicate the wide host cell range of the AIDS virus (Table 2–2).

Besides being found in several body tissues, HIV can be recovered from many body fluids (Table 2–3). In initial studies, we found infectious virus in 30% of plasma or serum samples of infected individuals.[54] We estimated the quantity present to be generally 10 to 50 infectious particles (IP)/ml. One individual had a titer as high as 25,000 IP/ml. Recent reports have found HIV in most plasma samples of infected individuals, with the highest levels ($>10^4$ IP/ml) in patients with AIDS.[26a] A small amount of freely circulating virus in the blood could explain the low risk of infection following needlestick injuries[21] compared with that of hepatitis B, which is present in the blood of infected individuals at 10^9 IPs/ml. Other body fluids, such as tears, saliva, and ear secretions, contain at least one-tenth to one-hundredth the amount of virus in the blood and plasma and at less frequency.[47] Thus they essentially present no source of contagion. Genital secretions (vaginal or cervical and seminal fluids) vary in virus quantities but generally have much less than blood.[47,76,81] CSF appears to yield high levels of virus (up to 1000 IPs/ml), reflecting good replication of HIV in certain brain cells. However, this body fluid would not be a natural source of infection.

TABLE 2—3.   ISOLATION OF HIV FROM BODY FLUIDS

	ISOLATION (POSITIVE/ATTEMPTS)
Readily Detectable Virus	
Plasma	3/9
Serum	20/78
Cerebrospinal fluid	27/37
Low Quantities of Virus	
Tears	2/5
Urine	1/5
Saliva	2/39
Vaginal or cervical secretions	6/16
Ear secretions	1/8
Breast milk	1/1
Virus in Infected Cells	
Peripheral blood mononuclear cells	87/92
Saliva	3/20
Vaginal or cervical fluid	7/16
Semen	11/28
Bronchial fluid	3/24

Results reflect number of specimens that contained HIV as determined by standard virologic procedures.[47,48]

Because of the relatively low level of infectious HIV particles present in body fluids, transmission of the virus in a free state seems less likely than transmission by the infected cells also present.[41] Certain body fluids, particularly genital secretions, can contain substantial numbers of virus-infected cells.[41] In studies conducted in our laboratory, we found variations in the number of infected cells in these fluids among seropositive individuals. We believe this factor relates directly to the ability to transfer the virus to others. In Africa, sexually transmitted diseases are clearly a cofactor in the transmission of HIV, particularly in the case of genital ulcers caused by *Haemophilus ducreyi* or herpesvirus.[5,60,70] These infections produce open lesions that would permit contact of virus-infected cells with susceptible host cells. This emphasis on the virus-infected cell as the major source of infection cannot be overstated. These cells pose a major problem in attempts at antiviral therapy and development of a vaccine. Probably only mechanisms that destroy HIV-carrying cells will lead to prevention and elimination of this viral infection.

HOW DOES HIV INFECT CELLS?

Retroviruses from all animal species require a cell surface receptor for attachment and penetration of the cell. It is generally accepted that HIV binds to the cell membrane primarily via the CD4 antigen complex. This protein was first recognized as a surface marker on T-helper cells. It has now been found on a variety of hematopoietic cells, including B lymphocytes and macrophages, as well as some brain cells. The presence of the CD4 antigen therefore appears to explain the susceptibility of many cells to HIV. However, as noted later, the virus also infects some cells lacking CD4 protein expression.

A direct interaction of viral gp120 with the CD4 molecule has been demonstrated by showing that both proteins are required for infection.[13,32,37,53] Monoclonal antibodies to specific epitopes on the CD4 protein block HIV infection, and antibodies to either CD4 or viral gp120 precipitate both proteins in a complex.[32,53] Nevertheless, work in our laboratory with cultured human fibroblasts,[73] as well as certain brain cells, has indicated that CD4 is not the only receptor for HIV; these cells lack any evidence of CD4 protein or RNA expression, but can be infected by the virus.[9,73] Moreover, even CD8+ lymphocytes lacking the CD4 molecule can be infected if they are coinfected by another retrovirus such as HTLV-I[14] (C. Walker and J.A. Levy, unpublished observations). Clearly, other mechanisms for HIV entrance into a cell are involved.

Evidence from some laboratories has shown that antibodies to gp41, the transmembrane protein of HIV, can prevent virus infection.[28] This observation suggests that the virus may interact with the cell surface at two sites. The HIV envelope gp120 appears to attach to the CD4 protein, whereas gp41 could act as a fusion protein and interact with a separate cellular receptor (Fig. 2–2). Thus both proteins working in concert permit the most

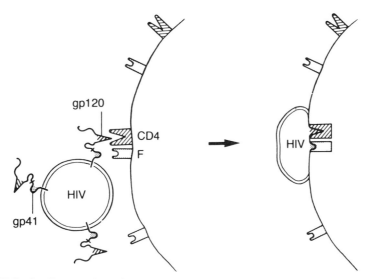

FIGURE 2–2. Proposed mechanism for HIV infection of a cell. The outside viral envelope protein, gp120, attaches to a cell surface receptor, most likely the CD4 antigen. The external portion of the transmembrane protein, gp41, attaches to a specific fusion receptor on the cell surface. Either receptor may permit viral entry into the cell, but both together would make this event more efficient.

efficient entrance of HIV into a cell. A similar mechanism of infection has been shown for the paramyxoviruses.[59] Further work on this model must be conducted, but perhaps the CD4-lacking cells (cited earlier) are infected via the gp41 receptor-fusion mechanism.

Once the virus enters the cell, its RNA, inside the central core, begins the process of reverse transcription that produces double-stranded DNA that circularizes and goes to the nucleus. This cDNA integrates into the host chromosome, where it then exists as a proviral DNA. The infected cell can remain in this latent state in which it makes little or no viral RNA or proteins. The cell can thus elude the host immune system possibly for years—a potential reason for long incubation periods.

Alternatively, the infected cell enters active virus production in which the proviral DNA makes the viral RNA and proteins, leading to release of infectious progeny. These infected cells can then spread the virus through production of infectious progeny or by fusion with uninfected cells.[50] This latter cell-to-cell interaction is important because it permits the transfer of viral information into an uninfected cell by a mechanism unaffected by neutralizing antibodies. The hypothetical fusion mechanism would occur between HIV gp41 and a cell receptor (see Fig. 2–2) and might also mediate cell-to-cell contact. Both viral envelope proteins (gp41, gp120) are found on the surface of HIV-infected cells.[20] Finally, the cell latently infected by HIV may later become activated in the host by still undefined factors and enter into a virus-productive state.

ARE ALL HIV STRAINS THE SAME?

Soon after the identification of the three prototypes of HIV, it became clear, based on molecular studies, that a heterogeneity of HIV strains existed. Whereas LAV and HTLV-III were very similar, ARV, as well as two other San Francisco isolates studied (ARV-3 and ARV-4), were quite distinct.[52,61] The genome of ARV versus LAV/HTLV-III differed by at least 6 percent; the predicted amino acid differences could be as high as 27 percent. Each HIV isolate has its own distinct restriction enzyme pattern and sequence identity. The major modifications in HIV occur in the envelope region[71] for reasons that are unknown. Perhaps the accumulation of unintegrated proviral DNA copies of HIV in the cells during virus infection[47] permits this effect because mutations and recombinations could occur more easily than if the virus were in an integrated state. This possibility is now under study.

HIV isolates can be distinguished not only by molecular but also by biologic features. They can differ in their ability to replicate in established T, B, and macrophage cell lines, as well as PMCs and primary macrophages.[2,3,17,19,43,44] Moreover, the ability of HIV isolates to induce plaques in the MT4 T cell line appears to correlate with differences in their cyto-

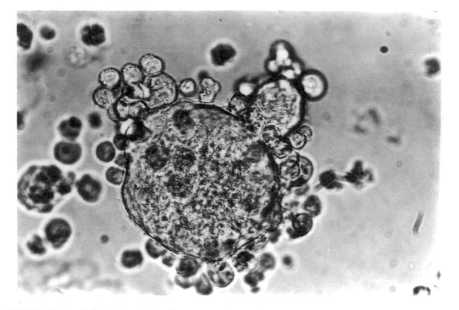

FIGURE 2–3. Infected peripheral mononuclear cells showing cytopathic effects from HIV. Note the multinucleated cell caused by cell fusion and the large balloon forms (×40).

pathic properties and replicating abilities in established T cell lines.[72] Those viruses that cause typical cytopathic effects, including formation of multinucleated cells and balloon degeneration leading to cell death (Fig. 2–3) and that replicate best in T cell lines readily induce plaques in the MT4 cells.

By performing a variety of tissue culture studies in the laboratory, we have been able to identify specific biologic properties of HIV that distinguish the strains associated with neurologic findings from those linked to immune suppression.[7] Those recovered from the brain do not replicate well in T cells but prefer primary macrophages. They are not neutralized efficiently by sera from HIV-infected individuals, and they are not very cytopathic in T cells and thus do not induce plaques in MT4 cells. These initial studies suggest that other HIV strains may be found that will selectively grow in B cells or brain cells. Their disease-causing properties could be determined by their specific host range and biologic features and may differ from the initially recognized T cell–tropic virus subtypes.

We have also demonstrated that the biologic properties of HIV can change in viruses recovered at different times from the same individual.[8] For example, one HIV isolate obtained from a patient with oral candidiasis was compared with an isolate recovered 5 months later from the same infected individual, who by that time had Kaposi's sarcoma and *Pneumocystis carinii* pneumonia. The second isolate showed greater replicating ability, a wider host range in cell culture, and more cytopathic changes, including the induction of MT4 cell plaques, than the initial HIV recovered. Yet both virus isolates are sensitive to neutralization by the same sera. Moreover, molecular studies strongly suggest that the sequences of these HIV are related, since few differences are observed in restriction enzyme analyses. These results and others with sequential HIV isolates emphasize the possibility that disease progression may occur with the emergence of more virulent strains of HIV in the individual.

Another subtype of HIV has been recovered from AIDS patients in West Africa. This virus, called HIV-2, had been suspected to exist because antibodies to it, unlike those against HIV-1, cross-react with the simian immunodeficiency virus (SIV).[10,35] Molecular studies have indicated that its sequence differs from HIV-1 by 55 percent, with changes noted primarily in the envelope region.[22] Antibodies to HIV-2 have been found primarily in West Africa and in some individuals in Europe and South America. The virus was also detected recently in the United States. Most tests for antibodies to HIV-1 can detect antibodies to HIV-2 unless only antibodies to HIV-2 envelope proteins are present in the serum. For this reason, screening tests for infection by an HIV should include the envelope protein of HIV-2 to detect exposure to either of these HIV subtypes. In our laboratory Evans, in collaboration with Moreau and Odehouri,[15] has evaluated patients from the Ivory Coast. She has isolated several strains of HIV-2 and has identified individuals in Abidjan with antibodies to both HIV-1 and HIV-2.[15] In one individual studied, both HIV-1 and HIV-2 subtypes were recovered from the blood.[16] These results indicate that some individuals may be infected by both types of HIV.

In our laboratory we have characterized eight strains of HIV-2 recovered from patients infected in the Ivory Coast. We have found the same kind of heterogeneity observed with HIV-1 strains, particularly in terms of cellular tropism and cytopathologic characteristics. One of the isolates, HIV-2_{UC1}, is noncytopathic in cell culture. It does not kill cells or induce cell fusion when infected cells are mixed with uninfected white blood cells from seronegative individuals.[15] Nevertheless, this HIV-2 strain was recovered from an individual who subsequently died of AIDS. This finding indicates that a noncytopathic HIV strain (perhaps attenuated) may be emerging in some parts of the world. Whether the individual at death had a more virulent form of this HIV-2 strain, as we have noted in HIV-1-infected individuals in whom AIDS later developed,[8] could not be determined.

HOW DOES THE HOST RESPOND TO HIV?

The outcome of any viral infection depends not only on the virulence of the virus, but also on the relative strength of the host's antiviral immune response. Because HIV attacks immune cells, its control poses an even greater challenge to an intact immune system.

The defense mechanism used by the host against viral infections consists of both humoral and cellular immune responses. B lymphocytes are a major arm of the humoral response. Through their interactions with macrophages and T-helper lymphocytes, they make antibodies to foreign proteins, including invading organisms. For HIV these include antibodies to the major structural and functional proteins of the virus that can be detected by standard immunoblot procedures.[56] Some of these antibodies can neutralize the virus; the titer depends on the specific B cell response of the infected individual. We have demonstrated wide differences in serum levels of neutralizing antibodies among individuals.[6] Some investigators suggest that this antibody response decreases as the clinical state worsens.[62] This was not found, however, in longitudinal studies of infected individuals in our laboratory. In any case, neutralizing antibodies do not appear to be protective once the viral infection has taken place. Thus vaccines made to induce these antibodies may help block initial infection by free virus but cannot change the disease course after infection is established. Most important, because the virus-infected cell is a major source of transmission,[41] neutralizing antibodies in this situation would not protect an individual from infection.

Homsy in our laboratory has detected the presence of antibodies to HIV that enhance virus infection.[30,31] These were first noted in guinea pigs immunized with selected HIV-1 strains in attempts to induce type-specific neutralizing antibodies. Instead, antibodies that increased the ability of the virus to infect macrophages, T cells, and even fibroblasts were found. Subsequent studies indicated the presence of these antibodies in infected chimpanzees and in naturally infected human subjects. Enhancing antibodies have been demonstrated with infections by the flaviviruses, togaviruses, and other viral families,[24] but this is the first time such antibodies have been demonstrated for lentiviruses. The observation is important because vaccination with viral proteins must take into consideration the potential for inducing enhancing and not protective neutralizing antibodies. These enhancing antibodies would not only increase the ability of the virus to infect T cells but might also change a lymphotropic virus into a macrophage-tropic virus. Laboratory studies have indicated that the mechanism for HIV entry into the macrophages and T cells after mixing with serum is the Fc receptor and does not depend on the CD4 molecule.[31] Thus enhancement is another mechanism by which HIV can enter cells without using the CD4 receptor (see the preceding). Robinson and colleagues[63] noted this enhancement of HIV infection in studies with complement-reconstituted serum and suggested that another mechanism is through the complement receptor.

The other major arm of the immune system, the cellular immune response, is often the most important defense against virus infections; with HIV this is also the case. This immune response is mediated primarily by T lymphocytes, macrophages, and natural killer (NK) cells. The T lymphocytes can be divided phenotypically into two major subgroups, T-helper (CD4+) and T-suppressor/cytotoxic (CD8+) cells. As noted earlier, the T-helper lymphocytes are a major target for HIV, and T-suppressor cells are rarely if ever infected by the virus. Macrophages are susceptible to HIV[19,47,49]; whether NK cells can be infected is not yet known. The T-suppressor or T-cytotoxic cells and the macrophages can function either by suppressing virus replication or by killing the infected cell. In several laboratories cytotoxic responses have been observed with cells of infected individuals.[58,77] However, these studies have used systems in the laboratory that may not mimic the natural state. Thus we cannot yet be certain that HIV infection induces a protective cytotoxic response in the host.

Studies in our laboratory have indicated that in some individuals replication of HIV in PMCs can be suppressed by CD8+ T cells.[78] This suppression does not involve cell killing but is mediated in part by a diffusible factor (or cytokine) released by the CD8+ cells.[79] In comparing asymptomatic individuals with those who have active disease, we have found that the suppression by CD8+ cells can be observed best in the healthy individuals. In one case, that of an AIDS patient whose Kaposi's sarcoma lesions had gone into remission, this antiviral reaction was also noted.[78] We are attempting to identify the cytokine produced by the CD8+ cells and develop methods to sustain CD8+ cell control of HIV replication.

Although the immune system may limit virus replication either through neutralizing antibodies or through T-suppressor or cytotoxic cells, viral infection often leads to other types of disarray in immune function. For instance, infection with many herpesviruses (for example, Epstein-Barr) leads to activation of B cells with resulting hypergammaglobulinemia and production of antibodies to a variety of cellular antigens.[26] In many individuals infected with HIV, a similar response can be seen with proliferation of B cells and production of antibodies. This feature is particularly found in newborn infants and young children.[1] In some individuals the antibodies directed against normal cellular proteins induce an autoimmune state. A variety of autoimmune syndromes have been observed in AIDS patients (Table 2–4). Each of them has been linked to an antibody to a normal protein present on the target cell.[42] Thus HIV infection may lead to the

TABLE 2–4. AUTOANTIBODIES IN HIV INFECTION

TARGET	CLINICAL SIGN
Platelet	Immune thrombocytopenic purpura
Red blood cell	Anemia
Neutrophil	Neutropenia
Peripheral nerve	Neuropathy
Lymphocyte	Immune deficiency
Lupus anticoagulant (phospholipid)	? Neurologic disease
Nucleus (antinuclear antibody)	Autoimmunity

production of autoantibodies that further compromise the immune system and contribute to the progression to disease.

SUMMARY

This chapter reviews briefly the important characteristics of the AIDS virus, the parameters of HIV infection, and the fact that this virus, upon infection of the host, can spread to many body tissues. Its major mode of transmission appears to be via virus-infected cells that must be destroyed or controlled by a strong cellular immune system. The ultimate outcome of the infection depends on the host's immune reaction to the virus either through suppression of HIV replication or through killing of the infected cell. In some individuals an active immune system has prevented development of the disease for more than 9 years (J.A. Levy, unpublished observations). The factors important in maintaining this immune response are not yet known and merit close attention. In some individuals, for example, the immune system appears to make enhancing antibodies to HIV, and we recently noted that this phenomenon occurs particularly with progression of disease.[30.] It is related to changes in the antibodies made and in some cases to modifications in the virus so that it is more sensitive to enhancing antibodies.[30] Moreover, the immune system can hyperreact with production of autoantibodies that can also hasten the development of disease. Clearly, then, changes in the virus and the immune response of the host play important roles in the ultimate steps leading to AIDS.

We have come a long way in understanding AIDS and its causative agent, HIV. Only through continued studies of its biologic, serologic, and molecular properties can we hope to learn the approaches that will eventually lead to effective antiviral therapy and a vaccine.

REFERENCES

1. Ammann A, Levy JA: Laboratory investigation of pediatric acquired immunodeficiency syndrome. Clin Immunol Immunopathol 40:122, 1986
2. Anand R, Reed C, Forlenza S, et al: Non-cytocidal natural variants of human immunodeficiency virus isolated from AIDS patients with neurological disorder. Lancet 2:234, 1987
3. Asjo B, Albert J, Karlsson A, et al: Replicative capacity of human immunodeficiency virus from patients with varying severity of HIV infection. Lancet 2:660, 1986
4. Barre-Sinoussi F, Nugeyre M, Dauguet C, et al: Isolation of a T-lymphotropic retrovirus from a patient at risk for acquired immune deficiency syndrome. Science 220:868, 1986
5. Cameron DW, Simonsen JN, D'Costa LJ, et al: Female to male transmission of human immunodeficiency virus type 1: Risk factors for seroconversion in men. Lancet 2:403, 1989
6. Cheng-Mayer C, Homsy J, Evans LA, et al: Identification of HIV subtypes with distinct patterns of sensitivity to serum neutralization. Proc Natl Acad Sci USA 85:2815, 1988

7. Cheng-Mayer C, Levy JA: Distinct biologic and serologic properties of HIV isolates from the brain. Ann Neurol 23:S58, 1988
8. Cheng-Mayer C, Seto D, Levy JA: Biologic features of HIV that correlate with virulence in the host. Science 240:80, 1988
9. Cheng-Mayer C, Rutka JT, Rosenblum ML, et al: The human immunodeficiency virus (HIV) can productively infect cultured human glial cells. Proc Natl Acad Sci USA 84:3526, 1987
10. Clavel F, Guetard D, Brun-Vezinet F, et al: Isolation of a new human retrovirus from West African patients with AIDS. Science 233:343, 1986
11. Cohen AH, Sun NCJ, Shapshak P, et al: Demonstration of human immunodeficiency virus in renal epithelium in HIV-associated nephropathy. Mod Pathol 2:125, 1989
12. Coffin J, Haase A, Levy JA, et al: Human immunodeficiency viruses. Science 232:697, 1986
13. Dalgleish A, Beverley P, Clapham P, et al: The CD4 (T4) antigen is an essential component of the receptor for the AIDS retrovirus. Nature 312:763, 1984
14. de Rossi A, Franchini G, Alsovini A, et al: Differential response to the cytopathic effects of human T cell lymphotropic virus type III (HTLV-III) superinfection in T4+ (helper) and T8+ (suppressor) T-cell clones transformed by HTLV-I. Proc Natl Acad Sci USA 83:4297, 1986
15. Evans LA, Moreau J, Odehouri K, et al: Characterization of a noncytopathic HIV-2 strain with unusual effects on CD4 expression. Science 240:1522, 1988
16. Evans LA, Moreau J, Odehouri K, et al: Simultaneous isolation of HIV-1 and HIV-2 from an AIDS patient. Lancet 2:1389, 1988
17. Evans LA, McHugh TM, Stites DP, et al: Differential ability of human immunodeficiency virus isolates to productively infect human cells. J Immunol 138:3415, 1987
18. Gallo R, Salahuddin S, Popovic M, et al: Frequent detection and isolation of cytopathic retrovirus (HTVL-III) from patients with AIDS and at risk for AIDS. Science 224:500, 1984
19. Gartner S, Markovits P, Markovitz DM, et al: The role of mononuclear phagocytes in HTLV-III/LAV infection. Science 233:215, 1986
20. Gelderblom HR, Hausmann EHS, Ozel M, et al: Fine structure of human immunodeficiency virus (HIV) and immunolocalization of structural proteins. Virology 156:171, 1987
21. Gerberding JL, Bryant-LeBlanc CE, Nelson K, et al: Risk of human immunodeficiency virus, cytomegalovirus, and hepatitis B virus transmission to health care workers exposed to patients with acquired immunodeficiency syndrome (AIDS) and AIDS-related conditions. J Infect Dis 156:1, 1987
22. Guyader M, Emerman M, Sonigo P, et al: Genome organization and transactivation of the human immunodeficiency virus type 2. Nature 326:662, 1987
23. Haase A: The slow infection caused by visna virus. Curr Top Microbiol Immunol 72:101, 1975
24. Halstead SB, O'Rourke EJ: Dengue viruses and mononuclear phagocytes. J Exp Med 146:201, 1977
25. Harper ME, Marselle LM, Gallo RC, et al: Detection of lymphocytes expressing human T-lymphotropic virus type III in lymph nodes and peripheral blood from infected individuals by in situ hybridization. Proc Natl Acad Sci USA 83:772, 1986
26. Henle G, Henle W: Immunology of Epstein-Barr virus. In Roizman B (ed): The Herpesviruses. New York, Plenum Press, 1982, p 209
26a Ho DD, Moudgil T, and Alam M: Quantitation of human immunodeficiency virus type 1 in the blood of infected persons. N Engl J Med 321:1621, 1989
27. Ho DD, Rota T, Schooley R, et al: Isolation of HTLV-III from cerebrospinal fluid and neural tissues of patients with neurologic syndromes related to the acquired immunodeficiency syndrome. N Engl J Med 313:1493, 1985
28. Ho DD, Sarngadharan MG, Hirsch MS, et al: Human immunodeficiency virus neutralizing antibodies recognize several conserved domains on the envelope glycoproteins. J Virol 61:2024, 1987
29. Hollander H, Levy JA: Neurologic abnormalities and human immunodeficiency virus recovery from cerebrospinal fluid. Ann Intern Med 106:692, 1987
30. Homsy J, Meyer M, Levy JA: Serum enhancement of HIV infection correlates with disease in HIV-infected individuals. J Virol 64:1437, 1990

31. Homsy J, Meyer M, Tateno M, et al: The Fc and not the CD4 receptor mediates antibody enhancement of HIV infection in human cells. Science 244:1357, 1989

32. Hoxie JA, Alpers JD, Rackowski JL, et al: Alterations in T4 (CD4) protein and mRNA synthesis in cells infected with HIV. Science 234:1123, 1986

33. Kalyanaraman VS, Cabradilla CD, Getchell JP, et al: Antibodies to the core protein of lymphadenopathy-associated virus (LAV) in patients with AIDS. Science 225:321, 1984

34. Kaminsky LS, McHugh T, Stites D, et al: High prevalence of antibodies to AIDS-associated retroviruses (ARV) in acquired immune deficiency syndrome and related conditions and not in other disease states. Proc Natl Acad Sci USA 82:5535, 1985

35. Kanki PJ, Barin F, M'Boup S, et al: New human T-lymphotropic retrovirus related to simian T-lymphotropic virus type III (STLV-III$_{agm}$). Science 232:238, 1986

36. Kiprov DD, Anderson RE, Morand PR, et al: Antilymphocyte antibodies and seropositivity for retroviruses in groups at high risk for AIDS. N Engl J Med 312:1517, 1985

37. Klatzmann D, Champagne E, Chamaret S, et al: T-lymphocyte T4 molecule behaves as receptor for human retrovirus LAV. Nature 312:767, 1984

38. Koenig RE, Pittaluga J, Bogart M, et al: Differences in prevalence of antibodies to the human immunodeficiency virus (HIV) in Dominicans and Haitians in the Dominican Republic. JAMA 257:631, 1987

39. Koenig S, Gendelman HE, Orenstein JM, et al: Detection of AIDS virus in macrophages in brain tissue from AIDS patients with encephalopathy. Science 233:1089, 1986

40. Levy JA: The multifaceted retrovirus. Cancer Res 46:5457, 1986

41. Levy JA: The transmission of AIDS: The case of the infected cell. JAMA 259:3037, 1988

42. Levy JA: Human immunodeficiency viruses and the pathogenesis of AIDS. JAMA 261:2997, 1989

43. Levy JA, Evans LA, Cheng-Mayer C, et al: The biologic and molecular properties of the AIDS-associated retrovirus that affect antiviral therapy. Ann Inst Pasteur 138:101, 1987

44. Levy JA, Evans LA, Pan L-Z, et al: The biologic heterogeneity of HIV and host immune response during HIV infection. In Ginsburg H, Lerner R, Chanock R (eds): Vaccines 1987. Cold Spring Harbor Laboratories, Cold Spring Harbor, 1987, p 168

45. Levy JA, Hoffman AD, Kramer SM, et al: Isolation of lymphocytopathic retroviruses from San Francisco patients with AIDS. Science 225:840, 1984

46. Levy JA, Hollander H, Shimabukuro J, et al: Isolation of AIDS-associated retroviruses from cerebrospinal fluid and brain of patients with neurological symptoms. Lancet 2:586, 1985

47. Levy JA, Kaminsky LS, Morrow WJW, et al: Infection by the retrovirus associated with the acquired immunodeficiency syndrome. Ann Intern Med 103:694, 1985

48. Levy JA, Shimabukuro J: Recovery of AIDS-associated retroviruses from patients with AIDS, related conditions, and clinically healthy individuals. J Infect Dis 152:734, 1985

49. Levy JA, Shimabukuro J, McHugh T, et al: AIDS-associated retroviruses (ARV) can productively infect other cells besides human T helper cells. Virology 147:441, 1985

50. Lifson JD, Feinberg MB, Reyes GR, et al: Induction of CD4-dependent cell fusion by the HTLV-III/LAV envelope glycoprotein. Nature 323:725, 1986

51. Lindenmann J: Viruses as immunological adjuvants in cancer. Biochem Biophys Acta 49:355, 1974

52. Luciw PA, Potter SJ, Steimer K, et al: Molecular cloning of AIDS-associated retrovirus. Nature 312:760, 1984

53. McDougal J, Kennedy M, Sligh J, et al: The binding of HTLV-III/LAV to T4+ T cells by a complex of the 110 kD viral protein (gp110) and the T4 molecule. Science 231:382, 1986

54. Michaelis B, Levy JA: Recovery of human immunodeficiency virus from serum. JAMA 257:1327, 1987

55. Nelson JA, Wiley CA, Reynolds-Kohler C, et al: Detection of the human immunodeficiency virus in bowel epithelium. Lancet 1:259, 1988

56. Pan L-Z, Cheng-Mayer C, Levy JA: Patterns of antibody response in individuals infected with the human immunodeficiency virus. J Infect Dis 155:626, 1987

57. Pape JW, Liautaud B, Thomas F, et al: The acquired immunodeficiency syndrome in Haiti. Ann Intern Med 103:674, 1985

58. Plata F, Autran B, Martins LP, et al: AIDS virus-specific cytotoxic T lymphocytes in lung disorders. Nature 328:348, 1987
59. Protner A, Scroggs RA, Naeve CW: The fusion glycoprotein of Sendai virus: Sequence analysis of an epitope involved in fusion and virus neutralization. Virology 157:556, 1987
60. Quinn TC, Mann JM, Curran JW, et al: AIDS in Africa: An epidemiologic paradigm. Science 234:955, 1986
61. Rabson A, Martin M: Molecular organization of the AIDS retrovirus. Cell 40:477, 1985
62. Robert-Guroff M, Giardina PJ, Robey WG, et al: HTLV-III neutralizing antibody development in transfusion-dependent seropositive patients with B-thalassemia. J Immunol 138:3731, 1987
63. Robinson WE Jr, Montefiori DC, Mitchell WM: Antibody-dependent enhancement of human immunodeficiency virus type 1 infection. Lancet 1:790, 1988
64. Salahuddin SZ, Markham PD, Popovic M, et al: Isolation of infectious human T-cell leukemia/lymphotropic virus type III (HTLV-III) from patients with acquired immunodeficiency syndrome (AIDS) or AIDS-related complex (ARC) and from healthy carriers: A study of risk groups and tissue sources. Proc Natl Acad Sci USA 82:5530, 1985
65. Sarin PS, Sun DK, Thornton AH, et al: Neutralization of HTLV-III/LAV replication by antiserum to thymosin alpha-1. Science 232:1135, 1986
66. Sarngadharan MG, Popovic M, Bruch L, et al: Antibodies reactive with human T-lymphotropic retroviruses (HTLV-III) in the serum of patients with AIDS. Science 224:506, 1984
67. Schupbach J, Haller O, Vogt M, et al: Antibodies to HTLV-III in Swiss patients with AIDS and pre-AIDS and in groups at risk for AIDS. N Engl J Med 312:265, 1985
68. Serwadda D, Mugerwa RD, Sewandambo NK: Slim disease: A new disease in Uganda and its association with HTLV-III infection. Lancet 2:849, 1985
69. Shaw G, Harper M, Hahn B, et al: HTLV-III infection in brains of children and adults with AIDS encephalopathy. Science 227:177, 1985
70. Simonsen JN, Cameron DW, Gaknya MN, et al: Human immunodeficiency virus infection among men with sexually transmitted diseases. N Engl J Med 319:274, 1988
71. Starcich BR, Hahn BH, Shaw GM, et al: Identification and characterization of conserved and variable regions in the envelope gene of HTLV-III/LAV, the retrovirus of AIDS. Cell 45:637, 1986
72. Tateno M, Cheng-Mayer C, Levy JA: MT-4 plaque formation can distinguish cytopathic subtypes of the human immunodeficiency virus (HIV). Virology 167:299, 1988
73. Tateno M, Gonzalez-Scarano F, Levy JA: The human immunodeficiency virus can infect CD4-negative human fibroblastoid cells. Proc Natl Acad Sci USA 86:4287, 1989
74. Tschachler E, Groh V, Popovic M, et al: Epidermal Langerhans cells: A target for HTLV-III/LAV infection. J Invest Dermatol 88:233, 1987
75. Van de Perre P, Lepage P, Kestelyn P, et al: Acquired immunodeficiency syndrome in Rwanda. Lancet 2:62, 1984
76. Vogt M, Craven D, Crawford D, et al: Isolation of HTLV-III/LAV from cervical secretions of women at risk for AIDS. Lancet 1:525, 1986
77. Walker B, Chakrabarti S, Moss B, et al: HIV-specific cytotoxic T lymphocytes in seropositive individuals. Nature 328:345, 1987
78. Walker C, Moody D, Stites DP, et al: CD8+ lymphocytes can control HIV infection in vitro by suppressing virus replication. Science 234:1563, 1986
79. Walker CM, Levy JA: A diffusible lymphokine produced by CD8+ T lymphocytes suppresses HIV replication. Immunology 66:628, 1989
80. Wiley CA, Schrier RD, Nelson JA, et al: Cellular localization of the AIDS retrovirus infection within the brains of acquired immune deficiency syndrome patients. Proc Natl Acad Sci USA 83:7089, 1986
81. Wofsy CB, Cohen JB, Hauer LB, et al: Isolation of the AIDS-associated retrovirus from vaginal and cervical secretions from women with antibodies to the virus. Lancet 1:527, 1986

3

PREVENTION OF HIV TRANSMISSION

CONSTANCE B. WOFSY, MD

Prevention of HIV transmission through blood and blood products, tissue and organ donations, and health care exposure rests largely with the medical and scientific community in providing the most up-to-date testing, policies, and health delivery safety. Prevention of HIV transmission by sexual contact and needle sharing, an issue of behavior change and behavior initiation, is a shared responsibility of legislative bodies, religious organizations, public health administrators, the medical community, and the individual. Sexually active persons and intravenous drug users have a responsibility to themselves, their sexual partners, and potential offspring to avoid unsafe activities. Information is everywhere, but comprehension and application are in short supply. Since sex and drug sharing are consensual acts, health care providers must obtain the attention of those at risk, make sure they hear the facts, and motivate them to change privately conducted, high-risk behavior. The challenge is difficult because such changes are perceived to be inconvenient, to decrease pleasure, and to interfere with the spontaneity of sex or the urgent need for a fix. Since most adults have been, will be, or are sexually active, the "they" who have to change may in fact be "us."

Physicians are accustomed to being prevention counselors in health decisions. For example, they encourage patients with impaired liver function to use indicated anticoagulants, caution patients with infectious mononucleosis to avoid sports during the course of the disease, or admonish patients to lose weight, avoid red meat, or drink less alcohol. Since the patient's health is the target of these preventive efforts, the responsibility for implementation rests with the patient. Societal consequences, such as the prevention of auto accidents caused by alcohol abuse, are a secondary goal of physicians' counseling. The physician shares responsibility for prevention of communicable diseases with the public health department after appropriate reporting. In AIDS care, however, the enormousness of the

38

population at potential risk, the fear and stigma of the disease, its complexity, discomfort with discussing sex and death, the patient's extraordinary expectations of the physician, and the time and patience required in discussion interfere with counseling efforts. The physician is assumed to be equipped for a role he or she may not be prepared to play. When personal risk and emotions are concerned, the most dedicated physician must work through these issues before he or she can adequately fulfill the role of health provider. Ambivalence about care of AIDS patients was reflected in a survey of nursing students: 70 percent thought that AIDS patients deserve the same care as any other patients, but only 9 percent strongly agreed that they should be assigned to AIDS patients and 33 percent did not believe that student nurses should be assigned to AIDS patients.[52]

Most people pass through five stages in becoming comfortable talking about HIV: (1) avoidance, (2) demand for a risk-free environment, (3) recognition that AIDS exists, (4) interest in self-education, and (5) concern for the person with HIV.[87] A health professional in the second stage may have trouble giving unbiased counseling to an equally frightened patient. As AIDS is becoming incorporated in training of health professionals, they are finding the disease easier to discuss.

MECHANISMS OF AIDS TRANSMISSION

Mechanisms of AIDS transmission are outlined in Table 3–1. Sexual transmission is responsible for 73 percent of AIDS cases; 68 percent of AIDS patients are homosexual or bisexual and 27 percent are heterosexual although only 5 percent acquire HIV through heterosexual activities.[3] It is estimated that up to 15 percent of homosexual men have female partners. These sexual partners and their offspring are also at risk for infection. Fully 94 percent of adults with AIDS acquired their infection through a consensual act, either sex or intravenous drug use, often without knowledge or acknowledgment of risk. Among children with AIDS under 13 years of age, 80 percent acquired the disease from an infected mother.[36] Receptive anal intercourse confers the greatest risk of infection to homosexual men[45] and female partners of bisexual men.[66] However, heterosexual infection in either direction is almost always the result of vaginal intercourse.[65] Several reports of lesbian-to-lesbian transmission suggest a role of vaginal secretions alone in HIV transmission,[35,56] and HIV has been cultured in vaginal secretions and menstrual blood, although in low titer.[82,88] Transfusion of infected blood or blood products accounts for only 2 percent of all reported AIDS cases, and hemophilia or coagulation disorders account for 1 percent. An infected woman has a 30 to 50 percent chance of giving birth to a child who is also infected with HIV.[9] HIV has been identified in vitro in breast milk,[78] and breast-feeding has been implicated as the sole means of

TABLE 3—1.   PREVENTION OF HIV TRANSMISSION

TRANSMISSION ROUTE	TRANSMISSION MECHANISM	FLUID OR TISSUE IMPLICATED	PREVENTION
Sex	Male to male, heterosexual, woman to woman	Semen, vaginal or cervical secretions	Careful partner selection; HIV discussion with potential partner; abstinence; latex condoms used properly; water-based lubricants; nonoxynol-9
Intravenous drug use	Needle sharing	Blood	Not starting drug use; getting drug treatment; not sharing needles; cleaning injection implements; cleaning skin; avoiding "shooting galleries"
Blood and blood products	Transfusion, hemophilia, treatment	Blood clotting factors	Voluntary donor exclusion; HIV testing; heat treatment
	Needlestick exposures	Blood	Avoiding recapping needles; using puncture-proof containers; following CDC guidelines
Maternal (seropositive mother)	Transplacental, birth	?Blood, fetal tissue, amniotic fluid	Avoiding conception if HIV positive; terminating of pregnancy; anticipating care of infected child
		Breast milk	Avoiding breast-feeding (in United States)
Sperm donation		Semen	Voluntary donor exclusion; reputable donor center; donor HIV test at 0 and 6 months; freezing sperm
Organ donation		Various organs	HIV testing before donor receives any transfusion; risk-benefit analysis

transmission from postnatally infected mothers to their infants.[19,51,91] Donor semen was a source of infection in four women who received sperm from a single infected man.[75] HIV transmission by transplantation of kidney, liver, bone, and other organs has been confirmed.[4,11]

CHANGING BEHAVIOR

The steps in changing behavior are common to many situations (Table 3—2). The physician's opinion can be a powerful impetus to change. However, the physician may need training in motivating patients. In smoking cessation programs, physicians who received several hours of training in smoking cessation and discussed the subject with patients for several minutes at routine office visits effected a small but significant increase in

TABLE 3–2. STEPS TO BEHAVIOR CHANGE

1. Understanding that the behavior is risky
   (Smoking causes cancer; intravenous drugs can cause AIDS.)
2. Acknowledgement that it could be *personally* risky
   (*I* could get lung cancer; *I* could get AIDS.)
3. Intent to change; commitment
   (I will stop smoking on May 6; I will enroll in drug treatment on Pine Street on June 4.)
4. Tools to change
   (nicotine gum, condoms, bleach, safe sex workshops)
5. Involvement and commitment of peers
   (the family, school curricula, consensus agreement to change as by using condoms,
   support groups, peer counselors)

1-year smoking free rates. Giving patients nicotine gum and reminder stickers enhanced efficacy,[18,24] although setting a specific date to stop smoking was the most effective tool. Such interventions were highly cost effective.[23]

Wearing seat belts decreased the severity of injury for people who were in accidents and resulted in substantial cost savings.[67] Legislation establishing fines for nonwearers enhanced seat belt use.[15] Behavior modification programs are particularly effective when legislation is combined with a public information campaign.[74] In contrast to legislation attempting to modify private behavior, however, legislation mandating seat belt use does not infringe on personal rights, since cars are driven on public roads. Furthermore, education about seat belts does not touch on societal taboos. Attempts to legislate mandatory HIV testing as a means of inducing behavior change have been costly. Six months of premarital testing in Illinois cost $2.5 million and led to a 22 percent reduction in marriage license applications and significant increase in licenses granted in surrounding states.[16,79]

When the scientific and medical communities fail to control or contain dangerous behavior, legislators attempt to fill the void. Most states have laws that attempt to change behavior by coercion.[32] Only when such laws are coupled with effective public education and acceptance, antidiscrimination, and recognized benefit to the affected or exposed person is legislation likely to help change behavior for the better.

PREVENTING SEXUAL TRANSMISSION

The standard recommendations for avoiding sexual transmission, in order of ensuring safety, are abstinence, mutually monogamous relationship with a partner since the mid-1970s, monogamous relationship with someone who has been HIV antibody negative for at least 6 months, avoidance of vaginal or anal intercourse with a person known to be seropositive, and use of latex condoms with nonoxynol-9 for insertive vaginal or anal sex.[28,76] This assumes that people can select sex partners dispassionately. Adherence to these guidelines depends on the perceived risk associated with the partner and the benefit and worth of applying the intervention. Moreover, both partners have to agree to the conditions for safe sex. Since partners change over time, the behavior of an entire peer group, such as adolescents or homosexuals in a specific city, must be modified. Control measures for sexually transmitted diseases, such as genital ulcers, which have a strong association with HIV transmission, are essential to control such transmission.[34]

Changing Sexual Behavior in Specific Populations

Male Homosexuals

Striking evidence of sexual behavior changes among homosexual men is found in the marked reductions in the incidence of rectal gonorrhea, hepatitis A acquisition, and number of sexual partners and in the leveling off of annual HIV infection rates measured by seroconversion. In major cities gay organizations, gay newspapers, gay men's health clinics, an army of volunteers, safe sex campaigns, and the tragedy of friends and lovers dying have contributed to the spread of information and presumably to changes in behavior. One program to train homosexual men in using condoms resulted in a 44 percent increase in condom use, compared with an 11 percent increase in a control group without the intervention.[80]

Heterosexuals

Widespread perception of AIDS risk among heterosexuals has not occurred although many excellent articles on this subject have appeared in the lay press.[9,49,77] However, incidence rates in the military have remained stable for 24 months,[10] and heterosexual clients of HIV testing sites in New York City increased from 39.4 to 58.7 percent between January 1986 and December 1987.[33] A prospective study in Florida evaluated sexual behavior change in 32 couples in which one partner was seropositive for HIV and the other seronegative. Eight couples (25 percent) became abstinent, 10 (31 percent) chose to use condoms consistently, and a striking 14 (44 percent) continued their sexual practices unchanged with an 86 percent seroconversion rate of the negative partners over 18 months.[27] This indicates that sexual habits are hard to change even among couples who have been adequately counseled with direct and repeated access to skilled HIV counselors.

Condoms and Nonoxynol-9

Although condoms and spermicides reduce the risk of transmission of sexually transmitted diseases, the failure rate is 13 to 15 percent when condoms are used as the sole means of contraception.[44] Only 10 of 32 HIV-discordant couples, studied prospectively, consistently used condoms for vaginal intercourse. One seroconversion was reported in the initial 18 months' follow-up, and two additional seroconversions have subsequently been reported. Latex and natural skin condoms have been tested in the laboratory for efficacy in preventing the passage of HIV,[21,81] cytomegalovirus,[43] hepatitis B virus,[63] and herpes simplex virus[20] across the condom material (Table 3–3).[69] Latex condoms subjected to simulated rigors of intercourse in the laboratory prevented transmission in all cases; natural skin condoms, however, allowed late passage of both hepatitis B virus[63] and HIV[81] through the material and thus are considered unsafe.

Condom ineffectiveness is less likely to be the result of microscopic holes than of episodic use, improper placement, or rupture or falling off during intercourse. This is particularly true of anal sex whether for gay or straight couples. Since condoms are designed for birth control and vaginal sex, they are not well suited for rectal sex. In one study condom breakage increased with increasing number of acts of rectal sex by gay men.[31] Nevertheless, in the Multi-Center AIDS Cohort Study, consistent use of condoms for insertive sex significantly reduced seroconversion.[25] In a study of consenting male homosexual couples, a condom specially designed for the rigors of anal intercourse was found to have the highest safety but the lowest availability.[85] *Consumer Reports* has listed condom brands specifically designed for rectal sex. Since petroleum-based lubricants make a latex condom more likely to rupture, water-soluble lubricants such as K-Y Jelly are advocated. Some condoms are impregnated with nonoxynol-9, a viricidal spermicide. In vitro, nonoxynol-9 exhibits excellent HIV viricidal activity at a 0.05 percent concentration, but reduces lymphocyte viability at 5 percent.[37] The

TABLE 3–3.   IN VITRO STUDIES OF EFFECTIVENESS OF COMMERCIALLY AVAILABLE CONDOMS

AGENT	LATEX CONDOM	NATURAL SKIN CONDOM	SIZE (nm)	REFERENCES
HIV	Safe	Leaked	120	20,81
Hepatitis B	Safe	Leaked	42	63
Cytomegalovirus	Safe	—	150-130	43
Herpesvirus	Safe	—	100-115	19
Sperm	Safe	—	3000	20,81
Air, water	—	—	<0.1	

TABLE 3—4.   STEPS FOR RESPONSIBLE SEXUALITY

Before the Need Arises
1. Discuss condom use with partner when unaroused.
2. Use latex condoms, water-soluble lubricants, and nonoxynol-9 if tolerated.
3. Practice condom placement in advance.
4. Keep condoms in a readily accessible place.

Condom Placement
1. Pinch end of condom before placement to allow a reservoir for semen.
2. Fully unroll the condom onto erect penis.
3. Hold condom at base of penis on withdrawal.
4. Use a new condom for each act of intercourse.
5. *Never* use a condom twice.
6. *Never* use petroleum-based lubricants with a condom.

concentration used in the Today Contraceptive Sponge induced virus inactivation in vitro while preserving tissue culture cell viability.[68] The use of nonoxynol-9 impregnated condoms, lubricants, vaginal foams, and contraceptive sponges is strongly advocated as added protection to latex condoms.

Condoms add a measure of safety but by no means guarantee it. Proper use and planning are essential (Table 3—4). Public desensitization to embarrassment about condoms is facilitated by ads in magazines and on buses and by articles in the lay press such as *Consumer Reports*.[1] A superb Australian advertisement for condoms won a Clio Award for television advertising in 1989.

Oral Sex, Cunnilingus, and French Kissing

Isolated and often unsubstantiated reports of HIV transmission by oral sex appear periodically. No seroconversions occurred in 147 gay men who practiced only oral sex.[45] One of eight seroconversions among 290 initially seronegative men studied at the Fenway Community Health Center in Boston was attributed to oral exposure to semen.[60] In the several reported cases of HIV transmission in lesbians, oral contact with vaginal secretions was implicated and in one case was suggested as the sole mode of transmission.[35,56] Thus prevention strategies must incorporate the possibility of oral sexual transmission. Condoms should be worn for fellatio, and cunnilingus should be avoided or performed with artful use of latex patches (dental dams).

Saliva has never been implicated in transmission, but large cohorts of couples who engage in French kissing as their sole means of sexual expression are hard to find. HIV was isolated in low titer from saliva in only one of 83 infected men.[39] However, deep prolonged kissing could be associated with rupture of small blood vessels and could result in the exchange of relatively large volumes of saliva.[58,67] Thus French kissing must be considered possibly unsafe in couples discordant for HIV infection.

TRANSMISSION BY NEEDLE SHARING

The message for avoiding needle transmission of HIV is: Don't experiment with intravenous drugs; get drug treatment if you're a user; don't share needles; clean your equipment (works); clean your skin; and avoid "shooting galleries."[55] HIV seroprevalence in intravenous drug users in major cities varies widely and is as high as 56 percent in certain treatment centers in New York.[55,72] The intensive education network and volunteerism of the gay community are absent among intravenous drug users. Professionals skilled at dealing with drug users representing a wide variety of ethnic groups and community organizations have made inroads in attempts to provide information, but they face a difficult battle. Seroprevalence among intravenous drug users is strongly associated with number of persons with whom needles are shared, nonwhite race, use of shooting galleries, and injection of cocaine.[12,13,55] Addicts often consider AIDS to be a gay disease, and nonwhites consider it a white disease. The sharing of drugs is social as well as convenient. Thus effective interventions for behavior change must be culturally and ethnically directed, must be accessible, and must involve the entire peer network.

Interventions that have altered risk of HIV in drug users are shown in Table 3–5. In a Boston study of 193 male intravenous drug abusers in an inpatient drug treatment program, 68 percent shared needles during 40 percent of their drug use episodes. Although 77 percent reported sharing only with relatives or close friends, 23 percent shared with casual acquaintances and strangers.[38] In a subsequent study in New York, sharing with strangers was strongly predictive of seropositivity.[72] It is a commonly held misconception that a person who appears healthy or is one's personal partner or relative must be safe. The message is: Don't share; use clean needles; and, if you share, clean your needles with bleach. The San Francisco AIDS

TABLE 3–5.   FACTORS SHOWN TO CHANGE HIV RISK IN INTRAVENOUS DRUG USERS

1. Cleaning of needles
2. Enrollment in treatment programs
3. Bleach distribution
4. Skill of the counselor
5. Needle exchange

Foundation has distributed 15,000 vials of household bleach with simple bilingual instructions to addicts through street outreach programs in conjunction with a poster and billboard campaign.[14] Needle sharing was reported by 71 percent of intravenous drug users studied. In 1985 only 6 percent usually or always sterilized with bleach, but by 1987, 47 percent of the 172 individuals evaluated reported that they sterilized. Bleach is an excellent choice because it is an inexpensive, fast-acting, accessible agent that is viricidal in a dilution of 1:100 and deactivates within 1 minute. (Not surprisingly, a case of an attempted suicide by injection of household bleach has been reported.[29]) In New York similar hard-won inroads into safer needle use through needle exchange have occurred.[61] These "best case" successes with aggressive intervention suggest that change is possible and support continued drug treatment programs and street outreach efforts that induce drug users to avoid sharing and to clean their equipment.

BLOOD AND BLOOD PRODUCT TRANSMISSION

Although transmission via blood and blood products accounts for only 2 percent of AIDS cases, people must accept this small risk because they have no alternative to these lifesaving measures. When 203 living recipients of HIV-infected blood were evaluated, 59 percent were HIV antibody positive or had AIDS. Transmission risk increased to 95 percent if the donor had previously infected a recipient.[83] The risk of receiving infected blood that is HIV antibody negative when tested (assuming an 8-week window period for a donor to develop seropositivity) is estimated at 1:153,000 per unit transfused or 1:28,000 per transfusion that averages 5.4 units.[9,22] Since 1983 the risk of transmission by blood products has been made negligible by aggressive efforts to encourage at-risk blood donors to defer donation and by HIV antibody testing of donated blood.[3] Steps to further reduce infected units and transmission include more careful assessment of need, fewer units per transfusion, and recruitment of more women donors, since blood from a repeat female donor is nine times as likely to be safe as that from a new male donor.[22] Although voluntary donor deferral has helped, some at-risk individuals still donate because of denial about their risk, pressure to donate, or desire to use the blood bank for testing. A face-to-face private interview with prospective donors might eliminate some infected volunteers.[50] In 1984 a process for heat inactivation of cryoprecipitate or factor VIII was instituted, and this has virtually eliminated new seroconversions in hemophiliacs. Immune serum globulin, RhoGam, and hepatitis B vaccines have never been reported to transmit HIV, and the methods of preparation have always inactivated infectious particles.

Needlestick Injuries

Despite the thousands of health care workers exposed to needlestick injuries or blood from HIV-infected or risk group patients, only a few cases have been confirmed as likely health care–associated infections (see Chapters 4 and 25).[6,30] The risk of HIV transmission from a single needlestick injury is negligible compared with the 20 percent risk of hepatitis B after a stick with a hepatitis B virus–contaminated needle. A small risk multiplied many times, however, is a very real risk, and rigorous attention to protection of health care workers is mandatory. Efforts to prevent HIV infection in health care workers include readily available instructional materials, repeated educational efforts, rigorous adherence to CDC infection control guidelines, impermeable needle disposal units, avoidance of recapping of needles, and appropriate use of eye protection, gowns, and gloves when in contact with body secretions or when exposed to potentially infectious fluids by splash. The adoption of universal blood and body fluid precautions will significantly enhance protection of health care workers,[6,54] since many infected persons do not know that they are infected and the results of antibody testing, even if more widely used, are not available in the emergency setting. Further efforts at worker safety focus on identifying and correcting behaviors associated with needlestick injuries and identifying the safest injection products[41] and glove materials.[90]

MATERNAL TRANSMISSION

Seventy-seven percent of AIDS patients under 13 years of age acquired HIV from an infected mother.[36] To interrupt the transmission pattern, men and women known or perceived to be at risk of HIV infection should be counseled, tested, and encouraged to avoid pregnancy. For those who are already pregnant, all information that would allow a woman and her partner to make an informed decision about abortion should be made available.[8,71] HIV infection, however, may not be a major stimulus for pregnancy termination. In one study termination choices of female intravenous drug users were the same regardless of HIV status (50 percent of 28 HIV antibody positive and 44 percent of 36 HIV antibody negative). Prior abortion was the major determining factor in choosing to abort. Knowledge of AIDS or fear of contracting HIV did not influence termination choice regardless of HIV status.[73]

A question is how accurately designated risk group categories identify women likely to pass HIV to an infant. In inner city hospitals the answer appears to be not very. In a study reported in November 1987, 2 percent of cord blood samples from 602 infants delivered at an inner city municipal hospital in New York were seropositive for HIV.[48] Five of the 12 seropositive mothers denied having a risk factor. Risk factor designations were broad and included intravenous drug use; a sex partner who used intravenous drugs, was bisexual, or had received a transfusion; residence in an endemic area for HIV; or past receipt of a transfusion. In the Bronx 2.6 percent of 353 women attending an abortion clinic were HIV positive.[72] Since the samples were anonymous, the incidence of risk factors was unknown. These findings of a high rate of unsuspected HIV infection parallel studies of hepatitis B. Risk factors for hepatitis B were elicited in only 10 (45 percent) of 22 hepatitis B surface antigen–positive women at the Cleveland Metropolitan General Hospital,[47] and 47 percent of hepatitis B–infected women would have been missed by routine risk assessment in a similar study at the University of Miami School of Medicine.[42]

Stemming the tide of pediatric AIDS infection requires the availability of ironclad confidentiality so women can be tested and make informed judgments about conception and childbearing. Seropositive women are often viewed as pariahs infecting their children; their needs and special issues must be carefully considered.[89] Premarital screening has been advocated as a means of preventing sexual and subsequent perinatal transmission. However, a pilot program was expensive, decreased the number of marriage license applications, and increased applications in neighboring states.[79]

Breast-Feeding

Postnatal transmission of HIV from mothers infected by transfusion at the time of birth to their infants by breast-feeding has been reported.[19,51,91] In all instances the relationships were monogamous, the father was seronegative at the time the mother proved seropositive, and the mother denied any history of other risk exposure. HIV has been cultured from breast milk.[78] In the United States a number of policymaking bodies advocate avoidance of breast-feeding by infected mothers.[8,71] The breast-feeding policy has generated considerable controversy, particularly in Third World countries. The relative protection of colostrum may outweigh the potential small added risk of transmission of HIV by breast-feeding to a child born to a mother who was infected throughout the gestation period. Milk banks are now pasteurizing donated milk.

DONOR SPERM INSEMINATION

Four of eight recipients of high intravaginal insemination with cryopreserved semen from an HIV-infected asymptomatic carrier became seropositive. Three subsequently gave birth to naturally conceived children, all of whom are seronegative as are the husbands.[75] In these instances semen had been stored for at least 3 months, but glycerol cryopreservation is now thought insufficient to inactivate HIV. The CDC has developed guidelines for donor insemination indicating that, after voluntary exclusion of men with any risk factor for HIV, semen will be frozen for at least 6 months until the donor has been retested and the semen deemed appropriate for use.[7,59] Frozen semen offers the advantages of convenience, time to evaluate the presence of pathogens and genetic abnormalities, and use of the same donor for subsequent pregnancies. However, frozen semen lowers the pregnancy rate by 10 to 15 percent and requires more inseminations per cycle. Unfortunately, many semen donation arrangements are made privately and outside established semen banks, and not all donation facilities adhere to the advocated standards. Only 44 percent of obstetrician-gynecologists surveyed in 1988 said that they tested donors for HIV antibody.[57] Couples should be encouraged to use reputable insemination centers and to inquire about HIV screening policies.[4,12]

ORGAN DONATION

Organ donation decisions are often made in a situation of urgency. The donor is often a trauma victim who received multiple transfusions before death was determined to be inevitable. A tragic case of HIV transmission by an infected donor whose antibody test was negative because of multiple transfusions underscores the need to test a pretransfusion blood sample from the donor. Guidelines for organ donation have been established.[4,11]

GUIDELINES FOR INFORMATION COUNSELING AND TESTING FOR HIV

The decision to test for HIV is now a medical one and is based on the need to implement antiviral therapy and *Pneumocystis* prophylaxis in seropositive persons, determination of candidacy for research studies, advisability of testing for tuberculosis and syphilis, and protection of potential partners and offspring.[26,53] Those tested must be counseled, informed of the possible consequences, and assured of confidentiality. The CDC has recommended that certain groups be targeted for information, counseling, and possible testing (Table 3–6).[5] A busy clinician can refer to a succinct summary of issues to be raised before and after testing, such as that displayed on a laminated card used by the HIV testing and counseling service at San Francisco General Hospital (Table 3–7).

To prevent transmission of other sexually transmitted diseases, pilot programs for partner notification have been undertaken with the goals of treating the index case and exposed individuals, decreasing disease ex-

TABLE 3–6.   SUMMARY OF HIV COUNSELING

Pretest Counseling
1. Review risk behaviors, transmission, incubation and latency, and counseling and testing program.
2. Explain test and meaning of positive and negative results.
3. Describe risk reduction (safer sex, condoms, needles [no sharing, bleach]).
4. Explain confidentiality procedure and risk of disclosure.
5. Obtain written informed consent and complete demographic form.
6. Make appointment for result disclosure.

Posttest Counseling
1. Assess mental status.
2. Inform patient in person.
3. Review transmission, risk behaviors, and meaning of test.
4. Provide community referrals for psychosocial help, social services, drug treatment, and medical treatment.

Modified from San Francisco General Hospital Testing and Counseling Services, 1989.

TABLE 3–7.   POPULATIONS TARGETED FOR INFORMATION AND COUNSELING

1. Homosexual men
2. Intravenous drug users
3. Persons with other sexually transmitted diseases
4. Women of childbearing age
5. Persons with multiple or anonymous partners
6. Prostitutes
7. Persons receiving transfusions mid-1970s to 1985
8. Persons planning marriage or childbearing
9. Persons with an obscure medical diagnosis
10. Hospital admissions
11. Persons in correctional institutions

Modified from Centers for Disease Control: MMWR 36:509, 1987.

posure, promoting condom use, and limiting transmission into the community. Because HIV itself is not treatable and the stigma of infection is far greater than with other sexually transmitted diseases, even greater care must be given to teach as well as to test. A question is whether a person's knowledge of his or her serologic status will change behavior and whether individuals will inform their sexual partners of their serologic status and institute behavioral changes. As noted earlier in Fischl's study of 32 heterosexual couples, 75 percent of HIV-discordant couples chose a safer form of sexual activity (abstinence or condoms) when informed of their serologic status. In our study of sexually active women, six (21 percent) of 29 seropositive women chose abstinence and those who remained sexually active substantially increased use of condoms for sexual activity.[17] Thus, in the highly restricted situation of seroepidemiologic studies, behavior definitely changes. In such epidemiologic studies, however, subjects have a very direct relationship with study investigators, teaching is repetitive, confidentiality is highly guarded, and subjects may well have less direct societal risk than when tested in the more routine and busier health care setting.

SUGGESTIONS FOR BROACHING THE SUBJECT OF HIV

Broaching the Subject

The physician could open with a general statement such as, "I am making it a habit to review HIV as part of my usual routine of health care maintenance, and I want to discuss with you whether anything in your life-style or medical past could have exposed you to HIV or the AIDS virus. The way most people become infected is through sex, especially with other men [for male patients], use of intravenous drugs, or a previous sexual partner who was bisexual or used intravenous drugs. If you have had any of these possible exposures or had a blood transfusion between 1978 and 1985, you could be at risk and we should talk about it further."

Providing Pamphlets and AIDS Information Numbers

The physician can acknowledge that a frank discussion of sexual issues may be a new role for him or her and the patient. The physician should rehearse the conversation and have AIDS pamphlets available with hot line numbers and other referral resources. The availability of printed material validates the issue as a real one in the medical care community, and giving a patient pamphlets sponsored by the appropriate ethnic or sexual orientation group suggests that this is a real and widely recognized issue for that population.

Dealing with Specific Groups

All Patients

Physicians should allay fears, dispel myths, and answer questions factually. They should confirm that AIDS cannot be transmitted by casual contact. Patients should be cautioned to avoid or postpone sex with people whose past habits they do not know well and to realize that people may not tell about their previous high-risk behavior. Health providers should avoid being judgmental, since their goal is to keep people as healthy as possible, not to judge behavior. A sensitively expressed professional opinion about the health risk of certain behaviors, however, could be lifesaving.

Sexually Active, Nonmonogamous Persons

A patient who has any doubts about a partner should insist on the use of a condom in conjunction with nonoxynol and water-based lubricants. The health care provider should have a condom sample available for demonstration if needed. Copies of the *Consumer Reports* condom article or a synopsis should also be available.[1] Women should be informed that they can enhance their protection by using a foam, jelly, or contraceptive sponge containing nonoxynol-9. Women and men who might conceive a child should be told that up to a 50 percent chance exists that HIV could be passed to a child conceived.

Intravenous Drug Users and Those Who Might Experiment With Drugs

The best advice is not to start using drugs. Those who have started should be referred to drug treatment. If that is not possible or desired, they should be instructed about cleaning needles and the risk of sharing.

Persons with Possible Past Exposures

If a patient has been involved in high-risk activity since the late 1970s, the physician should let the person think about the possibility of testing, give a brochure, discuss the pros and cons of testing, and refer the patient to hot line information.

Society

Physicians should provide a leadership role, give talks at schools, teach young family members to be safe, and not tolerate homophobic or AIDS jokes. They should be role models for openness and honesty and should set ethical standards.[46]

SUMMARY

With screening of the blood supply and effective heat and chemical treatment of blood product derivatives, the overwhelming majority of future adult HIV infection will result from consensual acts involving the exchange of blood, sexual secretions, or other body fluids. Societal relaxation about discussion of sex, death, homosexuality, drugs, and abortion is essential to prevent further deaths. Careful partner selection, use of condoms in conjunction with nonoxynol-9 (a viricidal spermicide), and selected confidential HIV antibody testing could decrease the number of infected persons. Efforts to discourage people from starting drug use, make drug treatment more accessible, and provide clean needles or simple techniques for cleaning needles, such as a quick rinsing with bleach and water, as well as drumming in the message not to share, could decrease the exponential rise of HIV infection in intravenous drug users. A substantial percentage of women infected with both HIV and hepatitis B are unaware of their infection. Prenatal counseling and antibody testing of men and women and presentation of information about options to those who are seropositive could reduce the risk of perinatal transmission. Health professionals must deal with their own fears and possible discomfort with various life-styles to function effectively as providers of care to HIV-infected persons.

REFERENCES

1. Can you rely on condoms? Consumer Reports, March 1989, pp 135-141
2. Centers for Disease Control: HIV-AIDS Surveillance Report. pp 1-16, Sept 1989
3. Centers for Disease Control: Human immunodeficiency virus infection in transfusion recipients and their family members. MMWR 36:137-139, 1987
4. Centers for Disease Control: Semen banking, organ and tissue transplantation, and HIV antibody testing. United States. MMWR 37(4), 1988
5. Centers for Disease Control: PHS guidelines for counseling and antibody testing to prevent HIV. MMWR 36:509, 1987
6. Centers for Disease Control: Recommendations for prevention of HIV transmission in health-care settings. MMWR 36:3s, 1987
7. Centers for Disease Control: Testing donors of organs, tissues, and semen for antibody to human T-lymphotropic virus type III/lymphadenopathy-associated virus. MMWR 34:294, 1985
8. Centers for Disease Control: Recommendations for assisting in the prevention of perinatal transmission of human t-lymphotropic virus type III/lymphadenopathy-associated virus and acquired immunodeficiency syndrome. MMWR 34:721-732, 1985
9. Centers for Disease Control: Update: Heterosexual transmission of acquired immunodeficiency syndrome and human immunodeficiency virus—United States. MMWR 38:423-434, 1989
10. Centers for Disease Control: Trends in human immunodeficiency virus among civilian applicants for military service—United States, October, 1985–March, 1988. MMWR 37:677-679, 1988
11. Centers for Disease Control: Transmission of HIV through bone transplantation: Case report and public health recommendations. MMWR 37:597-599, 1988
12. Chaisson R, Bacchetti P, Osmond D, et al: Cocaine use and HIV infection in intravenous drug users in San Francisco. JAMA 261:561-565, 1989
13. Chaisson RE, et al: Human immunodeficiency virus infection in heterosexual intravenous drug users in San Francisco. Am J Public Health 177:169-171, 1987
14. Chaisson RE, Osmond D, Moss AR, et al: HIV, bleach and needle sharing. (Letter.) Lancet 2:1430, 1987
15. Chorba TL, Reinfurt D, Hulka BS: Efficacy of mandatory seat-belt use legislation: The North Carolina experience from 1983 through 1987. JAMA 260:3593-3597, 1988
16. Cleary PD, Barry MJ, Mayer KH: Compulsory premarital screening for the human immunodeficiency virus. JAMA 258:1757-1762, 1987
17. Cohen JB, Lyons CA, Lockett GJ, et al: Emerging patterns of drug use, sexual behavior, HIV infection, and STDs in high-risk San Francisco areas from 1986-1989. Presented at the Fifth International Conference on AIDS, Montreal, Canada, June 4–9, 1989
18. Cohen SJ, Stookey GK, Katz BP, et al: Encouraging primary care physicians to help smokers quit. Ann Intern Med 110:648-652, 1989

19. Colebunders R, Kapita B, Nekwei W, et al: Breastfeeding and transmission of HIV. (Letter.) Lancet 2:1487, 1988
20. Conant MA, Spicer DW, Smith CD: Herpes simplex virus transmission: Condom studies. Sex Transm Dis 11:94-95, 1984
21. Conant M, Hardy D, Sernatinger J, et al: Condoms prevent transmission of AIDS-associated retrovirus. (Letter.) JAMA 255:1706, 1986
22. Cumming PD, Wallace EL, Schorr JB, et al: Exposure of patients to human immunodeficiency virus through the transfusion of blood components that test antibody negative. N Engl J Med 321:941-946, 1989
23. Cummings SR, Rubin SM, Oster G: The cost effectiveness of counseling smokers to quit. JAMA 261:75-79, 1989
24. Cummings SR, Coates TJ, Richard RJ, et al: Training physicians in counseling about smoking cessation. Ann Intern Med 110:640-647, 1989
25. Detels R, English P, Visscher B, et al: Seroconversion, sexual activity, and condom use among 2915 HIV seronegative men followed for up to 2 years. J AIDS 2:77-83, 1989
26. Drotman DP: Earlier diagnosis of human immunodeficiency virus (HIV) infection and more counseling. Ann Intern Med 110:680-681, 1989
27. Fischl MA, Dickinson GM, Scoh GB, et al: Evaluation of heterosexual partners, children, and household contacts of adults with AIDS. JAMA 257:640-644, 1987
28. Friedland GH, Klein RS: Transmission of the human immunodeficiency virus. N Engl J Med 317:1125-1135, 1987
29. Froner GA, Rutherford GW, Rokeach M: Injection of sodium hypochlorite by intravenous drug users. (Letter.) JAMA 258:325, 1987
30. Gerberding JL, Bryant-Leblanc CE, Nelson K, et al: Risk of transmitting the human immunodeficiency virus, cytomegalovirus, and hepatitis B virus to health care workers exposed to patients with AIDS and AIDS-related conditions. J Infect Dis 156:1-8, 1987
31. Golombok S, Sketchley J, Rust J: Condom failure among homosexual men. J AIDS 2:404-409, 1989
32. Gostin LO: Public health strategies for confronting AIDS. JAMA 261:1621-1630, 1989
33. Grabau JC, Morse DL: Seropositivity for HIV at alternate sites. (Letter.) JAMA 260:3128, 1988
34. Greenblatt, RM, Lukehart SA, Plummer FA, et al: Genital ulceration as a risk factor for human immunodeficiency virus infection. AIDS 2:47-50, 1988
35. Greenhouse P: Female-to-female transmission of HIV. (Letter.) Lancet 486:401-402, 1987
36. Guinan ME, Hardy A: Epidemiology of AIDS in women in the United States. JAMA 257:2039-2042, 1987
37. Hicks DR, Martin LS, Getchell JP, et al: Inactivation of HTLV-III/LAV-infected cultures of normal human lymphocytes by nonoxynol-9 in vitro. (Letter.) Lancet 1422-1423, 1985
38. Himmelstein DU, Woolhandler S: Sharing of needles among users of intravenous drugs (Letter.) N Engl J Med 1:446
39. Ho DD, Byington RE, Schooley RT, et al: Infrequency of isolation of HTLV-III virus from saliva in AIDS. N Engl J Med 313:1606, 1985
40. Hoffmann AF, Popper H: Breast feeding and HIV infection. (Letter.) Lancet 2:400-401, 1987
41. Jagger J, Hunt E, Brand-Elnaggar J, et al: Rates of needle injury caused by various devices in a university hospital. N Engl J Med 319:284-288, 1988
42. Jonas MM, Schiff ER, O'Sullivan MJ, et al: Failure of Centers for Disease Control criteria to identify hepatitis B infection in a large municipal obstetrical population. Ann Intern Med 107:335-337, 1987
43. Katznelson S, Drew WL, Mintz L: Efficacy of the condom as a barrier to the transmission of cytomegalovirus. J Infect Dis 150:155-157, 1984
44. Kelly JA, St Lawrence JS: Cautions about condoms in prevention of AIDS. (Letter.) Lancet 1:323, 1987
45. Kingsley LA, et al: Risk factors for seroconversion to human immunodeficiency virus among homosexuals. Lancet 1:345-348, 1987
46. Koop CE: Physician leadership in preventing AIDS. JAMA 258:2111, 1987

47. Kumar ML, Dawson NV, McCullough AJ, et al: Should all pregnant women be screened for hepatitis B? Ann Intern Med 107:273-277, 1987
48. Landesman S, Minkoff H, Holman S, et al: Serosurvey of human immunodeficiency virus infection in parturients. JAMA 258:2701-2703, 1987
49. Leishman K: Heterosexuals and AIDS. Atlantic Monthly, Feb. 1987, pp 39-58
50. Leitman S, Klein H, Melpolder J, et al: Clinical implications of positive tests for antibodies to human immunodeficiency virus type I in asymptomatic blood donors. N Engl J Med 321:917-924, 1989
51. Lepage P, Van de Perre P, Carael M, et al: Postnatal transmission of HIV from mother to child. (Letter.) Lancet 2:400-401, 1987
52. Lester LB, Beard BJ: Nursing attitudes toward AIDS. J Nurse Educ 27:399, 1988
53. Lo B, Steinbrook R, Cooke M, et al: Voluntary screening for human immunodeficiency virus (HIV) infection. Ann Intern Med 110:727-733, 1989
54. Lynch P, Jackson MM, Cummings MJ, et al: Rethinking the role of isolation practices in the prevention of nosocomial infections. Ann Intern Med 107:243-246, 1987
55. Marmor M, Des Jarlais DC, Friedman SR, et al: The epidemic of acquired immuno-deficiency syndrome (AIDS) and suggestions for its control in drug abusers. J Subs Abuse Treat 1:237-247, 1984
56. Marmor M, Weiss LR, Lyden M, et al. Possible female-to-female transmission of human immunodeficiency virus. (Letter.) Ann Intern Med 105:969, 1986
57. Marwick C: Artificial insemination faces regulation, testing of donor semen, other mea-sure. JAMA 260:1339-1340, 1988
58. Marzili TJ: The biologic possibility of HIV transmission during passionate kissing. (Let-ter.) JAMA 262:2230, 1989
59. Mascola L, Guinan ME: Screening to reduce transmission of sexually transmitted diseases in semen used for artificial insemination. N Engl J Med 314:1354-1359, 1986
60. Mayer KH, DeGruttola V: Human immunodeficiency virus and oral intercourse. (Letter.) Ann Intern Med 107:428-429, 1987
61. Medical news and perspectives: US cities struggle to implement needle exchanges despite apparent success in European cities. JAMA 260:2620-2621, 1988
62. Minkoff HL: Care of pregnant women infected with human immunodeficiency virus. JAMA 258:2714-2717, 1987
63. Minuk GY, Bohme CE, Bowen TJ: Condoms and hepatitis B virus infection. (Letter.) Ann Intern Med 104:584, 1986
64. Orsay EM, Turnbull TL, Dunne M, et al: Prospective study of the effect of safety belts on morbidity and health care costs in motor-vehicle accidents. JAMA 260:3598-3603, 1988
65. Padian NS: Heterosexual transmission of acquired immunodeficiency syndrome: Inter-national perspectives and national projections. Rev Infect Dis 9:947-960, 1987
66. Padian NS, Marquis L, Francis DP, et al: Male-to-female transmission of human im-munodeficiency virus. JAMA 258:788-790, 1987
67. Piazza M, Chirianni A, Picciotto L, et al: Passionate kissing and microlesions of the oral mucosa: Possible role in AIDS transmission. JAMA 261:244-245, 1989
68. Polsky B, Gold JWM, Baron PA, et al: Inactivation of human immunodeficiency virus (HIV) by the Today Contraceptive Sponge (TCS). Presented at an International Con-gress of Antimicrobial Agents and Chemotherapy (ICAAC), New York, 1987, p 161
69. Rietmeijer CA, Krebs JW, Feorino PM, et al: Condoms as physical and chemical barriers against human immunodeficiency virus. JAMA 259:1851-1853, 1988
70. Rhame FS, Maki DG: The case for wider use of testing for HIV infection. N Engl J Med 320:1248-1254, 1989
71. Rutherford GW, Oliva GE, Grossman M, et al: Guidelines for control of perinatally transmitted human immunodeficiency virus infection and care of infected mothers, infants and children. West J Med 147:104-108, 1987
72. Schoenbaum E, Hartel D, Selwyn P, et al: Risk factors for human immunodeficiency virus infection in intravenous drug users. N Engl J Med 321:874-879, 1989
73. Selwyn P, Carter R, Schoenbaum E, et al: Knowledge of HIV antibody status and de-cisions to continue or terminate pregnancy among intravenous drug users. JAMA 261:3567, 1989

74. Steed D: The case for safety belt use. (Editorial.) JAMA 260.3651, 1988
75. Stewart GJ, Tyler JPP, Cunningham AL, et al: Transmission of human T-cell lympho-tropic virus type III (HTLV-III) by artificial insemination by donor. Lancet 2:581-584, 1985
76. Surgeon General's report on acquired immune deficiency syndrome. JAMA 256:2784-2789, 1986
77. The big chill — how heterosexuals are coping with AIDS. Time Magazine, Feb 16, 1987
78. Thiry L, Sprecher-Goldbergers S, Jockheer T, et al. Isolation of AIDS virus from cell free breast milk of mice healthy virus carriers. Lancet 2:891-892, 1985
79. Turnock BJ, Kelly CJ: Mandatory premarital testing for human immunodeficiency virus. JAMA 261:3415-3418, 1989
80. Valdiserri R, Lyter D, Leviton L, et al: AIDS prevention in homosexual and bisexual men: Results of a randomized trial evaluating two risk reduction interventions. AIDS 3:21-26, 1989
81. Van de Perre P, Jacobs D, Sprecher-Goldberger S: The latex condom, an efficient barrier against sexual transmission of AIDS-related viruses. AIDS 1:49-52, 1987
82. Vogt MW, Witt DJ, Craven DE, et al: Isolation patterns of the human immunodeficiency virus from cervical secretions during the menstrual cycle of women at risk for the acquired immunodeficiency syndrome. Ann Intern Med 106:380-382, 1987
83. Ward J, Bush T, Perkins H, et al: The natural history of transmission-associated infections with human immunodeficiency virus. N Engl J Med 321:947-952, 1989
84. Ward JW, Holmberg SD, Allen JR, et al: Transmission of human immunodeficiency virus (HIV) by blood transfusions screened as negative for HIV antibody. N Engl J Med 318:473-478, 1988
85. Wigersma L, Oud R: Safety and acceptability of condoms for use by homosexual men as a prophylactic against transmission of HIV during anogenital intercourse. Br Med J 295:94, 1987
86. Winkelstein W, Samuel M, Padian NS, et al: Reduction in human immunodeficiency virus among homosexual/bisexual men, 1982-86: The San Francisco Men's Health Study: III. Am J Public Health, 76:685, 1987
87. Wofsy CB: AIDS — An Epidemic of Fear: AIDS in the Workplace. Videotape, Pacific Bell Telephone Co. (producer). Distributed by San Francisco AIDS Foundation
88. Wofsy CB, Cohen J, Hauer L, et al: Isolation of AIDS-associated retrovirus from genital secretions of women with antibodies to the virus. Lancet 1:527-529, 1986
89. Wofsy CB: Human immunodeficiency virus infection in women. JAMA 257:2074-2076, 1987
90. Zbitnew A, Greer K, Heise-Qualtiere J, et al: Vinyl versus latex gloves as barriers to transmission of viruses in the health care setting. J AIDS 2:201-204, 1989
91. Ziegler JB, Cooper DA, Johnson RO, et al: Postnatal transmission of AIDS-associated retrovirus from mother to infant. Lancet 1:896-897, 1985

4

OCCUPATIONAL HIV TRANSMISSION:
Issues for Health Care Providers

JULIE LOUISE GERBERDING, MD

Health care providers exposed to blood and other body fluids risk infection with HIV. Defining the risks of occupational HIV transmission and developing policies for protecting health care providers are important concerns in the AIDS era. Although progress has been made, these issues continue to stimulate controversy. This chapter provides an update of the status of risk assessment and risk reduction strategies for preventing occupational HIV infection.

RISK ASSESSMENT

The risk from occupational exposure to HIV has been evaluated prospectively in cohorts of intensively exposed health care providers at medical centers around the world. Since both the numerator (number of infections) and the denominator (number of exposures) are known, these studies allow estimates of the rate of transmission following various types of exposure. More than 4000 health care providers from a variety of occupations, including more than 1200 with a history of accidental parenteral inoculation with HIV-infected materials, have been enrolled in such studies and periodically tested for HIV antibody.[4,7,12,13,14,16,18,20,21,27]

In 5 years of observation, direct inoculation of infected material during accidental needlestick or similar parenteral injury has been the only mechanism of transmission observed among study subjects. The rate of nosocomial HIV transmission following parenteral exposure is approximately 0.4 percent (five infections of >1200 needlesticks involving HIV-infected blood).[4,5,7,12,13,14,16,18,20,21,27] The risk from mucous membrane contact or in-

57

TABLE 4−1.   CASES OF DOCUMENTED OCCUPATIONAL HIV TRANSMISSION REPORTED BY NOVEMBER 1989

11 needlestick (blood)
1 laceration (blood)
4 mucocutaneous (blood)
1 cutaneous (blood/body fluid)
1 parenteral (concentrated virus)
1 nonintact skin (concentrated virus)

Transmission was documented by seroconversion temporally related to exposure in 17 of 18 cases and by virus identity in 1 of 18. Cases were cited in references 1, 2, 4, 5, 7, 8, 10, 12, 13, 14, 16−18, 20−23, 27, 30, 32, 33, 35, and 36.

oculation of nonintact skin with HIV-infected blood or other body fluids is too low to be quantified in these studies to date, even though at least 1000 exposures of this type have been assessed.

Nineteen documented cases of occupational HIV transmission (including the five mentioned previously) have been reported in the world's medical literature since 1981 (Table 4−1). In the majority of these cases occupational transmission was proved by demonstration of seroconversion temporally related to a discrete accidental HIV exposure event.[1,2,5,8,12,17,20,22,23,27,30,32,33,35] Needlestick exposure or lacerations contaminated by infected blood produced infection in 12 health care workers.[1,2,8,12,20,22,23,27,32,33,35] In four, inapparent parenteral exposure to blood through breaks in the skin or mucous membrane inoculation with blood was the most likely route of transmission.[8,33] Two health care providers were infected via exposure to virus concentrate (parenteral and nonintact skin contamination) in research laboratories.[35] The mode of transmission is unknown in one health care provider with documented seroconversion who had extensive contact with infected blood and other body fluids without using appropriate infection control measures.[2] In at least six additional reported cases, occupational transmission is possible but was not proved by demonstration of seroconversion.[10,17,20,26,36] These anecdotal reports certainly do not include all cases of occupational infection because occupational infection is not a reportable condition until AIDS develops, and some cases may not yet be recognized or reported. Efforts to coordinate surveillance and reporting of occupationally acquired HIV infection are in progress and will permit a more complete assessment of the frequency of such events.

A variety of as yet poorly defined factors may influence the risk of transmission. Most authorities believe that the volume of the inoculum and the quantity of virus involved in the exposure influence the degree of risk. Deep (intramuscular) penetrations, large-bore hollow needles, and injections of blood are factors associated with most of the reported needlestick accidents causing infections. Large volumes of blood, prolonged duration of contact, and a portal of entry are common denominators in the reported mucocutaneous cases. The stage of infection in the source patient also may be linked to the probability of transmission. Circulating titers of HIV are believed to be highest at the time of seroconversion and later during advanced stages of symptomatic infection, but the relationship of this observation to the infectivity of occupational exposures remains speculative. The efficiency of transmission could also be increased by the presence of intracellular (as distinct from cell-free) virus in the inoculum. Finally, the immunolgic status of the recipient health care provider could influence the probability of infection.

Blood has been implicated as the source of the exposure in all infections occurring in clinicians. Other body fluids, including saliva, tears, and urine, may contain the virus, but the titer of HIV in these fluids is usually much lower than in blood and semen. Although HIV transmission through exposure to most nonbloody body fluids therefore is unlikely, these fluids could contain other viruses or pathogens and should be considered potentially infectious when infection control interventions are planned.

Cutaneous exposure involving normal skin has not been linked to HIV infection in any setting. Although in most infected patients Langerhans' cells and other subcutaneous cells possess CD4 receptors and contain HIV, these cells are protected from primary infection by an intact integument. However, transcutaneous inoculation during parenteral needlestick injury or contamination of skin lesions has been hypothesized to promote primary infection of subcutaneous target cells. No risk from close personal contact with patients, exposure to airborne droplets or aerosols, or contact with contaminated environmental surfaces or fomites has been observed.

Aerosols of infected blood or saliva can occur in dentists' offices, pathology departments, laboratories, and operating rooms. Because masks do not prevent exposure to aerosolized particles smaller than the pore diameter of the mask material, the possibility of aerosolized HIV transmission has alarmed some health care providers. Hepatitis B virus, which is present in much higher titers than HIV among infected patients, has not been recovered from aerosols during experiments performed in dental operatories and dialysis units.[24,25] The absence of HIV seroconversion in prospective studies of dentists practicing in areas where HIV is highly prevalent strongly suggests that aerosol transmission is unlikely to confer a measurable occupational hazard.[7] In fact, aerosols have not been associated with HIV infection in any setting to date. Even if aerosols contain viable HIV, the magnitude of risk is unlikely to be greater than the risk from mucous membrane splashes (see preceding discussion).

The cumulative professional risk from repeated exposure to HIV has not been adequately assessed. The overall risk to a given health care provider depends on the risk from discrete exposure events, as well as the frequency of exposure to body fluids and the prevalence of HIV in the work place. Health care providers such as nurses, dentists, surgeons, emergency care providers, and labor and delivery personnel are at highest risk for acquiring hepatitis B virus and also may be at higher risk for HIV infection over a lifetime of practice, particularly when practicing in areas with a high prevalence of HIV.[9,37] Large prospective studies of these individuals will be necessary to define the true magnitude of risk.

ALLAYING FEAR

Fear of AIDS may be masked by denial. Beliefs that HIV-infected patients are not present, that infected patients can be identified and avoided, or that transmission is impossible are often perpetuated until the reality of occupational risk becomes apparent. The first experience with occupational exposure or infection may precipitate a crisis. Anger, depression, surprise, and aggressiveness are reactions frequently described in this setting. Although a zero risk of infection is not a realistic possibility, a demand for excessive or unreasonable infection control measures often follows the initial crisis. Health care workers must recognize that some degree of risk is unavoidable and shared by all care providers. On the other hand, providers should be reassured that occupational infection is less likely when infection control procedures are implemented. Involving workers at risk for exposure in the development of precautions can help channel concern into constructive outlets.

Fear of acquiring HIV among clinicians who recognize their risk for exposure is not irrational when the degree of fear is appropriate to the degree of risk. Lack of knowledge about the magnitude of risk or routes of transmission, the epidemic nature of the disease, the high mortality rate, and the lack of effective treatment can amplify the perceived risk and should be addressed. In addition, the anxiety aroused by the complex psychologic issues related to homosexuality, morality, and mortality evoked by AIDS patients may be communicated as fear of infection. Some health care professionals find it easier to avoid AIDS patients altogether than to deal with the emotional conflicts encountered while providing care; fear of contagion provides a convenient and more publicly acceptable excuse. Constructive methods to acknowledge openly the stresses inherent in dealing with AIDS patients should be included in clinical training curricula and staff development programs.

RISK REDUCTION BY INFECTION CONTROL

Avoiding contact with potentially infected body fluids and tissues is an essential component of risk reduction for health care providers.[3,5,19,28,34] Preventing needlestick injuries and other parenteral exposures is likely to have the biggest impact on reducing HIV transmission in most health care settings.[15,28] Although blood is the only body fluid associated with occupational HIV transmission to date, common sense and concern for preventing transmission of other nosocomial pathogens dictate that other body fluids also should be considered potentially infectious.

The CDC has recommended universal precautions for all patients, regardless of diagnosis, to prevent transmission of bloodborne pathogens.[28] Additional isolation precautions are advised for patients with infections transmitted by other routes. The universal precautions include wearing gloves for procedures in which contact with blood, bloody body fluids, and certain other fluids (amniotic fluid, semen, vaginal fluid, cerebrospinal fluid, serosal transudates and exudates, and inflammatory exudates) might occur; wearing masks and protective eyewear when splatter of such body fluids is anticipated; and wearing gowns or other protective garments when clothing is likely to be soiled.[28]

Body substance precautions (BSP) (or body substance isolation [BSI]) is an alternative system of infection control practiced in a number of institutions.[3,19] A single standard of precautions, based on the anticipated degree of exposure to *all* body fluids and tissues, regardless of the infectious disease diagnosed or suspected, is implemented at the moment of initial contact with the patient.[15,19] The main difference between CDC and BSP infection control systems is that the CDC system considers the type of infection suspected, whereas BSP is based on the degree of contact anticipated. However, both universal precautions and BSP emphasize prevention of needlestick injury and barrier protection for avoiding exposure to potentially infectious materials, and neither requires labeling of patients or specimens for implementation. Compliance with either policy is likely to reduce exposure to bloodborne pathogens and should be encouraged in all health care settings.

HIV TESTING FOR INFECTION CONTROL

The list of valid indications for considering HIV testing continues to expand, especially since the advent of effective antiretroviral therapy and prophylaxis for pneumocystic pneumonia. Unlike most other laboratory tests, testing for HIV involves a degree of risk to the patient. Because effective antidiscrimination legislation has not yet been passed in most areas, many HIV-infected persons risk discrimination in employment, housing, insurance, and even medical care. Most states have recognized both the benefits and risks associated with HIV testing and require informed consent before the test is performed.

Testing for HIV to implement infection control procedures remains controversial. Some health care providers believe that identifying infected patients will improve compliance with infection control procedures or that surgical techniques safer for the surgical team should be selectively employed for those with diagnosed HIV infection. In some hospitals, such as San Francisco General Hospital (SFGH), surgeons can opt to test patients preoperatively (after informed consent is obtained) and adjust infection control practices accordingly. Other institutions prohibit HIV testing unless a medical indication is present, and a few routinely test all patients. Currently no evidence supports the validity of any of these approaches. Clearly more research is warranted to determine whether benefit (reduced exposure) at minimal risk to the patient (good surgical outcome, confidentiality) and cost to the institution (avoidance of excessive expenditures) can be achieved through identifying infected patients preoperatively.

MANAGING OCCUPATIONAL EXPOSURES TO HIV

The CDC has published guidelines for managing health care workers accidentally exposed to HIV.[28,32] Determining whether exposure has actually occurred is rarely simple. Health care workers may not report exposures for a variety of reasons or may underestimate or overestimate the severity of the exposure. A careful history usually permits categorization of the exposure route into one of the following broad categories: (1) needlestick (or similar injury resulting in direct transcutaneous exposure), (2) mucous membrane inoculation, (3) contamination of open skin wound or lesion, or (4) contamination of nonintact skin. Needlesticks and other percutaneous accidents should be further characterized by the size and type of needle or instrument involved (suture, hollow, scalpel, etc.), approximate depth of penetration, volume of blood injected (if any), site, wound appearance, amount of bleeding produced, and time during which the contaminating fluid was ex vivo before the exposure occurred. The type, volume, and duration of contact should be estimated for mucous membrane and skin wound contacts.

A system for estimating exposure severity developed at SFGH classifies exposures as "massive" (transfusions, parenteral exposure to HIV concentrates), "definite parenteral" (intramuscular parenteral inoculations or injections of blood or bloody fluids), "possible parenteral" (subcutaneous or superficial percutaneous exposures, mucous membrane splashes, contamination of open wounds), "doubtful parenteral" (exposures involving nonbloody body fluids such as saliva, urine, or tears), and "nonparenteral" (contamination of normal skin) (Table 4–2).[11] Although the relationship of these designations to the actual risk of transmission remains unproved, clinicians have found the classification scheme useful in counseling exposed workers and planning follow-up interventions (see the following).

Establishing the presence of infection in the source patient is often difficult but can help clarify the degree of risk induced by the exposure event. Obviously the presence of HIV infection can be assumed when patients are found to have AIDS or ARC or are known to be HIV infected. Institutions vary in testing policies for source patients whose HIV status is less clear. In most the probability of HIV infection is assessed on the basis of

TABLE 4–2. ZIDOVUDINE PROPHYLAXIS FOR OCCUPATIONALLY EXPOSED HEALTH CARE PROVIDERS

EXPOSURE LEVEL	TREATMENT RECOMMENDATION
Massive exposure (transfusion)	Recommended
Definite parenteral (intramuscular injection)	Endorsed
Possible parenteral (subcutaneous or mucosal)	Available
Doubtful parenteral (nonbloody fluid)	Discouraged
Nonparenteral (cutaneous)	Not provided

Interim protocol at San Francisco General Hospital, 1989, is zidovudine 200 mg q.4h. 5 times a day for 4 weeks, ideally started within 1 hour of exposure.

clinical and epidemiologic criteria. Patients perceived to be at risk are counseled and asked to consent to testing. Routine testing of all source patients is gaining acceptance, although mandatory testing (without informed consent) to identify a source patient is not yet widespread. Regardless of the testing strategy employed, every effort must be made to protect the confidentiality of the source patient.

The exposed health care worker should be encourage to undergo baseline HIV testing or at least have serum banked as soon as possible after exposure has occurred. Without a negative baseline HIV test, proving that infection was temporally related to the exposure event is impossible. Consequently, the worker's ability to claim workers' compensation and other benefits may be seriously jeopardized. Subsequent HIV testing, usually performed 6 weeks, 3 months, and 6 months after exposure, is recommended when HIV is present or potentially present in the exposure source. Sequential testing is extremely useful in allaying fear, documenting seronegativity, and, rarely, diagnosing HIV infection.

Because symptoms of acute retroviral infection (fever, lymphadenopathy, rash, headache, profound fatigue) have been associated with the majority of reported occupational infections, exposed persons should be advised to return for evaluation if a compatible illness occurs.[32] Enzyme-linked immunosorbent assay (ELISA) HIV antibody tests are negative or indeterminate during the early phases of seroconversion illness. The Western blot test, virus cultures, or HIV p24 antigen tests may be more sensitive methods for detecting early infection. The value of gene amplification technology (polymerase chain reaction [PCR]) in identifying infection in seronegative health care workers remains unproved, but preliminary studies suggest that latent infections detected by PCR rarely if ever are detected in seronegative health care workers.[6]

Postexposure counseling by experienced care providers familiar with the special medical and psychologic needs of exposed health care providers is essential. Counseling should provide information about the degree of risk present, options for follow-up, a description of the confidentiality procedures in place, and infection control procedures to prevent similar occurrences. Counselors should be alert to the concerns of the sexual partners, co-workers, and friends of the exposed worker.

The CDC recommends "safer" sexual practices and other behavior changes to minimize the potential for transmission until a negative antibody test 6 months after the exposure rules out infection. Unfortunately, offering this advice frequently produces confusion and anxiety in the exposed person. Counselors are faced with the difficult task of communicating a mixed message about the risk of infection: reassurance that occupational transmission is statistically unlikely, yet advocacy of behaviors to prevent exchange of body fluids, avoid pregnancy, and defer blood donation until infection has been ruled out. In some medical centers advice is individualized to the specific situation. For example, persons sustaining trivial punctures with small-bore nonhollow needles minimally contaminated by blood from a low-risk, untested patient may decide to return for follow-up HIV testing for 6 months but to comply with safer sex guidelines for a shorter interval. In contrast, recipients of deep intramuscular injections of infected blood may be cautioned to follow guidelines for preventing transmission compulsively for more than 6 months and to continue follow-up for 12 months.

Postexposure Chemoprophylaxis

Interest in postexposure chemoprophylaxis for occupationally exposed health care workers has increased since zidovudine was licensed for palliating HIV infection in persons with advanced disease. Theoretically, when zidovudine or other nucleoside analogs are administered soon after exposure, they could prevent HIV infection by preventing HIV replication in the initial target cells.

The relevance of animal models of retrovirus infection to human infection with HIV has not been established. Experiments with murine, feline, and simian retrovirus in animals inoculated with high titers of virus indicate that zidovudine can prevent viremia and illness under some conditions.[29,31] However, the efficacy of zidovudine in preventing the establishment of asymptomatic latent infection has not yet been evaluated in these models. Protection is most apparent when treatment is started within 24 hours of exposure.

The efficacy of zidovudine for preventing latent infection in exposed health care workers will be difficult to assess because the low rate of seroconversion mandates an extremely large sample. Furthermore, detecting infection in treated individuals may be complicated by delayed seroconversion related to drug-induced inhibition of virus replication. Anecdotal experience with zidovudine for short intervals in healthy health care workers indicates that reversible hematologic toxic effects occur rarely but that less serious subjective symptoms of intolerance such as fatigue, insomnia, and flulike symptoms are common.

Investigators at the National Institutes of Health (NIH), CDC, and SFGH are developing collaborative efforts to evaluate the safety of prophylactic zidovudine. In the meantime, some institutions (including the NIH and SFGH) have developed protocols for offering prophylactic zidovudine to selected health care workers exposed to HIV.[11] Until more information is available, protocols for prophylactic treatment should be considered experimental therapy requiring written informed consent from the health care worker electing treatment.

At SFGH and the NIH the option of taking zidovudine is discussed with all exposed health care providers, and expert consultation is readily available. Although the decision to take zidovudine is ultimately left to the health care worker, the advice given at SFGH depends on the severity of exposure. For example, zidovudine is strongly encouraged for "massive exposures," endorsed for "definite parenteral exposures," not routinely recommended but available for "possible parenteral exposures," and discouraged for "doubtful" or "nonparenteral exposures" (Table 4–2). This approach assumes that exposure severity is a major predictor of infection risk and that the benefit from prophylactic zidovudine is most evident for high-risk exposures.

Most authorities believe that prophylactic zidovudine treatment should be started as soon as possible (within minutes to hours) after the exposure to maximize the chance of efficacy. The optimal dosage and duration for chemoprophylaxis have not been established, but most protocols employ conventional doses used to treat AIDS patients for 2 to 6 weeks. Treatment of pregnant women or persons not practicing effective contraception should be discouraged. Close monitoring for hematologic, hepatic, renal, and neurologic dysfunction is essential. Adverse reactions should be reported to the Food and Drug Administration.

Clearly, further in vitro and animal research on chemoprophylaxis with zidovudine and other antiretroviral agents is warranted. Until efficacy and toxicity of any agent are established, chemoprophylaxis will remain a promising but unproven strategy for preventing HIV infection in health care providers.

REFERENCES

1. Anonymous: Needlestick transmission of HTLV-III from a patient infected in Africa. Lancet 2:1376-1377, 1984
2. Apparent transmission of human T-lymphotropic type III/lymphadenopathy-associated virus from a child to a mother providing health care. MMWR 35:76-79, 1986
3. Gerberding JL, University of California, San Francisco, Task Force on AIDS: Recommended infection-control policies for patients with human immunodeficiency virus infection: An update. N Engl J Med 315:1562-1564, 1986

4. Gerberding JL, Bryant-LeBlanc CE, Nelson KN, et al: Risk of transmitting the human immunodeficiency virus, cytomegalovirus, and hepatitis B virus to health care providers exposed to patients with AIDS and AIDS-related conditions (ARC). J Infect Dis 156:1-8, 1987
5. Gerberding JL, Henderson DK. Design of rational infection control guidelines for human immunodeficiency virus infection. J Infect Dis 156:861-864, 1987
6. Gerberding JL, Littell C, Louie P. Gene amplification to detect latent HIV in health care workers at risk for low inoculum exposures (Abstract No. 1171). In Programs and abstracts of the 29th Interscience Conference on Antimicrobial Agents and Chemotherapy. Washington, DC, American Society for Microbiology, 1989
7. Gerberding JL, Nelson K, Greenspan D, et al: Risk to dentists from occupational exposure to human immunodeficiency virus (HIV): Followup (Abstract No. 698). In Programs and abstracts of the 27th Interscience Conference on Antimicrobial Agents and Chemotherapy. Washington, DC, American Society for Microbiology, 1987
8. Gioannini P, Sinicco A, Cariti G, et al: HIV infection acquired by a nurse. Eur J Epidemiol 4:119-120, 1988
9. Grady GF, Lee VA, Prince AM, et al: Hepatitis B immune globulin for accidental exposures among medical personnel: Final report of a multicenter controlled trial. J Infect Dis 138:625-638, 1978
10. Grint P, McEvoy M: Two associated cases of the acquired immunodeficiency syndrome (AIDS). PHLS Commun Dis Rep 42:4, 1985
11. Henderson DH, Gerberding JL: Post-exposure zidovudine chemoprophylaxis for health care workers occupationally exposed to the human immunodeficiency virus: An interim analysis. J Infect Dis 160:321-327, 1989
12. Henderson DK, Fahey BS, Saah AJ, et al: Longitudinal assessment of the risk for occupational/nosocomial transmission of human immunodeficiency virus, type 1 in health care workers (Abstract No. 634). In Programs and abstracts of the 28th Interscience Conference on Antimicrobial Agents and Chemotherapy. Washington, DC, American Society for Microbiology, 1988
13. Henderson DK, Saah AJ, Zak BJ, et al: Risk of nosocomial infection with human T-cell lymphotropic virus type III/lymphadenopathy-associated virus in a large cohort of intensively exposed health care providers. Ann Intern Med 104:644-647, 1986
14. Health and Welfare Canada: National surveillance program on occupational exposure to HIV among health care workers in Canada. Can Dis Wkly Rep 13-37:163-166, 1987
15. Jagger J, Hunt EH, Bland-Elnaggar J, et al: Rates of needlestick injury caused by various devices in a university hospital. N Engl J Med 319:284-288, 1988
16. Joline C, Wormser GP: Update on a prospective study of health care providers exposed to blood and body fluids of acquired immunodeficiency syndrome patients. Am J Infect Control 15:86, 1987
17. Klein RS, Phelan JA, Freeman K, et al: Low occupational risk of HIV infection among dental professions. N Engl J 318:86-90, 1988
18. Kuhls TL, Viker S, Parris NB, et al: Occupational risk of HIV, HBV, and HSV-2 infections in health care personnel caring for AIDS patients. Am J Pub Health 77:1306-1309, 1987
19. Lynch P, Jackson MM, Cummings MJ, et al: Rethinking the role of isolation practices in the prevention of nosocomial infections. Ann Intern Med 107:243-246, 1987
20. Marcus R, The Cooperative Needlestick Surveillance Group: Surveillance of health care workers exposed to blood from patients infected with the human immunodeficiency virus. N Engl J Med 319:1118-1123, 1988
21. McEvoy M, Porter K, Mortimer P, et al: Prospective study of clinical, laboratory, and ancillary staff with accidental exposures to blood or other body fluids from patients infected with HIV. Br Med J 294:1595-1597, 1987
22. Neisson-Verant C, Arfi S, Mathez D, et al: Needlestick HIV seroconversion in a nurse. Lancet 2:814, 1986
23. Oskenhendler E, Harzic M, Le Roux JM, et al: HIV infection with seroconversion after a superficial needlestick injury to the finger. N Engl J Med 315:582, 1986
24. Petersen NJ: An assessment of the airborne route in hepatitis B transmission. Ann NY Acad Sci 253:157-166, 1980

25. Petersen NJ, Bond WW, Favero MS: Air sampling technique for hepatitis B surface antigen in a dental operatory. J Am Dent Assoc 99:465-467, 1979
26. Ponce de Leon RS, Sanchez-Mejorada G, Zaidi-Jacobson M: AIDS in a blood bank technician in Mexico City. (Letter.) Infect Control Hosp Epidemiol 9:101-102, 1988
27. Ramsey KM, Smith EN, Reinarz JA: Prospective evaluation of 44 health care workers exposed to human immunodeficiency virus-1, with one seroconversion. (Abstract.) Clin Res 36:22A, 1988
28. Recommendations for prevention of HIV transmission in health-care settings. MMWR 36(suppl 2S):3S-18S, 1987
29. Ruprecht RM, OBrien LG, Rossoni LD, et al: Suppression of mouse viraemia and retroviral disease by 3'-azido-3'-deoxythymidine. Nature 323:467-469, 1986
30. Stricof RL, Morse DL: HTLV-III/LAV seroconversion following a deep intramuscular needlestick injury. (Letter.) N Engl J Med 314:1115, 1986
31. Travares L, Roneker C, Johnston K, et al: 3'-Azido-3'-deoxythymidine in feline leukemia virus–infected cats: A model for therapy and prophylaxis of AIDS. Cancer Res 47:3190-3194, 1987
32. Update: Acquired immunodeficiency syndrome and human immunodeficiency virus infection among health care workers. MMWR 37:229-239, 1988
33. Update: Human immunodeficiency virus infections in health care workers exposed to blood from infected patients. MMWR 36:285-289, 1987
34. US Department of Labor, US Department of Health and Human Services: Joint advisory notice: Protection against occupational exposure to hepatitis B virus (HBV) and human immunodeficiency virus (HIV). Fed Register 52:41818-41824, 1987
35. Weiss SH, Goedert JJ, Gartner S, et al: Risk of human immunodeficiency virus (HIV-1) infection among laboratory workers. Science 239:68-71, 1988
36. Weiss SH, Saxinger WC, Rechtman D, et al: HTLV-III infection among health care workers: Association with needlestick injuries. JAMA 254:2089-2093, 1985
37. Werner BJ, Grady GF: Accidental hepatitis-B-surface antigen-positive inoculations: Use of e antigen to estimate infectivity. Ann Intern Med 97:367-369, 1982

5

PRIMARY HIV INFECTION:

Clinical, Immunologic and Serologic Aspects

BRETT TINDALL, BAppSc, MSc
ALLISON IMRIE, BSc
BASIL DONOVAN, MB, BS, Dip Ven (Lond), FAC Ven
RONALD PENNY, MD, DSc, FRACP, FRCPA
DAVID A. COOPER, BSc(Med), MD, FRACP, FRCPA

The CDC's clinical definition of primary HIV infection is a mononucleosis-like syndrome, with or without aseptic meningitis, associated with seroconversion for HIV antibody.[18] This syndrome was first recognized in 1985[23,40] following the identification in 1984 of HIV as the etiologic agent of AIDS and the development of serologic tests for the detection of antibodies to HIV,[7,34,52] which had the potential to identify seroconversion. In this chapter we review the characteristic clinical, serologic, and immunologic response to primary HIV infection and speculate on possible therapeutic strategies.

CLINICAL DESCRIPTION

Features

In March 1985 we first reported the clinical illness associated with primary HIV infection.[21] Of 12 homosexual men with documented HIV seroconversion, 11 had an illness characterized as mononucleosis-like, with fever, sweats, lethargy, malaise, myalgia, arthralgia, headache, photophobia, diarrhea, sore throat, lymphadenopathy, and a truncal maculopapular

68

rash (Color Plate IA). The illness was of sudden onset and lasted 3 to 14 days. In a subsequent report Gaines et al[32] found that the illness had a median duration of 12.7 days (range 5 to 44). Since this illness was first recognized, it has been reported in association with primary HIV infection in all major groups at risk for HIV infection, including homosexual men,[11,15,32,36,46,54,88,96] intravenous drug users,[40,44,66] persons with hemophilia,[90,97] recipients of blood and blood component transfusions,[6,12,79] transplant recipients,[47,71,81] heterosexual men and women,[9,17,19,61,98] and health care workers who had received significant needlestick injuries.[62,64,85] Similar manifestations of primary HIV infection have been reported in children who acquired infection through transfusion of HIV-contaminated blood.[20]

In addition to this mononucleosis-like illness, primary HIV infection has also been reported with a wide range of neurologic manifestations, including meningoencephalitis,[16,39,40] myelopathy,[25] peripheral neuropathy,[69] brachial neuritis (neuralgic amyotrophy,[13,15] facial palsy,[69,98] and Guillain-Barré syndrome.[37] Headaches and photophobia are not uncommon during primary HIV infection,[11,14,21,25,40,54,97] and these may reflect the initial phase of central nervous system infection.[29] Although neurologic manifestations are generally self-limited, persistent neurologic deficit has been reported.[15] The reports of neurologic involvement and the isolation of HIV from cerebrospinal fluid during the acute illness[39] indicate that central nervous system infection may occur soon after exposure to HIV. Studies reporting depression, irritability, and mood changes during primary HIV infection[16,87] suggest that early central nervous system infection may also manifest as cognitive or affective impairment.

Febrile pharyngitis was the main sign of primary infection in two reports,[11,92] and sore throat or pharyngeal edema, or both, has been reported in other cases.[9,11,21,24,25,32,46,63,78] Several studies have reported gingival or palatal,[9,11,21,24,25,32,54,57,95] esophageal,[32,46] or genital ulceration.[9,32] Typically no virus has been isolated from these ulcers,[32] and their cause remains unclear.

Although gastrointestinal manifestations of primary HIV infection are uncommon, diarrhea[11,14,17,21,37,54,69] nausea, and vomiting[9,17,21,64,78,79] have been reported. Conjunctivitis has been reported in nine cases,[24,32] and pneumonitis in one case.[17]

In many cases lymphadenopathy develops coincidentally with primary HIV infection, most commonly in the second week of the illness.[23,87] The axillary, occipital, and cervical nodes are involved most commonly, but lymphadenopathy may be generalized. Although the lymph nodes tend to decrease in size after the acute illness, lymph node enlargement remains detectable for many months and even years after primary infection. Splenomegaly has also been reported.[21,32,69,79,90,98] Since changes in the titers of antibodies to cytomegalovirus (CMV) or Epstein-Barr virus (EBV) have not usually been detected during primary HIV infection,[11,19,22,58,66,69,85] nor have heterophil antibodies or autoantibodies such as rheumatoid factor, the development of lymphadenopathy appears to be a response to HIV infection alone. Biopsy studies of enlarged lymph nodes during primary HIV infection typically show follicular hyperplasia and immature sinus histiocytosis indicative of HIV infection.[19]

An erythematous, maculopapular rash is common during primary HIV infection and usually affects the face or trunk but can involve the extremities (including the palms and soles) or be generalized.[9,11,21,24,25,32,40,46,63,66,69,79,85,90,96,97] The lesions vary in size but are typically 5 to 10 mm in diameter. The rash generally resolves within a week. Immunohistologic features of this rash have been reported for one patient.[57] The cell infiltrate around the superficial dermal vessels was predominantly CD4 +. HIV p24 antigen was detected in occasional cells (possibly Langerhans' cells) of the infiltrate. Their presentation of HIV antigen to local CD4 + lymphocytes may lead to a delayed-type hypersensitivity reaction. Such a histologic pattern is not specific for HIV, and infection with other bacteria and viruses may lead to lesions with similar histologic features. Other skin lesions noted during primary HIV infection have included a roseola-like rash,[54] a vesicular, pustular exanthem and enanthem,[15] diffuse urticaria,[40] desquamation of the palms and soles,[21,76] and alopecia.[17,46]

Abnormal findings of liver function tests, particularly elevated levels of alkaline phosphatase and aspartate transaminase, have frequently been reported in patients with the primary HIV illness.[9,11,14,16,25,64,69] In only one of these cases were the abnormal results associated with clinical hepatitis.[64] One subject had an increased serum level of creatine kinase associated with a clinical presentation of myalgia and muscle weakness that improved with resolution of the acute illness.

AIDS-associated opportunistic infections may also occur during primary HIV infection, presumably as a result of the severe immunodepression that may be present at this stage of infection.[88] Seven cases of esophageal candidiasis in association with primary HIV infection have been reported,[19,66,88] and in five of these the patient had a low absolute number of CD4 + cells. Perhaps the development of esophageal candidiasis at this stage of infection is related to the esophageal ulceration found in some patients.[32,46] Such ulceration may provide a local environment that favors proliferation of *Candida albicans;* other contributory factors may include the inappropriate use of antibiotics to treat the symptoms of primary HIV infection, as well as severe anorexia, nausea, and vomiting, which could alter normal oropharyngeal flora. Serologic tests may be necessary to differentiate clinical illnesses associated with primary HIV infection from AIDS in individuals not known to be previously HIV seropositive. The increasing documentation of such cases, together with a wide range of neurologic presentations other than aseptic meningitis, suggests that the CDC clinical definition of primary HIV infection[18] may not encompass all aspects of this stage of infection.

Prevalence and Characteristics of Symptomatic Seroconversion

To define further the prevalence and pattern of clinical features of the acute seroconversion illness and its consistency and reliability as an indicator of primary HIV infection, we conducted a retrospective study of 39 homosexual men with documented HIV seroconversion.[87] During the period in which seroconversion occurred, these patients were significantly more likely than a group of seronegative control subjects to have had an acute clinical illness (93 percent compared with 40 percent). The true prevalence of an acute clinical illness associated with primary HIV infection would therefore lie between 53 percent of subjects (if the total background level of control subjects' illnesses were deducted) and 93 percent of subjects (if all the subjects' illnesses were related to primary HIV infection). Given the distinct nature of the symptoms reported by the seroconverters, we believe the prevalence lies toward the top of this range. The symptoms that most clearly differentiated patients with seroconversion from control subjects were swollen lymph nodes, truncal or generalized rash, depression, irritability, anorexia, weight loss, and retro-orbital pain. Lymphadenopathy developed in 75 percent of seroconverters compared with four percent of control subjects. The duration of the illness was longer in the seroconverters (mean ± standard deviation 18 ± 9.9 days) than in the control subjects (10 ± 4.4 days). Several subjects also reported chronic lethargy for weeks to months after the acute illness. Medical attention for the illness was sought by 87 percent of the seroconverters (including 13 percent who were admitted to hospitals) compared with 20 percent of control subjects, reflecting the greater severity of illness in the seroconverters. Indications for hospitalization included extreme lethargy, dehydration, and neurologic involvement. These findings were supported in a prospective study of homosexual men in which 22 seroconverted subjects were more likely to report fever, swollen lymph nodes, night sweats, and headaches in the seroconversion period than were a group of 44 matched seronegative subjects. Of the seroconversions, 55 percent were associated with symptoms lasting 3 days or more.[29] In a further study 37 (74 percent) of 50 men who had seroconversion reported an illness characteristic of primary HIV infection in the 4-month period preceding HIV seroconversion.[50]

Incubation Period

In case reports the time from exposure to HIV until the onset of the acute clinical illness has ranged from 5 days[21] to 3 months,[69] with most reporting an incubation period of 2 to 4 weeks.[5,16,17,32,76,78,90,92] The varying incubation periods between individuals might reflect differences in the route, dose, and frequency of viral inoculum or individual differences in host responses to exposure.

Differential Diagnosis and Investigation

The main clinical syndromes associated with primary HIV infection reflect both the lymphocytopathic and neuropathic effects of HIV (Table 5–1). Although typically referred to as "mononucleosis-like," the characteristic clinical presentation of primary HIV infection is different from EBV mononucleosis in many respects and the illness should be appreciated as a distinct clinical entity. The major clinical differences between EBV mononucleosis and primary HIV infection were detailed by Gaines et al[32] and are summarized in Table 5–2. The other major differential diagnoses that should be considered are presented in Table 5–3.

The skin rash associated with primary HIV infection is a valuable aid in establishing the diagnosis. Skin eruptions are rare in EBV infection (unless antibiotics are given), toxoplasmosis, and CMV infection and spare the palms and soles in rubella; secondary syphilis can be rapidly excluded by serologic assays. In some cases the rash appears like pityriasis rosea, and the systemic symptoms can be similar, but the rash of pityriasis rosea is usually scaly and pruritic.

In a patient with a history of recent or probable exposure to HIV, the presence of a febrile illness with a maculopapular rash, lymphadenopathy, retro-orbital pain, fatigue, cognitive or affective impairment, or neurologic

TABLE 5–1. CLINICAL MANIFESTATIONS OF PRIMARY HIV INFECTION

Mononucleosis-Like	**Dermatologic**
Fever	Erythematous maculopapular rash
Pharyngitis	Roseola-like rash
Lymphadenopathy	Diffuse urticaria
Arthralgia/myalgia	Desquamation
Headache/retro-orbital pain	Alopecia
Lethargy/malaise	Palatal/gingival ulceration
Anorexia/weight loss	
Nausea/vomiting	
Diarrhea	
Neuropathic	
Meningitis	
Encephalitis	
Peripheral neuropathy	
Radiculopathy	
Brachial neuritis	
Guillain-Barré syndrome	
Cognitive/affective impairment	

TABLE 5–2. CLINICAL FACTORS DIFFERENTIATING EBV MONONUCLEOSIS FROM PRIMARY HIV INFECTION

EBV MONONUCLEOSIS	PRIMARY HIV INFECTION
Insidious onset	Sudden onset
Marked tonsillar hypertrophy	Little or no tonsillar hypertrophy
Enanthema on border of hard and soft palate	Enanthema on hard palate
Exudative pharyngitis common	Exudative pharyngitis unknown
No oral ulcers	Oral ulcers common
Rash rare unless antibiotics given	Rash common
8% jaundiced	Jaundice unknown
Diarrhea unknown	Diarrhea can occur

TABLE 5–3. DIFFERENTIAL DIAGNOSES

Primary HIV infection
Epstein-Barr virus mononucleosis
Cytomegalovirus mononucleosis
Toxoplasmosis
Rubella
Viral hepatitis
Syphilis
Disseminated gonococcal infection
Herpes simplex virus
Other viruses
Drug reaction

signs should alert the clinician to the possibility of primary HIV infection. Our diagnostic approach to a patient who was recently exposed to HIV and has a febrile illness is presented in Table 5–4.

Prognostic Factors

Evidence from some other viral infections suggests that the nature of the initial clinical response to infection may influence the subsequent course of disease. For example, patients with sudden onset of acute hepatitis B virus (HBV) infection in whom deep jaundice develops usually recover completely,[83] and progressive disease rarely develops in survivors of fulminant viral hepatitis.[45] Possibly in such persons the cytotoxic immunologic response to HBV-infected hepatocytes is effective in clearing infection and this is reflected in the severity of the clinical illness.

In a study of 86 homosexual men with documented HIV seroconversion, the 3-year progression rate to CDC group IV HIV disease was eight times higher among subjects who had long-lasting primary illness (greater than 14 days) than in those with briefer illnesses (78 percent versus 10 percent).[67]

TABLE 5—4.   ASSESSMENT OF FEBRILE ILLNESS

Clinical history
Physical examination
Complete blood count and erythrocyte sedimentation rate
Monotest
Liver function tests
HIV antibody
HIV p24 antigen
T-cell subsets
CMV, EBV, toxoplasmosis, hepatitis, and syphilis serologic tests
Performed as Needed
Total IgG, IgA, and IgM
Throat swab
Blood cultures
Cerebrospinal fluid examination
Stool and urine examination

All six patients in whom AIDS developed had long-lasting illnesses. Three-year progression rates to low numbers of CD4+ cells or to recurrence of HIV antigenemia were significantly greater in subjects with long-lasting illnesses. The exact nature of the association between primary infection and subsequent disease progression remains to be determined. A severe primary illness could be related to an early and extensive spread of HIV owing to a defective host immune response. The documentation of fatal primary HIV infection in two immunocompromised patients[6,81] suggests that this may be a factor. Future studies on the pathogenesis of primary HIV infection should provide a better understanding of progressive clinical disease during HIV infection.

SEROLOGIC PROFILE

Antibody

After primary HIV infection, specific antibodies develop that are directed against the major structural gene products of HIV: *gag* (p55, p24, p18), *pol* (p68, p53, p34), and *env* (gp160, gp120, gp41). The early diagnosis of HIV infection has been aided by the characterization of the order in which these antibodies appear and the development of sensitive tests for their detection.

Several reports have examined the time from onset of the primary HIV illness to appearance of antibodies to the major structural proteins of HIV.[22,33] In each study specific HIV antibodies were detectable within 2 weeks of onset of the acute illness. Antibodies are generally first detected by immunofluorescent assay (IFA) or enzyme-linked immunosorbent assay (ELISA) for immunoglobulin M (IgM) antibody within the first 2 weeks after onset of the primary HIV illness. Immunoglobulin G (IgG) antibody is detected generally 2 to 6 weeks after onset of the illness. Western blot (WB) analysis typically first detects antibodies to p24/gp41.[10,28,49,91]

Differences between studies in the time taken to identify subjects as seropositive on the basis of screening test results emphasize the need for consistent use of sensitive screening tests. Supplementary tests (antigen detection, WB analysis, IFA for IgM) should be performed on all sera from persons with an illness typical of primary HIV infection.

In addition to the structural gene products, the HIV provirus codes for several major regulatory proteins that influence the production of infectious virions (*nef, tat, rev, sor,* and so forth). The *nef* gene product (3' orf, negative factor, or F protein) downregulates viral expression and may therefore participate in the establishment and maintenance of viral latency. Anti-*nef* antibodies are elicited early in infection, generally concomitantly with *gag/env* seroconversion but before it in a few cases.[4,26,75] One study found antibodies to *nef* months to years before seroconversion to the structural gene products in almost 50 percent of subjects,[72] but these findings appeared to result from the use of an ELISA with poor sensitivity.[26] Antibodies to *tat* (a protein that accelerates the production of viral particles) and *rev* (a protein that negatively regulates *nef*) have been found in up to 3 percent and 10 percent of subjects, respectively, as much as 6 months before *gag/env* seroconversion.[74]

Some studies have reported subjects who were persistently antibody negative but had virus isolated from their peripheral blood mononuclear cells (PBMCs)[42,60,80] or demonstrated by the enzymatic amplification of viral DNA with the use of a polymerase chain reaction.[41,55,99] HIV p24 antigen was typically undetectable in the serum during this period.[99] In some cases WB analysis showed restricted antibody response to structural proteins, but this was not diagnostic. Although these studies have indicated that a prolonged latency period may occur in some instances, whether persons are infectious during this stage of infection is not clear.

IgM Antibody

The early production and subsequent rapid disappearance of IgM[22] is typical of primary exposure to an infectious agent. In chimpanzees IgM synthesis has been detected approximately 30 to 40 weeks after inoculation with HIV.[4] In humans HIV-specific IgM usually appears within 2 weeks of the onset of the acute clinical illness[31,38] and may circulate for up to 41 weeks,[8] although it usually becomes undetectable by 3 months.[31,50] The early IgM response has been found to be directed against the *gag* proteins (p17, p24, p55) and the *env* proteins (gp41, gp120).[31,44] IgM antibody decreases concomitantly with an increase in HIV-specific IgG.[8,65] The detection of HIV-specific IgM is therefore a sign of recent infection, and the test might be used clinically, in seroepidemiologic studies examining the frequency of recent infection in populations,[1] or in differentiating congenital infection from antibody passively acquired in utero.[35] However, a test for IgM antibody is not always positive in the first few weeks after infection,[50] and a negative result is therefore inconclusive.

In a report of the characteristic neonatal antibody response to HIV infection, HIV-specific IgM was absent at birth, appeared at 4 weeks of age, peaked at 8 weeks of age, and then disappeared.[70] This IgM response was followed by a rise in the serum level of IgG3 antibodies, an IgG subclass response characteristic of the infant population. The detection of IgM or IgG3 HIV antibodies in a neonate indicates perinatal infection. Antigen detection and viral isolation should be used as complementary tests.

Antigen

HIV p24 antigen can be detected by enzyme immunoassay (EIA) in both serum and cerebrospinal fluid in the period before seroconversion[3,15,36,43,46,84,93,95] and has been detected as early as 24 hours after onset of the acute illness.[46,93] In one study HIV p24 antigen was detected in all of 13 subjects for whom serum samples were available during the first 18 days after the onset of the acute illness,[93] suggesting that HIV antigenemia occurs consistently during this period of infection. These data indicate that tests for the detection of HIV antigen should be routinely performed in patients with an illness typical of primary HIV infection. Detecting HIV antigen in a person recently exposed to HIV who has a characteristic acute illness allows rapid diagnosis of infection and appropriate counseling to prevent further spread of HIV.

In most persons a rise in the serum level of HIV antibodies is accompanied by a decrease in the serum HIV p24 antigen level.[36,43,46,93] Persistent antigenemia after primary infection or the reappearance of antigenemia later in the course of infection is associated with a poor clinical outcome.[23,27,36,51,68]

Virus Isolation

HIV has been isolated from PBMCs,[2,33,40,43,79,84] cell-free plasma,[2,33] bone marrow cells,[79] and cerebrospinal fluid[39,79] during primary HIV infection. These findings suggest that the antigenemia found during this period reflects a true viremia. The frequency and ease with which virus can be isolated decreases after resolution of the clinical illness and seroconversion.[2,46] These results indicate that persons are potentially highly infectious between onset of the primary illness and the point of seroconversion.

IMMUNOLOGIC RESPONSE

Predisposing Immune Status

In a group of patients with hemophilia, HIV seroconversion after administration of HIV-infected factor VIII preparation was more likely in patients who had a preexisting reduced CD4+ cell count or CD4+ :CD8+ ratio.[56] To examine this possibility further, we compared the antecedent T-cell profiles of 45 homosexual men who had had seroconversion with those of 90 matched seronegative homosexual men.[21] We found no significant differences between the two groups in the absolute numbers of CD4+ or CD8+ cells or the CD4+ :CD8+ ratio, indicating that an abnormal number of T-cell subsets is not a prerequisite for the establishment of HIV infection in this population. A subsequent study confirmed that antecedent T-cell subset enumeration did not predict seroconversion but found that anergy to dinitrochlorobenzene (DNCB), a novel antigen, predicted subsequent seroconversion.[59] In contrast, anergy to three recall antigens was not associated with seroconversion, suggesting that persons who could not mount an adequate primary immune response were at increased risk of HIV infection. These data imply that an impaired host response may be associated with an increased risk of HIV infection and that HIV may be an opportunistic agent in an immunocompromised host.[53] However, they do not indicate that absolute resistance to HIV infection occurs.

T-Cell Response

Few case reports detail the T-cell changes associated with primary HIV infection.[11,14,21] Different findings between these reports relate to the rapidly changing T-cell pattern in this period and indicate the need to monitor subjects frequently. The recognition of the characteristic acute clinical illness associated with primary HIV infection has permitted early identification of infected persons and regular monitoring of their T-cell subsets. In a study of six seroconverted patients who had multiple enumerations of T-cell subsets at the time of seroconversion and for 300 days after, we documented a characteristic four-phase T-cell response to primary HIV infection.[23] The typical pattern of response is presented in Figure 5–1.

A reduction in the peripheral lymphocyte count characterized the initial phase of reaction to infection in all patients. The relative percentages of CD4+ and CD8+ lymphocytes did not decrease during this initial phase, but a decrease in their absolute numbers occurred as a result of the reduced lymphocyte count. The lowest median value for CD4+ and CD8+ lymphocytes was found a median of 9 days after the onset of the acute clinical illness. This acute phase was characterized by the development of the first

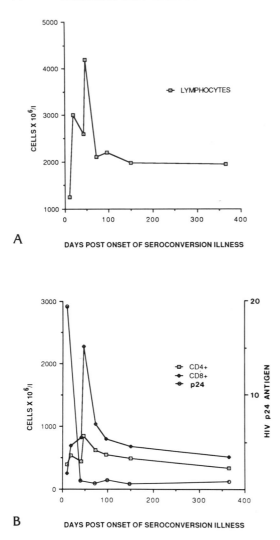

FIGURE 5–1. Changes in number of lymphocytes *(A)* and numbers of CD4+ and CD8+ cells and serum HIV p24 antigen level *(B)* in typical subject according to time from onset of seroconversion illness. (From Cooper DA, Tindall B, Wilson E, et al: Characterization of T lymphocyte responses during primary HIV infection. J Infect Dis 157:889-896, 1988.)

symptoms of the acute illness. The decrease in the absolute number of CD4+ cells occurring during this period is transient and recovers rapidly.

The main feature of the second phase of response to infection, occurring a median of 16 days after the onset of the acute illness, was an inversion of the normal CD4+ :CD8+ ratio to a median value of 0.70. This was noted as the number of CD8+ cells increased relative to the number of CD4+ cells. This period was marked by the development of lymphadenopathy.

The third phase of reaction to infection was characterized by an appreciable increase in the absolute number of CD8+ cells, which led to a further inversion of the CD4+ :CD8+ ratio. The CD8+ response peaked a median of 33 days after the onset of the acute illness. This high CD8+ response to primary HIV infection has previously been described in both humans[11,21] and nonhuman primates.[30] Atypical lymphocytes similar to those seen with the mononucleosis of EBV and CMV infection appeared concomitant with the development of lymphocytosis and generally resolved as the peripheral CD8+ lymphocyte count fell from its peak levels.[21]

The main feature of the fourth phase of response to infection was a resolution of the elevated levels of circulating lymphocytes and their subsets. The level of CD8+ cells remained higher than the level of CD4+ cells, and the inverted ratio was maintained in four of the six patients but was not as low as during the third phase. In the other two patients the ratio reverted to a value greater than 1.00 for a brief period before inverting again. Data obtained on the six patients a median of 100 days after the onset of the clinical illness showed that the numbers of circulating cells were relatively stable.

Role of CD8+ Cells in Controlling Viremia

Sufficient sera were available from five of the foregoing six patients to assay for HIV p24 antigen.[23] In three of these patients the characteristic rise in the absolute number of CD8+ cells was associated with a decrease in the detectable level of serum HIV p24 antigen. This relationship is shown in Figure 5–1 for a typical patient. In the fourth patient the rise in CD8+ cells was associated with an increase rather than a decrease in the level of antigen. This patient was of interest because he died of AIDS 530 days after the onset of his acute illness. Antibody to gp41 was not detectable in his serum between the time of primary HIV infection and the time of death. The fifth patient was not antigen positive at any time during the course of his primary infection, and his results were therefore not informative.

The temporal association between a rise in CD8+ cells and a decrease in serum HIV p24 antigen indicates that the CD8+ response may have a role in suppressing expression of HIV p24 antigen in vivo, as it has been shown to do in vitro.[94] In EBV infection the proliferating CD8+ cells have been shown to be suppressor-cytotoxic[89] and to control infection by killing virally infected B lymphocytes.[86] The availability of reagents that reliably distinguish CD8+ lymphocytes as suppressor or cytotoxic may enable further study of this CD8+ response in primary HIV infection.

Effects on Lymphocyte Function

Studies of lymphocyte function during primary HIV infection are available for one person who was being prepared as a bone marrow donor at the time of his primary infection.[23] Lymphocyte responsiveness to both mitogen (phytohemagglutinin) and antigen (keyhole limpet hemocyanin and tetanus toxoid) decreased markedly with the onset of the seroconversion illness. In particular, antigen-specific response almost disappeared and had not recovered 50 days after the onset of the illness. The mechanism for this hyporesponsiveness is unclear. Diminished lymphocyte responsiveness during acute EBV and CMV infection is well documented and has been shown to be related to an increased number of CD8+ cells, which suppress autologous T-cells.[58,73] Lymphocyte hyporesponsiveness in primary HIV infection could also be a direct effect of the independent action of HIV inhibiting the antigen-specific proliferative responses of PBMCs.[48]

THERAPEUTIC STRATEGIES

The mainstays of treatment of primary HIV infection are early recognition and diagnosis and symptomatic therapy. Recognition and early diagnosis of HIV infection are important to institute appropriate counseling and prevent further spread of the virus. Moreover, an early diagnosis obviates the need for further investigations or empiric therapy, which may not be appropriate. This is especially important when neurologic signs are present. Therapy for the acute illness itself is directed mainly at the symptoms.

In the future, therapeutic strategies might specifically target persons who have a characteristic primary HIV illness and in whom viral infection may not be well established. In adult mice, long-term administration of zidovudine (AZT) has been shown to prevent viremia and retroviral disease if begun soon after inoculation with Rauscher's murine leukemia virus.[77] Oral zidovudine therapy begun shortly after inoculation can also shorten the course of neurologic disease in mice infected prenatally or postnatally with the murine neurotropic type C retrovirus Cas-Br-E.[82] These studies suggest a potential role for zidovudine and other antiretroviral drugs or perhaps hyperimmune HIV immunoglobulin in the early management of HIV-infected persons and urge the prompt establishment of postexposure prophylaxis and early intervention trials in humans.

SUMMARY───────────────────────────

The identification of characteristic clinical, serologic, and immunologic responses to primary HIV infection has contributed greatly to our understanding of the natural history of HIV infection. Initially infected persons usually have a mononucleosis-like illness, and during the period of primary infection they have a characteristic four-phase T-cell response. Early serologic findings of infection include IgM antibody and free HIV p24 antigen.

We believe future research into primary HIV infection should have three primary goals: to further define the features of this phase of infection, to develop early intervention strategies effective against HIV, and to further develop and foster education strategies that will prevent primary HIV infection.

REFERENCES

1. Aiuti F, Rossi P, Sirianni MC, et al: IgM and IgG antibodies to human T cell lymphotropic retrovirus (HTLV-III) in lymphadenopathy syndrome and subjects at risk for AIDS in Italy. Br Med J 291:165-166, 1985
2. Albert J, Gaines H, Sonnerborg A, et al: Isolation of human immunodeficiency virus (HIV) from plasma during primary HIV infection. J Med Virol 23:67-73, 1987
3. Allain J-P, Laurian Y, Paul DA, et al: Serological markers in early stages of human immunodeficiency virus infection in haemophiliacs. Lancet 2:1233-1236, 1986
4. Alter HJ, Eichberg JW, Masur H, et al: Transmission of HTLV-III infection from human plasma to chimpanzees: An animal model for AIDS. Science 226:549-552, 1984
5. Ameisen J-C, Guy B, Chamaret S, et al: Antibodies to the *nef* protein and to *nef* peptides in HIV-1-infected seronegative individuals. AIDS Res Hum Retroviruses 5:279-291, 1989
6. Apperley JF, Rice SJ, Hewitt P, et al: HIV infection due to a platelet transfusion after allogeneic bone marrow transplantation. Eur J Haematol 39:185-189, 1987
7. Barre-Sinoussi F, Chermann JC, Rey F, et al: Isolation of a T-lymphotropic retrovirus from a patient at risk for acquired immune deficiency syndrome (AIDS). Science 220:868-871, 1983
8. Bedarida G, Cambie G, D'Agostino F, et al: Anti-IgM screening for HIV. Lancet 2:1456, 1986
9. Biggar RJ, Johnson BK, Musoke SS, et al: Severe illness associated with appearance of antibody to human immunodeficiency virus in an African. Br Med J 293:1210-1211, 1986
10. Biggar RJ, Melbye M, Ebbesen P, et al: Variation in human T lymphotropic virus III (HTLV-III) antibodies in homosexual men: Decline before onset of illness related to acquired immune deficiency syndrome (AIDS). Br Med J 291:997-998, 1985
11. Biggs B, Newton-John HF: Acute HTLV-III infection: A case followed from onset to seroconversion. Med J Aust 144:545-547, 1986
12. Boiteux F, Vilmer E, Girot R, et al: Lymphadenopathy syndrome in two thalassemic patients after LAV contamination by blood transfusion. N Engl J Med 312:648-649, 1985
13. Brew BJ, Perdices M, Darveniza P, et al: The neurological features of early and "latent" human immunodeficiency virus infection. Aust NZ J Med 19:700-705, 1989
14. Buchanan JG, Goldwater PN, Somerfield SD, et al: Mononucleosis-like-syndrome associated with acute AIDS retrovirus infection. NZ Med J 99:405-407, 1986
15. Calabrese LH, Proffitt MR, Levin KH, et al: Acute infection with the human immunodeficiency virus (HIV) associated with acute brachial neuritis and exanthematous rash. Ann Intern Med 107:849-851, 1987
16. Carne CA, Tedder RS, Smith A, et al: Acute encephalopathy coincident with seroconversion for anti-HTLV-III. Lancet 2:1206-1208, 1985
17. Case records of the Massachusetts General Hospital: Case 33-1989. N Engl J Med 321:454-463, 1989
18. Centers for Disease Control: Classification system for human T-lymphotropic virus type III/lymphadenopathy-associated virus infections. MMWR 35:334-339, 1986
19. Cilla G, Trallero EP, Furumdarena JR, et al: Esophageal candidiasis and immunodeficiency associated with acute HIV infection. AIDS 2:399-400, 1988

20. Colebunders R, Greenberg AE, Francis H, et al: Acute HIV illness following blood transfusion in three African children. AIDS 2:125-127, 1988
21. Cooper DA, Gold J, Maclean P, et al: Acute AIDS retrovirus infection: Definition of a clinical illness associated with seroconversion. Lancet 1:537-540, 1985
22. Cooper DA, Imrie AA, Penny R: Antibody response to human immunodeficiency virus after primary infection. J Infect Dis 155:1113-1118, 1987
23. Cooper DA, Tindall B, Wilson E, et al: Characterization of T lymphocyte responses during primary HIV infection. J Infect Dis 157:889-896, 1988
24. Denning DW, Amos A, Wall RA: Oral and cutaneous features of acute human immunodeficiency virus infection. Cutis 40:171-175, 1987
25. Denning DW, Anderson J, Rudge P, et al: Acute myelopathy associated with primary infection with human immunodeficiency virus. Br Med J 294:143-144, 1987
26. De Ronde A, Reiss P, Dekker J, et al: Seroconversion to HIV-1 negative regulation factor. Lancet 2:574, 1988
27. De Wolf F, Goudsmit J, Paul DA, et al: Risk of AIDS related complex and AIDS in homosexual men with persistent antigenaemia. Br Med J 295:569-572, 1987
28. Esteban JI, Shih JW-K, Tai C-C, et al: Importance of Western blot analysis in predicting infectivity of anti-HTLV-III/LAV positive blood. Lancet 2:1083-1086, 1985
29. Fox R, Eldred LJ, Fuchs EJ, et al: Clinical manifestations of acute infection with human immunodeficiency virus in a cohort of gay men. AIDS 1:35-38, 1987
30. Francis DP, Feorino PM, Broderson JR, et al: Infection of chimpanzees with lymphadenopathy-associated virus. Lancet 2:1276-1277, 1984
31. Gaines H, von Sydow M, Parry JV, et al: Detection of immunoglobulin M antibody in primary human immunodeficiency virus infection. AIDS 2:11-15, 1988
32. Gaines H, von Sydow M, Pehrson PO, et al: Clinical picture of primary HIV infection presenting as a glandular-fever-like illness. Br Med J 297:1363-1368, 1988
33. Gaines H, von Sydow M, Sonnerborg A, et al: Antibody response in primary human immunodeficiency virus infection. Lancet 1:1249-1253, 1987
34. Gallo RC, Salahuddin SZ, Popovic M, et al: Frequent detection and isolation of cytopathic retroviruses (HTLV-III) from patients with AIDS and at risk for AIDS. Science 224:500-503, 1984
35. Geroldi D, Arico M, Plebani A, et al: Western blot technique in the serological evaluation of three LAV/HTLV III-infected Italian families. Infection 14:60-63, 1986
36. Goudsmit J, De Wolf F, Paul DA, et al: Expression of human immunodeficiency virus antigen (HIV-Ag) in serum and cerebrospinal fluid during acute and chronic infection. Lancet 2:177-180, 1986
37. Hagberg L, Malmvall B-E, Svennerholm L, et al: Guillain-Barré syndrome as an early manifestation of HIV central nervous system infection. Scand J Infect Dis 18:591-592, 1986
38. Healey DS, Maskill WJ, Gust ID: Detection of anti-HIV immunoglobulin M by particle agglutination following acute HIV infection. AIDS 3:301-304, 1989
39. Ho DD, Rota TR, Schooley RT, et al: Isolation of HTLV-III from cerebrospinal fluid and neural tissues of patients with neurologic syndromes related to the acquired immunodeficiency syndrome. N Engl J Med 313:1493-1497, 1985
40. Ho DD, Sarngadharan MG, Resnick L, et al: Primary human T-lymphotropic virus type III infection. Ann Intern Med 103:880-883, 1985
41. Horsburgh CR Jr, Ou CY, Jason J, et al: Duration of human immunodeficiency virus infection before detection of antibody. Lancet 2:637-639, 1989
42. Imagawa DT, Lee MH, Wolinsky SM, et al: Human immunodeficiency virus type I infection in homosexual men who remain seronegative for prolonged periods. N Engl J Med 320:1458-1462, 1989
43. Isaksson B, Albert J, Chiodi F, et al: AIDS two months after primary human immunodeficiency virus infection. J Infect Dis 158:866-868, 1988
44. Joller-Jemelka HI, Joller PW, Muller F, et al: Anti-HIV IgM antibody analysis during early manifestations of HIV infections. AIDS 1:45-47, 1987
45. Karvountzis GG, Redeker AG, Peters RL: Long term follow-up of studies of patients surviving fulminant viral hepatitis. Gastroenterology 67:870-877, 1974
46. Kessler HA, Blaauw B, Spear J, et al: Diagnosis of human immunodeficiency virus infection in seronegative homosexuals presenting with an acute viral syndrome. JAMA 258:1196-1199, 1987

47. L'Age-Stehr J, Schwarz A, Offermann G, et al: HTLV-III infection in kidney transplant recipients. Lancet 2:1361-1362, 1985
48. Lane HC, Depper JM, Greene WC, et al: Qualitative analysis of immune function in patients with the acquired immunodeficiency syndrome: Evidence for a selective defect in soluble antigen recognition. N Engl J Med 313:79-84, 1985
49. Lange JMA, Couthino RA, Krone WJA, et al: Distinct IgG recognition patterns during progression of subclinical and clinical infection with lymphadenopathy associated virus/human T lymphotropic virus. Br Med J 292:228-230, 1986
50. Lange JMA, Parry JV, de Wolf F, et al: Diagnostic value of specific IgM antibodies in primary HIV infection. AIDS 2:31-35, 1988
51. Lange JMA, Paul DA, Huisman HG, et al: Persistent HIV antigenaemia and decline of HIV core antibodies associated with transition to AIDS. Br Med J 293:1459-1462, 1986
52. Levy JA, Hoffman AD, Kramer SM, et al: Isolation of lymphocytopathic retroviruses from San Francisco patients with AIDS. Science 225:840-843, 1984
53. Levy JA, Ziegler JL: Acquired immune deficiency syndrome (AIDS) is an opportunistic infection and Kaposi's sarcoma results from secondary immune stimulation. Lancet 2:78-81, 1983
54. Lindskov R, Lindhart BO, Weismann K, et al: Acute HTLV-III infection with roseola-like rash. Lancet 1:447, 1986
55. Loche M, Mach B: Identification of HIV-infected seronegative individuals by a direct diagnostic test based on hybridisation to amplified viral DNA. Lancet 2:418-421, 1988
56. Ludlam CA, Tucker J, Steel CM, et al: Human T-lymphotropic virus type III (HTLV-III) infection in seronegative haemophiliacs after transfusion of factor VIII. Lancet 2:233-236, 1985
57. McMillan A, Bishop PE, Aw D, et al: Immunohistology of the skin rash associated with acute HIV infection. AIDS 3:309-312, 1989
58. Mangi RJ, Niederman JC, Kelleher JE Jr, et al: Depression of cell-mediated immunity during acute infectious mononucleosis. N Engl J Med 291:1149-1153, 1974
59. Marion SA, Schechter MT, Weaver MS, et al: Evidence that prior immune dysfunction predisposes to human immunodeficiency virus infection in homosexual men. J AIDS 2:178-186, 1989
60. Mayer KH, Stoddard AM, McCusker J, et al: Human T-lymphotropic virus type III in high-risk, antibody-negative homosexual men. Ann Intern Med 104:194-196, 1986
61. Murphy S, Kitchen V, Harris JRW, et al: Rape and subsequent seroconversion to HIV. Br Med J 299:718, 1989
62. Needlestick transmission of HTLV-III from a patient infected in Africa. Lancet 2:1376-1377, 1984
63. Neisson-Vernant C, Arfi S, Mathez D, et al: Needlestick HIV seroconversion in a nurse. Lancet 2:814, 1986
64. Oskenhendler E, Harzic M, Le Roux J-M, et al: HIV infection with seroconversion after a superficial needlestick injury to the finger. N Engl J Med 315:582, 1986
65. Parry JV, Mortimer PP: Place of IgM antibody testing in HIV serology. Lancet 2:979-980, 1986
66. Pedersen C, Gerstoft J, Lindhardt BO, et al: *Candida* esophagitis associated with acute human immunodeficiency virus infection. J Infect Dis 156:529-530, 1987
67. Pedersen C, Lindhardt BO, Jensen BL, et al: Clinical course of primary HIV infection: Consequences for subsequent course of infection. Br Med J 299:154-157, 1989
68. Pedersen C, Nielsen CM, Vestergaard BF, et al: Temporal relation of antigenaemia and loss of antibodies to core antigens to development of clinical disease in HIV infection. Br Med J 295:567-569, 1987
69. Piette AM, Tusseau F, Vignon D, et al: Acute neuropathy coincident with seroconversion for anti-LAV/HTLV-III. Lancet 1:852, 1986
70. Pyun KH, Ochs HD, Dufford MTW, et al: Perinatal infection with human immunodeficiency virus: Specific antibody responses by the neonate. N Engl J Med 317:611-614, 1987
71. Quarto M, Germinario C, Fontana A, et al: HIV transmission through kidney transplantation from a living related donor. N Engl J Med 320:1754, 1989
72. Ranki A, Valle S-L, Krohn M, et al: Long latency period precedes overt seroconversion in sexually transmitted human-immunodeficiency-virus infection. Lancet 2:589-593, 1987

73. Reinherz EL, O'Brien C, Rosenthal P, et al: The cellular basis for viral-induced immunodeficiency: Analysis by monoclonal antibodies. J Immunol 125:1269-1274, 1980
74. Reiss P, de Ronde A, Dekker J, et al: Seroconversion to HIV-1 rev- and tat-gene-encoded proteins. AIDS 3:105-106, 1989
75. Reiss P, de Ronde A, Lange JMA, et al: Antibody response to the viral negative factor (nef) in HIV-1 infection: A correlate of levels of HIV-1 expression. AIDS 3:227-233, 1989
76. Romeril KR: Acute HTLV III infection. NZ Med J 779:401, 1985
77. Ruprecht RM, O'Brien LG, Rossoni LD, et al: Suppression of mouse viraemia and retroviral disease by 3'-azido-3'-deoxythymidine. Nature 323:467-469, 1986
78. Rustin MHA, Ridely CM, Smith MD, et al: The acute exanthem associated with seroconversion to human T-cell lymphotropic virus III in a homosexual man. J Infect 12:161-163, 1986
79. Ruutu P, Suni J, Oksanen K, et al: Primary infection with HIV in a severely immunosuppressed patient with acute leukemia. Scand J Infect Dis 19:369-372, 1987
80. Salahuddin SZ, Groopman JE, Markham PD, et al: HTLV-III in symptom-free seronegative persons. Lancet 2:1418, 1984
81. Samuel D, Castaing D, Adam R, et al: Fatal acute HIV infection with aplastic anaemia, transmitted by liver graft. Lancet 1:1221-1222, 1988
82. Sharpe AH, Jaenisch R, Ruprecht RM: Retroviruses and mouse embryos: A rapid model for neurovirulence and transplacental antiviral therapy. Science 236:1671-1674, 1987
83. Sherlock S: Predicting progression of acute type-B hepatitis to chronicity. Lancet 2:354-356, 1976
84. Stramer SL, Heller JS, Coombs RW, et al: Markers of HIV infection prior to IgG antibody seropositivity. JAMA 262:64-69, 1989
85. Stricof RL, Morse DL: HTLV-III/LAV seroconversion following a deep intramuscular needlestick injury. N Engl J Med 314:1115, 1986
86. Svedmyr E, Jondal M: Cytotoxic effector cells specific for B cell lines transformed by Epstein-Barr virus are present in patients with infectious mononucleosis. Proc Natl Acad Sci USA 72:1622-1626, 1975
87. Tindall B, Barker S, Donovan B, et al: Characterization of the acute clinical illness associated with human immunodeficiency virus infection. Arch Intern Med 148:945-949, 1988
88. Tindall B, Hing M, Edwards P, et al: Severe clinical manifestations of primary HIV infection. AIDS 3:747-749, 1989
89. Tosato G, Magrath I, Koski I, et al: Activation of suppressor T cells during Epstein-Barr-virus-induced infectious mononucleosis. N Engl J Med 301:1133-1137, 1979
90. Tucker J, Ludlam CA, Craig A, et al: HTLV-III infection associated with glandular-fever-like illness in a haemophiliac. Lancet 1:585, 1985
91. Ulstrup JC, Skaug K, Figenschau KJ, et al: Sensitivity of Western blotting (compared with ELISA and immunofluorescence) during seroconversion after HTLV-III infection. Lancet 1:1151-1152, 1986
92. Valle S-L: Febrile pharyngitis as the primary sign of HIV infection in a cluster of cases linked by sexual contact. Scand J Infect Dis 19:13-17, 1987
93. von Sydow M, Gaines H, Sonnerborg A, et al: Antigen detection in primary HIV infection. Br Med J 296:238-240, 1988
94. Walker CM, Moody DJ, Stites DP, et al: CD8+ lymphocytes can control HIV infection in vitro by suppressing virus replication. Science 234:1563-1566, 1986
95. Wall RA, Denning DW, Amos A: HIV antigenaemia in acute HIV infection. Lancet 1:566, 1987
96. Wantzin GRL, Lindhardt BO, Weismann K, et al: Acute HTLV III infection associated with exanthema, diagnosed by seroconversion. Br J Dermatol 115:601-606, 1986
97. White GC II, Matthews TJ, Weinhold KJ, et al: HTLV-III seroconversion associated with heat-treated factor VIII concentrate. Lancet 1:611-612, 1986
98. Wiselka MJ, Nicholson KG, Ward SC, et al: Acute infection with human immunodeficiency virus associated with facial nerve palsy and neuralgia. J Infect 15:189-194, 1987
99. Wolinsky SM, Rinaldo CR, Kwok S, et al: Human immunodeficiency virus type 1 (HIV-1) infection a median of 18 months before a diagnostic Western blot: Evidence from a cohort of homosexual men. Ann Intern Med 111:961-972, 1989

6

NATURAL HISTORY OF HIV INFECTION

JOHN P. PHAIR, MD

Following isolation of HIV types 1 and 2 (HIV-1, HIV-2) and the development of assays for antibody, it became possible to definitively identify infected individuals. With the recognition that a large number of individuals are asymptomatic and antibody-positive, identification of codeterminants of disease and prognostic indicators of progression or activity of the viral infection became a major focus of research activity. This chapter will review recent developments in this area. It should be noted that the widespread use of zidovudine and prophylaxis for *Pneumocystis carinii* pneumonia (PCP) will greatly alter the clinical manifestations of HIV-1 infection in Western countries.

It is apparent from a number of studies that the majority of individuals do not manifest signs or symptoms in the first months to years of infection with HIV-1.[16] However, following infection but before developing antibody, a significant number of individuals have a self-limited viral syndrome[2] that resembles mononucleosis in some instances. A smaller group will develop an aseptic meningitis that resolves within 1 to 2 weeks.

Recent seroconverters generally remain AIDS-free for months to years. Within the Multicenter AIDS Cohort Study (MACS) of approximately 5000 homosexual and bisexual men, only 21 of 318 newly antibody-positive men developed AIDS within 54 months of seroconversion. This group of 21 did not differ in age or in history of sexually transmitted disease from the AIDS-free seroconverters but did report a greater number of lifetime sexual partners. In a limited analysis of laboratory studies, there was no difference between groups in preseroconversion T-cell phenotyping, total white cell count, hemoglobin, or mean titer of antibody to cytomegalovirus. Following infection, this subgroup demonstrated a significantly greater rise in CD8-bearing T-suppressor lymphocytes and decline in CD4-bearing T-helper lymphocytes. The AIDS-defining illness in this small group of 21 seroconverters was similar to that in large-scale reports of the first AIDS-defining illness; 57 percent developed PCP, and 14 percent developed Ka-

85

posi's sarcoma.[18] The long incubation period has been reported from other incident cohorts[9] and in studies of seroprevalent cohorts infected for an unknown duration. Within the MACS, approximately 300 of 1628 antibody-positive men progressed to AIDS within the first 4 years of follow-up. Mathematical modeling of these data provides a projection that the median AIDS-free time following seroconversion will be approximately 11 years.

Two primary questions arise from these observations. First, are there cofactors which influence the rate of development of immunodeficiency due to HIV-1 infection, and second, are there markers that identify individuals at increased risk of earlier progression to AIDS?

Although there have been a number of investigations relevant to the first question, to date no cofactor has been definitively identified as playing a role in determining the rapidity of development of the opportunistic diseases which define AIDS. These studies include analysis of concomitant infections[23] as well as other environmental factors, such as recreational drug use.[6] A promising lead has been the information that progression of infection is associated with an increased viral burden in peripheral lymphocytes as indicated by enzymatic amplification of the provirus genome utilizing the polymerase chain reaction.[21]

However, whether or not this increased burden is secondary to genetic control of the immune response to the virus, the presence of a cofactor or alteration in the virulence or other characteristics of HIV-1 remains unknown. There are suggestions that biologic and genomic variations are present in HIV isolated from individuals with AIDS as compared to asymptomatic individuals.[3] Finally, there are preliminary data demonstrating associations of specific HLA type with declining immune function and development of AIDS. AIDS-free men were compared with persons with AIDS (PWA) in a cross-sectional analysis that revealed that HLA-Cw7 was found more frequently in PWA with opportunistic infections and HLA-DR1-DRw14 and -DQW1 was found more often in those with Kaposi's sarcoma. HLA-DR3 and HLA-DQw3 frequencies were decreased in men with Kaposi's sarcoma, and DRw53 was less frequent in PWA with opportunistic infections. Finally, AIDS developed in HLA-DR1–positive men significantly more often among a cohort followed for 43 months.[13]

Investigation of possible markers of increased risk of developing AIDS has been more productive. One of the first attempts at classification of HIV-1 infection, the Walter Reed Staging Classification, utilized measures of immunologic function and clinical status.[20] The two immunologic markers measured were the number of CD4+ (T-helper) lymphocytes in peripheral blood and the presence or absence of reactivity to a battery of skin-test antigens. Clinically patients were stratified by the presence of generalized lymphadenopathy and opportunistic but non-AIDS-defining infections, primarily oropharyngeal thrush. Implied in this scheme is the possibility of progression from one class to another, although it was not designed for that purpose. MacDonell et al stratified the Chicago MACS

Cohort using a modification of the Walter Reed System and correlated outcome among 459 seropositive homosexual and bisexual men over a 3-year period of follow-up.[11] There was clearly a significantly increased risk for men in class V (T-helper cells $\leq 400/mm^3$ with anergy and thrush) as compared with those in classes I, II, and III ($>400/mm^3$ T-helper cells and reactivity to skin-test antigens). However, stratification on the basis of T-helper cell numbers alone provided equally relevant prognostic information. Furthermore, the correlation of anergy with T-helper cell number was not good; a number of participants could not be classified using the Walter Reed System.

The data demonstrating that CD4 number is of critical prognostic importance are presented in several studies.[8,19] In addition to helper cell number, a case control study of the first 90 participants in the MACS who developed AIDS showed that high CD8+ cell number and IgA level, low platelet number, and higher titer of antibody to CMV were associated with progression to AIDS.[19]

The critical number of T-helper cells that identify individuals at risk of developing an AIDS-defining event appears to be $200/mm^3$. A more accurate method of evaluating risk may be the proportion or percentage of lymphocytes which bear the CD4 marker on their surface. The percentage of CD4 is less variable over time and provides significantly better prognostic information.[22] AIDS-defining events such as PCP are uncommon in individuals with more than 20 percent T-helper cells.[14] The rate of decline of these cells also has been cited as providing prognostic information. The various patterns of change in T-helper cell number over time have been cited as supporting evidence for a cofactor, such as a second viral infection, in determining outcome.[1]

The level of T-helper cell number at one point in time is not a totally reliable marker of risk. Some individuals with T-helper cell counts above $200/mm^3$ will be diagnosed within 3 months as having AIDS. In such patients the presence of HIV-1–related signs or symptoms such as thrush, unexplained fever, weight loss, and fatigue have been demonstrated to add to the risk of developing AIDS. It is important to note that a large proportion of individuals reach a level of immunosuppression (T-helper cell number $\leq 200/mm^3$) and have no signs of illness. The subsequent development of thrush or fever, however, greatly adds to the risk of progression of AIDS.[17]

More recently, there have been investigations of the use of markers reflecting viral replication or activation of the immune system as prognostic indicators. The first to be widely studied was the presence in serum of the core p24 antigen of HIV-1. This viral antigen is detected using an enzyme-linked assay with polyclonal or monoclonal antibody directed at the core viral protein(s). These studies indicate that months to years after onset of infection, antigen concentrations rise to detectable levels in approximately one fifth of antibody-positive individuals. Although detectable antigen is more frequently noted in persons with low T-helper cell number, antigenemia occurs in individuals with more than 400 per mm³ as well. The risk of progressing to AIDS is increased three- to fivefold in persons who are antigenemic over a 3-year period of follow-up.[10] It is presumed that rising levels of antigen reflect increased viral replication, although this has not been proven.

Preceding antigenemia, a decline in antibody specific for p24 has been noted. The initial indication that this decline was associated with a poor prognosis was the finding in PWA of an increased frequency of an absent band to p24 on Western blots.[12] In prospectively followed cohorts Western blots also indicated that anti-p24 bands became less dense or disappeared as an individual neared the onset of an AIDS-defining event. Recently, more quantitative assays for antibody have become available, and these tests confirm the impression that low levels or absent antibody to p24 are associated with AIDS or AIDS-related symptoms. The decline in the level of detectable antibody could be due to complexing of the specific immunoglobulin by excess antigen or by a loss of function or depletion of a specific clone of antibody-producing cells. Both antigenemia and the decline in antibody to the p24 protein are believed, therefore, to reflect augmented viral replication in the infected host.

Indirect measures of continued viral activity are those assays known to reflect activation of the immune system secondary to chronic infection or antigenemic stimulation, as seen in autoimmune diseases or graft rejection. Two measures which have been widely used are serum β_2-microglobulin and neopterin. Increases in serum levels of both have been associated with an increased risk of progressing to AIDS.[15] Similarly, increasing concentrations of tumor necrosis factor have been noted in patients with AIDS or constitutional symptoms as compared with asymptomatic seropositive individuals.[7]

The one agreed-upon determinant of progression of HIV is the duration of infection. A controversial aspect of this concept is the unknown effect of a prolonged latent period of infection. Data have been presented demonstrating that latent infection, defined as antibody-negative infection, can be present for months before seroconversion.[5,24] Conflicting information indicates that occurrence of latent infection is uncommon and that the majority of exposed individuals seroconvert within 12 weeks of inoculation.[4] Obviously, if a significant proportion of infected individuals develops latent infection for prolonged periods, and if duration of infection determines the rate of development of immunosuppression, latency could partially explain the differing patterns of response to this virus. Application of techniques which can be used to investigate the frequency of this phenomenon in cohorts followed prospectively is necessary to clarify this issue.

SUMMARY

The natural history of HIV infection is becoming clearer, but we do not understand the determinants of variations in responses to the virus. Results of investigations of host factors and alterations in the virus could provide important information relevant to this issue. A profile of infected individuals who are at greater risk of developing AIDS, however, has emerged. Loss of T-helper cells and antibody to p24, p24 antigenemia, and rising concentrations of CD8+ cells, IgA, antibody to CMV, β_2-microglobulins, and neopterin identify individuals who progress more rapidly to clinical illness.

REFERENCES

1. Detels R, English PA, Phair JP, et al: Patterns of CD4+ cell changes after HIV-1 infection indicate the existence of a codeterminant of AIDS. J AIDS 1:390-395, 1988
2. Fox R, Eldred LV, Fuchs EJ, et al: Clinical manifestations of acute infection with human immunodeficiency virus in a cohort of gay men. AIDS 1:35-38, 1987
3. Gupta P, Bolachendran R, Thompatty C, et al: HIV isolates from asymptomatic men are biologically and genetically different from those isolated from AIDS patients. Presented at V International Conference on AIDS, Montreal, 1989
4. Horsburgh CR, Jason J, Longini IM, et al: Duration of human immunodeficiency virus infection before detection of antibody. Lancet 2:637-639, 1989
5. Immagawa DT, Lee MH, Wolinsky SM, et al: Human immunodeficiency virus type 1 infection in homosexual men who remain seronegative for prolonged periods. N Engl J Med 320:1458-1462, 1989
6. Kaslow RA, Blackwelder WC, Ostrow DG, et al: No evidence for a role of alcohol or psychoactive drugs as cofactor for HIV-1 induced immunodeficiency. JAMA 261:3424-3429, 1989
7. Lahdevirta J, Maury CPJ, Teppo A-M, Repo H: Elevated levels of circulating cachectin/tumor necrosis factor in patients with acquired immunodeficiency syndrome. Am J Med 85:289-291, 1988
8. Lang W, Perkins H, Anderson RE, et al: Patterns of T-lymphocyte changes with human immunodeficiency virus infection. J AIDS 2:63-69, 1989
9. Luis KJ, Darrow WW, Rutherford GW: A model-based estimate of the mean incubation period for AIDS in homosexual men. Science 240:1335, 1988
10. MacDonell K, Byers E, Chmiel JS, et al: HIV antigenemia. Presented at the American Federation of Clinical Research, Washington, DC, 1988
11. MacDonell KB, Chmiel JS, Goldsmith J, et al: Prognostic usefulness of the Walter Reed Staging Classification of HIV infection. J AIDS 1:376-384, 1988
12. McHugh TM, Stites DP, Busch M, et al: Relation of circulating levels of human immunodeficiency virus (HIV) antigen, antibody to p24 and HIV-containing immune complexes in HIV-infected patients. J Infect Dis 158:1088-1091, 1988
13. Mann DL, Murray C, Yarchoan R, et al: HLA antigen frequencies in HIV-1 seropositive disease-free individuals and patients with AIDS. J AIDS 1:13-17, 1988
14. Masur H, Ognibene P, Yarchoan R, et al: CD4 counts as predictors of opportunistic pneumonias in human immunodeficiency virus (HIV) infection. Ann Intern Med 111:223-231, 1989
15. Moss AR, Bacchetti P: Natural history of HIV infection. AIDS 3:55-61, 1989
16. Munoz A, Wang M-C, Bass S, et al: Acquired immunodeficiency syndrome (AIDS)—free time after human immunodeficiency virus type 1 (HIV-1) seroconversion in homosexual men. Am J Epidemiol 130:530-539, 1989

17. Phair JP, Munoz A, Detels R, et al: Incidence of *Pneumocystis Carinii* pneumonia in men infected with human immunodeficiency virus type-1 (HIV-1). Presented at V International Conference on AIDS, Montreal, 1989
18. Phair JP, Munoz A, Kingsley L, et al: Incidence of AIDS in homosexual men developing HIV-1 specific antibody. Presented at V International Conference on AIDS, Montreal, 1989
19. Polk BF, Fox R, Brookmeyer R, et al: Predictors of acquired immunodeficiency syndrome developing in a cohort of seropositive homosexual men. N Engl J Med 316:61-66, 1987
20. Redfield RR, Wright DC, Tramont EC: The Walter Reed Staging Classification for HTLV-III/LAV Infection. N Engl J Med 314:131-132, 1986
21. Schruttman S: Personal communication
22. Taylor JM, Fahey JL, Detels R, et al: CD4 percentage, CD4 number and CD4 : CD8 ratio in HIV infection: Which to choose and how to use. J AIDS 2:114-124, 1989
23. Webster A, Lee CA, Cook DG, et al: Cytomegalovirus infection and progression towards AIDS in haemophiliacs with human immunodeficiency virus infection. Lancet 2:63-65, 1989
24. Wolinsky SM, Rinaldo CR, Kwok S, et al: HIV-1 infection a median of 18 months before a diagnostic Western blot: Evidence from a cohort of homosexual men. Ann Intern Med 111:961, 1989

II

MANAGEMENT OF HIV INFECTIONS AND ITS COMPLICATIONS

7

CARE OF THE INDIVIDUAL WITH EARLY HIV INFECTION:
Unanswered Questions, Including the Syphilis Dilemma

HARRY HOLLANDER, MD

Now that much has been learned about the natural history of HIV infection, the precarious nature of the asymptomatic stage is better appreciated. Early intervention is a laudable goal and aims to prevent the many organ-system complications of progressive HIV infection. With growing numbers of infected individuals, crucial questions arise which relate to the allocation of limited resources. There are many diagnostic tests and emerging treatment strategies which may be useful in given individuals. However, cost effectiveness studies in this area are nonexistent, and data regarding the efficacy of many potential interventions are not available. This chapter attempts to consider some of these issues and proposes a minimal level of care and investigation of individuals while awaiting further prospective data. Evaluation of new symptom complexes in previously healthy persons is covered in other chapters.

DISEASE MONITORING—HOW MUCH IS ENOUGH?

To adequately assess the risk of progression of HIV disease, both clinical and laboratory data are important. The initial and interval history should concentrate on the development of major symptoms and problems which

TABLE 7–1.   ESSENTIAL PORTIONS OF THE FOLLOW-UP PHYSICAL EXAMINATION

General
Overall well-being, weight
Skin
Seborrheic dermatitis, folliculitis, dermatophytosis, Kaposi's sarcoma
Mouth
Candidiasis (pseudomembranous and erythematous), hairy leukoplakia, aphthous ulcers, periodontal disease
Lymphatic
Localized lymphadenopathy,* splenomegaly
Neurologic or Psychologic
Mood or affect, psychomotor slowing, eye movement abnormalities, hyperreflexia (if feasible, simple motor tests such as timed gait and quantifiable neuropsychiatric tests like digit symbol substitution are more sensitive to early neurologic disease than is bedside examination)

*Generalized lymphadenopathy does not correlate with increased disease progression.

portend a poor outcome. These include constitutional complaints (especially fever and weight loss) and minor opportunistic infections, of which oral candidiasis, hairy leukoplakia, and cutaneous herpes zoster are most important.[14,19]

A complete baseline physical examination should be done. Repeated routine physical examinations have proven unhelpful in a variety of medical screening settings. Similarly, it is difficult to justify the time and expense of repeated full examinations in infected persons. Nevertheless, a focused examination may uncover important new data. The pertinent pieces of the examination with potential findings are listed in Table 7–1. It is important to reiterate that these abridged recommendations pertain only when there has been no change in clinical status. The interval development of significant symptoms dictates a complete reexamination.

Given the explosion of surrogate laboratory markers which (at least retrospectively) correlate with disease progression, a major challenge to the clinician is appropriate laboratory utilization.[4,9,11,15,16,17,18,19] Table 7–2 lists some of the tests which have been advocated as markers.

All these tests suffer from common drawbacks. First, data derived from epidemiologic cohorts have not been validated prospectively for individual patients. Second, normative values often have not been established for these tests in HIV-infected populations or in uninfected risk group members. Finally, laboratory variability and laboratory errors occur; *the reliance upon a single mistaken value may have profound implications for an individual.* Thus, any laboratory markers must be interpreted carefully in the context of clinical findings and repeated if any question exists about their validity.

Reviewing the list of potential tests, it can be seen that three types of test have been used. The hematocrit is an example of the first type, a completely nonspecific laboratory value that is abnormal in many disease states. The

TABLE 7–2.   LABORATORY MARKERS OF HIV DISEASE PROGRESSION

Nonspecific
Decreased hematocrit
Elevated erythrocyte sedimentation rate
Immunologic
Decreased CD4 lymphocytes
Decreased CD4/CD8 lymphocyte ratio
Elevated serum β_2 microglobulin
Elevated serum neopterin
Elevated serum acid labile interferon
Absent or decreased levels of anti-p24 antibody
HIV-Specific
p24 antigenemia
Positive serum HIV culture

TABLE 7–3.   SURROGATE MARKERS—HOW TO DECIDE

Specificity for HIV infection
Correlation with disease progression (sensitivity and predictive value)
Variability of results
    Temporally
    Inter/Intralaboratory
Availability
Cost
Applicability to clinical management

second type is defined by tests which attempt to quantify immunologic deficits or immunologic activation. Enumeration of lymphocyte subsets and measurement of β_2 microglobulin are examples of these surrogate markers. Finally, measurement of p24 antigenemia and HIV serum culture examine direct quantitative evidence of HIV infection.

Which of these tests should be chosen? None of the available surrogate markers is perfect. Table 7–3 outlines considerations that should drive the choice of laboratory markers. Certainly, the hematocrit is inexpensive, universally available, and an essential part of the general evaluation of an HIV-infected individual. Beyond ordering a complete blood count, however, there is a variety of potential strategies. Practically, lymphocyte subsets have been the most widely utilized of these markers. There is some debate about the relative predictive value of absolute CD4 numbers versus CD4/CD8 ratio. However, since absolute CD4 number is currently an important criterion in the prescription of medications such as zidovudine and inhaled pentamidine, the CD4 count should be an essential part of the evaluation of every infected individual. Nevertheless, this measure still has the relative drawbacks of expense, lack of universal availability, diurnal variability, and interlaboratory variability which make it an imperfect monitoring test.

Therefore, insofar as possible, one should perform the test serially in the same laboratory at the same time of the day.

Once the CD4 count is known, other laboratory markers should then be used very selectively, if at all. These may be most helpful in cases where the CD4 count indicates an intermediate prognosis for disease progression. Such an "intermediate" range might be 200 to 600 CD4 cells. There is little justification for ordering additional prognostic markers when CD4 cells are below 200 or greater than 600. The two best candidates as second line markers are β_2-microglobulin and p24 antigen. β_2-Microglobulin is a relatively inexpensive test that is widely available; in some studies it has had a higher correlation with disease progression than CD4 counts. Its main problem is poor specificity. On the other hand, p24 antigen is highly specific but relatively expensive and difficult to obtain. Furthermore, fewer than 70 percent of patients with full-blown AIDS will have p24 antigenemia, so this is not a highly sensitive marker of active disease. A final caveat is that approximately half of individuals without measurable antigenemia appear to have serum antigen bound in circulating immune complexes.[14] The prognostic significance of this finding is unknown. Despite these drawbacks, p24 antigenemia has been shown to correlate with a higher risk of disease progression in hemophiliacs and homosexual men.

Thus, there are still many questions remaining in the area of disease monitoring. It is clear that both clinical and laboratory assessment are important components, but the optimal visit interval and laboratory utilization have yet to be determined. One approach is to stratify asymptomatic individuals on a basis of complete blood count and CD4 studies. For those with normal results, an initial follow-up frequency of 6 to 12 months may be adequate. In contrast, individuals with low, intermediate, or rapidly declining CD4 values might be seen every 4 to 6 months, with a shorter follow-up period if additional surrogate markers such as β_2-microglobulin are found to be abnormal. Once the decision is made to embark upon medical therapy, follow-up recommendations intensify accordingly.

INSTITUTION OF ANTIRETROVIRAL THERAPY

Although this topic is discussed in more detail in Chapter 25 and data are rapidly accumulating, this section will briefly review the arguments for and against early institution of antiviral therapy in asymptomatic seropositive patients.

The strongest rationale for the early initiation of antiretroviral therapy is epidemiologic data that show that the majority of infected people will ultimately become ill due to HIV's effects. There is also evidence that drugs such as azidothymidine (AZT), which have significant toxicities in advanced disease, may be better tolerated by individuals who are healthier at the start of therapy. Preliminary data from a national trial of AZT for this indication suggest that this is true and also provide hope that AZT and other agents may delay the onset of HIV-related complications.

The drawbacks of early antiretroviral therapy involve three very different considerations. The first is the cost of such long-term therapy to individuals, their insurers, and society. Second, many clinical trials do not provide data about long-term toxicity of these agents. For example, myopathy associated with AZT was not appreciated until several years after the initial placebo-controlled trial was finished. It should be anticipated that AZT and other experimental antiretroviral agents will be associated with other idiosyncratic, unexpected side effects over time. Finally, there is the issue of development of drug resistance by HIV. To date, the only examples of resistance have occurred in people with advanced disease. However, chronic low-dose therapy provides a favorable milieu for resistant viruses to occur. One unsupported notion is that by treating HIV earlier in the course of the infection, when the overall viral burden is lower, the incidence of emerging resistance may be lower than in advanced disease. This awaits documentation.

In light of the above arguments and problems that exist in estimating a given individual's prognosis, the decision to initiate antiretroviral therapy in an asymptomatic seropositive person needs to be individualized and discussed fully with the patient. Besides the medical factors involved, cost of therapy will be a deciding factor for many patients. Without provision of unapproved drugs by federal or state governments or coverage of therapy by insurance carriers, many individuals may not be able to afford therapy which will ultimately prove to be medically indicated and beneficial.

PROPHYLAXIS OF OPPORTUNISTIC INFECTIONS

Experience with *Pneumocystis carinii* has reinforced the principle that, when possible, prophylaxis of opportunistic infection should be attempted in the setting of HIV infection (see Chapter 15). Table 7–4 lists issues to consider when planning prophylactic therapy. Several uncertainties are identified in the table. First, we still lack data that allow prediction of a

TABLE 7–4.   CRITICAL ISSUES IN OPPORTUNISTIC INFECTION PROPHYLAXIS

Likelihood of reactivation of the infection
Availability of effective, bioavailable antimicrobials
Acceptable long-term toxicity profile
Compatibility with other therapies, particularly antiretrovirals
Development of drug resistance
Cost of therapy

given infection in HIV-infected individuals. Thus, improved diagnosis is fundamental in the planning of rational prophylaxis. Second, efficacy or lack thereof in other treatment settings does not necessarily predict the outcome of prophylaxis. An example is the trend toward decreased CMV infection in HIV-infected persons receiving high doses of acyclovir. Third, prophylaxis may lead to undesirable therapeutic trade-offs. For example, a highly effective antimicrobial that has synergistic toxicity with an antiretroviral could, on balance, be detrimental. Fourth, the past several years have demonstrated the clinical significance of antimicrobial resistance in this population. One must ask if it is worth risking the development of resistance which could render later therapy useless. This is particularly germane for infections treatable with only one or few efficacious agents. Finally, cost of therapy is a major consideration.

Thus, at present, there are no ideal prophylactic agents. Even for the best studied infection, *P. carinii* pneumonia (PCP), major questions remain about initiation criteria and choices of drug, dosing, and route of administration. Other chapters specifically address prophylaxis prospects for other infections, but at present, nothing can be recommended to all individuals early in the course of disease. It is hoped that continued drug development will yield more prospects for successful and rational prophylaxis.

Vaccination

Several bacterial and viral infections may be preventable by vaccination. Clinical efficacy data are not available, but the majority of people with early HIV disease will mount an appropriate antibody response to some serotypes represented in pneumococcal vaccine. Since the incidence of adverse effects is no higher in this population, polyvalent pneumococcal vaccine should be administered to each HIV-infected person at the time of first contact. The need for booster doses is unknown. Since data on the antibody response to *Haemophilus influenzae* type B vaccine do not exist and the serotype distribution of *H. influenzae* in HIV-seropositives is unknown, widespread use of this vaccine cannot be generally recommended.

Seasonal influenza vaccination is recommended. However, there is no evidence that influenza is more severe in the face of concomitant HIV infection or that vaccination prevents disease. Finally, recombinant hepatitis B vaccine should be administered to those who have no prior exposure and who might continue behaviors which place them at risk for hepatitis B infection. Antibody to hepatitis B surface antigen declines more rapidly in an HIV-infected cohort, but the need for rechecking serology and booster doses has not been evaluated.

THE DILEMMA OF SYPHILIS AND HIV INFECTION

There has recently been renewed interest in syphilis and its interrelationships with HIV infection.[8] Issues of facilitation of HIV transmission and syphilis as a cofactor for HIV disease progression will not be covered here. The problems for the clinician revolve around recent observations that the natural history of syphilis and the ability to treat this infection may be substantially different in HIV-infected individuals.[1,9,13] For example, some case reports document an unusually rapid progression from primary infection to late disease; others raise the question of more frequent neurologic manifestations of syphilis in this setting. This latter observation becomes especially important in view of data that suggest treatment failures and neurologic relapse with standard therapeutic regimens.

Both diagnostic and therapeutic problems are commonly encountered. False positive nontreponemal tests such as the RPR (rapid plasma reagin) may be seen as part of the polyclonal B cell activation caused by HIV. Thus, any positive test result must be confirmed by a specific treponemal antibody test. There is also one reported case of false negative serologic studies in classic secondary syphilis in an HIV-positive person.[6] The frequency of this aberrant antibody response is unknown. In addition to these potential problems with peripheral serology, definitive diagnosis of central nervous system syphilis may be very difficult without the research tool of treponemal isolation. Again, problems may occur which could lead to either under- or over-diagnosis of this entity. If cerebrospinal fluid (CSF) has a positive VDRL test, it is assumed that neurosyphilis is present. However, the sensitivity of this test is not known. Conversely, one runs the risk of overdiagnosing neurosyphilis if nonspecific CSF abnormalities such as an elevated protein or lymphocytic pleocytosis are interpreted as evidence for syphilis.[7] Many HIV-infected people have these laboratory abnormalities noted without any current or past history of syphilis. The lack of clinical and laboratory gold standards for diagnosis lead to some of the therapeutic questions discussed below.

Given the limitations with current diagnostic testing and our understanding of the natural history of syphilis in the presence of HIV infection, it is most practical to consider several different clinical scenarios. The first is clinically apparent early syphilis *without* neurologic signs or symptoms. Current concerns dictate the choice of a regimen which achieves adequate CSF levels; however, the optimal agent and duration of therapy have not been defined. An individual *with* neurologic signs or symptoms and a positive CSF VDRL clearly deserves a prolonged course of intravenous penicillin; more difficult is the question of therapy for the person with similar neurologic problems and a positive peripheral RPR but a negative CSF VDRL. A conservative choice would be to treat with high-dose intravenous penicillin (12 to 24 million units every day for 10 to 14 days) if there has been no documented prior therapy for syphilis and no other etiology is found during the evaluation.

A different problem occurs in individuals who had previously been treated with benzathine penicillin regimens, are neurologically asymptomatic, and have persistently positive peripheral RPRs. If lumbar punctures were done in all of these patients, one would predict that many would be overtreated for "neurosyphilis" when, in fact, their CSF abnormalities are caused by HIV. One approach is to arbitrarily re-treat those who have a peripheral titer of 1:8 or greater with a neurologically efficacious regimen. If the titer is lower, no treatment is administered, and the peripheral RPR is repeated at 3- to 6-month intervals. CSF analysis could then be reserved for individuals who develop neurologic findings or have a fourfold or greater rise in peripheral RPR titer. This recommendation conflicts with current CDC guidelines, which advise lumbar puncture in all such patients.[2]

Finally, for the rare HIV-positive individual who has a clinical picture compatible with syphilis but negative serologies, biopsy of suspicious lesions may be helpful, but the institution of antibiotic therapy needs to be made upon clinical grounds.

SUMMARY

It is obvious that while more attention is being paid to the delivery of adequate care early in the course of HIV disease, many questions still remain. It is hoped that patients with HIV infection will have their care optimized and disease progression slowed by a combination of monitoring, preventive therapy, and well-timed intervention with antiretroviral agents.

TABLE 7–5.   BASIC CARE OF EARLY HIV DISEASE

Monitoring
Complete baseline history and physical examination; directed interval interview and
    examination approximately every 6 months
Baseline complete blood count and absolute CD4 cell count with repetition approximately
    every 6 months
Diagnosis and Therapy of Occult Infection
Baseline purified protein derivative (PPD)*
Baseline RPR; fluorescent treponemal antibody absorption test (FTA-ABS) or
    microhemiagglutination assay-*Treponema pallidum* test (MHA-TP) if negative
Health Care Maintenance
Assessment for ongoing counseling needs and referral for significant psychiatric or social
    problems
Pneumococcal vaccine
Hepatitis B vaccine if no prior exposure
Yearly influenza vaccine

*See Chapter 19 for discussion of the limitations of tuberculin skin testing.

It is increasingly clear that decisions made in the course of treating individuals cannot be made in vacuo, without consideration of the changing ecology of HIV infection and the potential costs of therapy to society. Practitioners must have the flexibility to manage individuals according to their unique needs. Table 7–5 summarizes the main points previously discussed and proposes a basic level of care for those with early HIV disease, but it is fully anticipated that these guidelines will soon change as more clinical questions are resolved and rapid drug development continues.

REFERENCES

1. Berry CD, Hooton TM, Collier AC, Lukehart SA: Neurological relapse after benzathine penicillin therapy for secondary syphilis in a patient with HIV infection. N Engl J Med 316:1587-1589, 1987
2. Centers for Disease Control: Recommendations for diagnosing and treating syphilis in HIV-infected patients. MMWR 37:601, 1988
3. Eyster ME, Ballard JO, Gail MH, et al: Predictive markers for the acquired immunodeficiency syndrome (AIDS) in hemophiliacs: Persistence of p24 antigen and low T4 cell count. Ann Intern Med 110:963-969, 1989
4. Goedert JJ, Biggar RJ, Melbye M, et al: Effect of T4 count and cofactors on the incidence of AIDS in homosexual men infected with the human immunodeficiency virus. JAMA 257:331-334, 1987
5. Greenspan D, Greenspan JS, Hegarst NG, Pan L, Conant MA, Abrams DI, Hollander H, Levy JA: Relation of oral hairy leukoplakia to infection with the human immunodeficiency virus and risk of developing AIDS. J Infect Dis 155:475-481, 1987
6. Hicks CB, Benson PM, Lupton GP, et al: Seronegative secondary syphilis in a patient infected with the human immunodeficiency virus (HIV) with Kaposi sarcoma: A diagnostic dilemma. Ann Intern Med 107:492-495, 1987
7. Hollander H: Cerebrospinal fluid normalities and abnormalities in individuals infected with human immunodeficiency virus. J Infect Dis 158:855-858, 1988
8. Hook EW: Syphilis and HIV infection. J Infect Dis 160:530-534, 1989
9. Johns DR, Tierney M, Felsenstein D: Alteration in the natural history of neurosyphilis by concurrent infection with the human immunodeficiency virus. N Engl J Med 315:1569-1572, 1987
10. Kaslow RA, Phair JP, Friedman HB: Infection with the human immunodeficiency virus: Clinical manifestations and their relationship to immune deficiency—a report from the multicenter AIDS cohort study. Ann Intern Med 107:474-480, 1987
11. Lange JM, Paul DA, Huisman HG, et al: Persistent HIV antigenemia and decline of HIV core antibodies associated with transition to AIDS. Br Med J 293:1459-1462, 1986
12. Larder BA, Darby G, Richman DD: HIV with reduced sensitivity to zidovudine (AZT) isolated during prolonged therapy. Science 243:1731-1734, 1989
13. Lukehart SA, Hood EW, Baker-Zander SA, et al: Invasion of central nervous system by treponema pallidum: Implications for diagnosis and treatment. Ann Intern Med 109:855-862, 1988
14. McHugh TM, Stites DP, Busch MP, Krowka JF, Stricker RB, Hollander H: Relationship of circulating levels of HIV antigen, anti-p24 antibody and HIV containing immune complexes in patients infected with HIV. J Infect Dis 158:1088-1091, 1988
15. Melbye M, Biggar R, Ebbesen P, et al: Long-term seropositivity for human T-lymphotropic virus type III in homosexual men without the acquired immunodeficiency syndrome: Development of immunologic and clinical abnormalities. Ann Intern Med 104:496-500, 1986
16. Melmed RN, Taylor JMG, Detels R, et al: Serum neopterin changes in HIV infected subjects: Indicator of significant pathology, CD4 T cell changes and development of AIDS. J AIDS 2:70-76, 1989

17. Moss AR, Bacchetti P, Osmond D, et al: Seropositivity for IIIV and the development of AIDS or AIDS related condition: Three year follow up of the San Francisco General Hospital cohort. Br Med J 296:745-750, 1988
18. Polk BF, Fox R, Brookmeyer R, et al: Predictors of the acquired immunodeficiency syndrome developing in a cohort of seropositive homosexual men. N Engl J Med 316:61-66, 1987
19. Taylor JMG, Fahey JL, Detels R, Giorgi JV: CD4 percentage, CD4 number, and CD4 : CD8 ratio in HIV infection: Which to choose and how to use. J AIDS 2:114-124, 1989

8

TREATMENT OF HIV INFECTION

MARGARET A. FISCHL, MD

Drug development for anti-HIV therapies hinges on knowledge of the replication cycle of the human immunodeficiency virus (HIV). Infection with HIV begins with the binding of envelope protein gp120 to the cellular receptor CD4. Virus core can then enter cells. Once in cells, the RNA genome of the virus is converted to a DNA copy via reverse transcriptase. A complementary-strand DNA copy of viral genomic RNA is made, and then a second, double-stranded DNA copy is made. This linear, double-stranded provirus is integrated into host chromosomes and transcribed into mRNA. mRNA is then translated to make precursor proteins which are specifically cleaved to form mature virus particles that reassemble with virus genome RNA to form new infectious virus particles. Thus, replication of HIV begins with binding to cells and integration into host-cell DNA. Transcription of HIV mRNA occurs with production of infectious virions. Agents that block the initial phases of viral replication will prevent infection of new cells but will not affect chronically infected cells. Agents that block the later phases of viral replication will block the chronic infection of cells but will not prevent uninfected cells from becoming infected.

A number of compounds under evaluation or development interfere with HIV replication. The best known of these agents are the dideoxynucleosides, which are potent inhibitors of HIV in vitro. As 5'-triphosphates, these agents exert anti-HIV activity at the reverse transcriptase level. Two mechanisms may contribute to dideoxynucleoside effects on reverse transcriptase. As triphosphates, they compete with cellular dideoxynucleoside-5'-triphosphates, which are essential substrates for the formation of proviral DNA by reverse transcriptase. They also act as chain terminators in the synthesis of proviral DNA. Mammalian DNA polymerase alpha is relatively resistant to the effects of this class of drugs, which accounts for the select anti-HIV activity of these compounds. However, mammalian DNA polymerase gamma, found in mitochondria, and DNA polymerase beta are sensitive to these compounds, which may account for their toxicities. Compounds approved or under evaluation include zidovudine (Retrovir) dideoxycytidine (ddC), dideoxyinosine (ddI), didehydro-dideoxythymidine (D4T), and phosphonoformate (foscarnet).

The target cells of HIV express the CD4 receptor. The region of CD4 that binds directly with the gp120 envelope protein of the virus has been mapped. Fragments of the CD4 molecule which exist in a soluble form can be used as viral inhibitors. Soluble CD4 can prevent HIV from binding to the cellular receptor. Anti-idiotypic antibodies to CD4, which mimic the CD4 molecule, should have similar effects. Soluble recombinant CD4, however, is not very stable in the blood and necessitates continuous infusion of the compound. The binding region of the CD4 molecule has been combined in a chimeric molecule containing an antibody chain (immunoglobulin IgG) which has resulted in a more stable compound. Phase I studies are being conducted to evaluate recombinant human CD4–immunoglobulin G alone and in combination with zidovudine.

HIV has several genes to moderate or down-regulate virus expression to prevent killing of infected host cells and persistent viral infection. At least three genes, *tat, nef,* and *rev,* have been identified to have a direct role in regulation. *tat* turns on all proteins forming the structure of virus particles and regulates growth. *nef* down-regulates both sets of proteins. *rev* is a differential regulator, and a threshold of *rev* is required for expression of viral structural proteins. When *rev* is overexpressed, it will shut down the other two proteins.

Therefore, the regulator genes of HIV are potential targets for inhibiting viral replication. Chronically infected cells cultured with an antisense oligonucleotide construct derived from the coding sequence of the *tat* and *rev* genes will result in a reduction of viral expression. Such compounds may also inhibit the replication of HIV in a manner that is not sequence-specific.

ZIDOVUDINE

Zidovudine is a thymidine analogue that inhibits the replication of HIV in vitro. Zidovudine is phosphorylated by cellular enzymes to the 5'-triphosphate, which interferes with HIV RNA-dependent DNA polymerase (reverse transcriptase) and elongation of the viral DNA chain, inhibiting viral replication.

On the basis of the pharmacologic properties of zidovudine, the initial dose tested in clinical trials for the treatment of patients with advanced HIV disease was 250 mg orally every 4 hours (1500 mg total daily dose).[4,10] Because of toxicity and formulation considerations, the current recommended dose is 100 mg every 4 hours (600 mg total daily dose). Although the serum half-life of zidovudine is 1 hour, the intracellular half-life of the 5'-triphosphate approaches 3 hours. A study evaluating lower daily doses

TABLE 8–1. BENEFICIAL EFFECTS ASSOCIATED WITH ZIDOVUDINE THERAPY

Prolongs survival	Increases CD4 cell numbers
Decreases frequency and severity of opportunistic infections	Increases CD8 cell numbers
Delays progression to AIDS	Increase skin-test reactivity
Delays progression to ARC	Decreases serum and CSF p24 antigen levels
Weight gain	Delays development of serum p24[1] antigen
Improved performance status	Increases platelet counts
Improved cognitive or neurologic function	

of zidovudine (100 mg every 4 hours versus 250 mg every 4 hours) has recently been completed through the NIAID AIDS Clinical Trials Group (ACTG). Preliminary data showed a statistically significant better survival and no difference in the time to the first opportunistic infection for the lower dose tested (600 mg per day) versus the previously recommended dose (1500 mg per day). In addition, the two treatment groups experienced a comparable degree of efficacy using either serum p24 antigen suppression of CD4 cell counts as indicators. A statistically significant lower incidence of hematologic toxicity, including both anemia and neutropenia, was noted among patients receiving 100 mg every 4 hours (presented ACTG meeting, Washington D.C., November 1989).

Another recent ACTG study revealed no difference in progression rates to AIDS or advanced ARC and significantly less toxicity in asymptomatic subjects with HIV infection who received 100 mg of zidovudine every 4 hours while awake (500 mg total daily dose) as compared with 300 mg every 4 hours while awake (1500 mg total daily dose) (presented ACTG meeting, November 1989). Ongoing studies in Europe and Australia have shown that 250 mg of zidovudine taken orally every 6 hours in patients with AIDS and ARC will decrease serum and cerebrospinal fluid p24 antigen, increase the number of CD4 lymphocytes, and have at least short-term efficacy similar to that seen in patients taking 200 to 250 mg every 4 hours. In another study, no differences in number of opportunistic infections, weight gain, or performance status were noted in patients taking 200 mg of zidovudine three times a day compared with patients taking 200 mg six times a day. Based on these data, a lower daily dose of zidovudine, 500 to 600 mg per day, seems warranted. It also appears that the dosing interval can be safely increased to every 6 to 8 hours without loss of efficacy.

Zidovudine has been shown in several studies to be beneficial (Table 8–1) in the treatment of patients with advanced HIV disease.[3,4,8,12] Beneficial effects have been seen among patients with AIDS-defining opportunistic infections, including *Pneumocystis carinii* pneumonia and *Toxoplasma* encephalitis. It is likely that zidovudine administration will also benefit patients with other AIDS defining infections. However, certain opportunistic infections remain difficult to treat, and patients who are terminally ill with these types of infections may not respond as well.

Zidovudine has been shown to benefit patients with advanced ARC as manifested by persistent fevers, unintentional weight loss, unexplained diarrhea, oral candidiasis, oral hairy leukoplakia, or herpes zoster, and a CD4 lymphocyte count $\leq 200/mm^3$. In addition, preliminary data from two recently terminated ACTG studies show that zidovudine is beneficial to patients with early ARC, defined as the presence of oral candidiasis, hairy leukoplakia, herpes zoster, chronic seborrheic dermatitis, moderate to severe fatigue, or mild unintentional weight loss and a CD4 cell count $\geq 200/mm^3$ but $<500/mm^3$ and patients with asymptomatic HIV infection and a CD4 lymphocyte count $<500/mm^3$.

On the basis of these data any patient with an AIDS-defining opportunistic infection, wasting syndrome (Slims disease), symptomatic HIV infection, and with a CD4 cell count $<500/mm^3$, or asymptomatic HIV infection and a CD4 cell count $<500/mm^3$ should be considered a candidate for zidovudine therapy.

Zidovudine has been administered to patients with HIV-related neurologic disease, including dementia, peripheral neuropathy, and myelopathy.[14] Patients with dementia have been noted to improve in neurologic dysfunction as assessed by clinical evaluations, neuropsychological testing, or positron-emission tomographic scans. Improvements have been noted soon after the initiation of zidovudine, and in approximately 50 percent of patients, sustained improvements for up to 18 months have been described. In a subgroup of patients, neurologic dysfunction reappears within several months of initiation of therapy. Less promising benefits have been described among patients with HIV-related peripheral neuropathy and myelopathy (Chapter 12).

Autoimmune thrombocytopenia has been described among patients with HIV infection. Administration of zidovudine will increase the mean platelet count within 1 to 2 weeks after the initiation of therapy.[5,7,9] This rapid increase in platelet count suggests that zidovudine may lead to diminished clearance of immunoglobulin-coated platelets or, alternatively, may stimulate platelet production by interfering with HIV infection in the bone marrow. Among patients with HIV-related autoimmune thrombocytopenia, a substantial improvement in the platelet count has been noted in at least 50 percent of patients receiving zidovudine, suggesting a beneficial effect of zidovudine in the treatment of HIV-associated autoimmune thrombocytopenia (Chapter 13).

The most common opportunistic infection noted among patients receiving zidovudine is *P. carinii* pneumonia. The greatest risk for recurrent *P. carinii* infection is within the first 9 months following diagnosis. Hemoglobin concentration, number of CD4 cells, and time interval since the diagnosis

TABLE 8–2.   ADVERSE EXPERIENCES ASSOCIATED WITH ZIDOVUDINE THERAPY

Malaise or fatigue	1-4 wk	Macrocytosis	4-12 wk
Nausea or vomiting	1-4 wk	Anemia	4-12 wk
Abdominal discomfort	1-4 wk	Neutropenia	4-24 wk
Headaches	1-4 wk	Hepatoxicity (uncommon)	>24 wk[2]
Confusion	1-2 wk	Myopathy	>24 wk
Fever or rash (rare)	1-2 wk	Nail pigmentation	>24 wk

of *P. carinii* pneumonia correlate with the early development of recurrent *P. carinii* pneumonia following initiation of zidovudine therapy. Concomitant therapy with zidovudine and an antimicrobial agent effective in the prevention of *P. carinii* pneumonia is likely to further improve survival benefits. Patients receiving zidovudine who are at an increased risk for *P. carinii* pneumonia should be placed on chemoprophylaxis for the prevention of *P. carinii* infection. Any of the currently effective antimicrobial agents can be used, as long as patients are monitored carefully (Chapter 15). If additive toxicities are seen and if lower doses of zidovudine are not tolerated, another antimicrobial agent for the prevention of *P. carinii* pneumonia should be chosen.

Adverse reactions reported during the first several weeks of zidovudine therapy include headache, insomnia, nausea, vomiting, abdominal discomfort, diarrhea, malaise, myalgias, rash, and fever (Table 8–2).[10] Headache, nausea, and malaise are the most common early adverse experiences, especially in patients with early HIV infection. Symptoms generally subside with ongoing therapy. Occasionally symptoms will persist or be severe enough to require interruption of therapy. Rarely does zidovudine therapy have to be discontinued. Rare reports of rash and fever have been described that necessitated discontinuing zidovudine. Anaphylaxis has not been noted.

An association has been described between long-term zidovudine therapy and the development of a myopathy characterized by myalgias, proximal muscle weakness, and wasting and elevation in serum creatine kinase values. Development of myopathy is associated with prolonged therapy and has not been described during the first 6 months of treatment. The lower extremities are disproportionately effected. Temporary interruption of therapy and use of nonsteroidal anti-inflammatory agents may be helpful. Patients should be started on reduced doses of zidovudine to delay or prevent long-term debilitation. Doses as low as 100 mg every 8 hours can be tried.

The major toxicity or adverse reaction associated with zidovudine administration is bone marrow toxicity.[10] Both anemia and neutropenia have

TABLE 8–3.   CLINICAL ENDPOINTS AND ADVERSE EXPERIENCES ASSOCIATED WITH ZIDOVUDINE THERAPY IN PATIENTS WITH ASYMPTOMATIC HIV INFECTION*

	PLACEBO GROUP (N = 428)	ZIDOVUDINE GROUP 500 mg/d (N = 453)	ZIDOVUDINE GROUP 1500 mg/d (N = 457)
Clinical Endpoints			
AIDS or ARC	38	17 ($P = 0.006$)	19 ($P = 0.05$)
AIDS	33	11 ($P = 0.001$)	14 ($P = 0.02$)
Adverse Reactions			
Anemia (Hgb < 8 g/dl)	1	5 ($P = 0.010$)	29 ($P < 0.0001$)
Neutropenia (<750/mm^3)	7	8 ($P = 0.7$)	29 ($P < 0.0001$)

*Preliminary data from a multicenter study of the NIAID AIDS Clinical Trials Group.

TABLE 8–4.   CLINICAL ENDPOINTS AND ADVERSE EXPERIENCES ASSOCIATED WITH ZIDOVUDINE THERAPY IN PATIENTS WITH MILDLY SYMPTOMATIC HIV INFECTION[1]

	PLACEBO GROUP	ZIDOVUDINE GROUP	P VALUE
Clinical Endpoints			
CD4 cells >200-800/mm^3	N-361	N-360	
AIDS/ARC	26	15[2]	0.0013
CD4 cells >200-500/mm^3	N-253	N-260	
AIDS/ARC	34	12	0.0002
CD4 cells >500-800/mm^3	N-98	N-100	
AIDS/ARC	2	3	0.63
Adverse Reactions	N-361	N-360	
Anemia (Hgb < 8 g/dl)	0	17	0 < 0.0001
Neutropenia (cells < 750/mm^3)	5	15	0.03

[1]Preliminary data from a multicenter study of the NIAID AIDS Clinical Trials Group.
[2]Two deaths occurred without progressive HIV disease.

been described and, less commonly, thrombocytopenia (Tables 8–3 and 8–4). A macrocytosis with moderate elevations in the mean corpuscular volume (MCV) of 25 to 40 units has been seen in approximately 75 percent of patients receiving zidovudine. Increases in the MCV can be appreciated as early as 6 to 8 weeks after initiation of therapy and are most prominent after 16 to 24 weeks of therapy. In the majority of patients, this macrocytosis is not associated with anemia; if anemia is seen, it is frequently mild, and reductions in the dose of zidovudine may not necessarily be required.

In a subgroup of patients, a more severe anemia secondary to suppression of erythropoiesis has been noted.[13] Occasionally, a mild to moderate elevation in the MCV may also be seen. Serum folate levels are generally normal or elevated, and vitamin B_{12} levels are normal to low normal. The reticulocyte count is frequently depressed (to less than 0.5%) and may be the first sign of bone marrow toxicity and developing anemia. A decrease or absence of red cell precursors is frequently seen on bone marrow evaluation. Erythropoietin levels are commonly elevated, suggesting that the erythroid hypoplasia or aplasia seen is not due to an interference with erythropoietin production. These findings suggest that zidovudine may inhibit commitment of cells into the erythroid line or may have a direct toxic effect on committed erythroid stem cells. Interruption of therapy will result in increases in the levels of hemoglobin and resolution of erythroid hypoplasia or aplasia findings in the bone marrow. However, in one third of patients with advanced HIV disease, blood transfusions may be needed, and in 10 percent of patients repeated blood transfusions may be necessary to maintain patients on long-term zidovudine therapy. Several studies have demonstrated that recombinant human erythropoietin (r-HuEPO) is safe and will decrease blood transfusion needs in patients receiving zidovudine who do not have an elevation in endogenous erythropoietin levels (Chapter 13). Lower doses of zidovudine may also be helpful in decreasing the incidence and severity of anemia. Patients with anemia should be maintained on no more than 500 to 600 mg of zidovudine per day.

Neutropenia has also been described with zidovudine therapy and is usually the dose-limiting factor for long-term treatment. Neutropenia can be seen as early as 4 weeks but is most common after 12 weeks of therapy. Mild to moderate neutropenia (neutrophil count $750-1000/mm^3$) is seen in the majority of patients with advanced HIV disease during initial therapy with 1000 to 1500 mg per day and is typically well tolerated. Moderate to more severe neutropenia (cell count $500-750/mm^3$) occurs in 50 percent of patients and is more common among patients with advanced HIV disease receiving zidovudine for more than 16 to 24 weeks, especially among those patients also receiving other medications known to cause neutropenia. Decreasing the dose of zidovudine is essential in limiting neutropenia and should be considered early in therapy.

Zidovudine inhibits replication of HIV in vitro at concentrations of <0.1 μmol/L (<0.37 μg/ml). The development of reduced viral sensitivity after 6 months or more of zidovudine therapy has been shown in HIV isolates from patients with AIDS and ARC.[6] Sequential isolates from patients on zidovudine therapy typically show a stepwise decrease in sensitivity over time. Isolates obtained from patients late in therapy have had up to a hundredfold reduction in sensitivity. Cross-resistance to other nucleosides (ddC, ddI, d4T) or nonnucleoside anti-HIV drugs has not been seen. No apparent correlation between reduced sensitivity in vitro and clinical outcome has been documented to date. However, further careful, prospective studies are still needed. Until such data are available, no change in current patient management is suggested.

DIDEOXYCYTIDINE

ddC inhibits replication of HIV at concentrations of 0.01 to 0.5 μmol/L in vitro. ddC is rapidly absorbed from the gastrointestinal tract with a mean ddC half-life of approximately 1 hour. Mean steady-state plasma peak concentrations of ddC following oral administration of 0.03 mg/kg of body weight is 0.1 to 0.2 μmol/L. ddC has been detected in cerebrospinal fluid (CSF), although penetration into the CSF is not optimal.

In phase I studies, ddC doses of 0.03 to 0.06 mg/kg per day resulted in significant decreases in serum p24 antigen levels and less prominent increases in the number of CD4 T-lymphocytes in the majority of subjects. At lower doses of ddC tested (0.01 to 0.005 mg/kg per day), decreases in serum p24 antigen levels still occurred but were less prominent.

The major toxicities associated with ddC include maculovesicular cutaneous eruptions, aphthous oral ulcerations, and fevers during the first 4 weeks of therapy. The occurrence of this constellation of symptoms was both less frequent and less severe at lower daily doses of ddC tested, ≤0.01 mg/kg per day. Resolution of these symptoms is also common without interruption of therapy. During long-term follow-up of subjects in phase I studies, the major dose-limiting toxicity proved to be a pain sensory-motor peripheral neuropathy, involving predominantly the lower extremities. Both the incidence and severity of peripheral neuropathy decreased with decreasing daily doses of ddC. Problems with peripheral neuropathy were uncommon, for example, among subjects receiving daily doses of less than 0.01 mg/kg per day of ddC.

Currently, the efficacy and toxicities of ddC are being evaluated in the treatment of patients with advanced HIV disease. The combination of ddC and zidovudine in vitro has been shown to have synergistic inhibitory activity against HIV. A phase I study evaluating the combination of both drugs is also being done.

DIDEOXYINOSINE

ddI is a nucleoside analogue that inhibits the replication of HIV in vitro. After single oral doses of 0.8 to 22.8 mg/kg, the mean half-life was 1.6 hours. Mean steady-state plasma peak concentrations following oral administration of ddI was 244 to 4163 ng/ml. The mean bioavailability was 40 percent in dose ranges of 0.8 to 10.2 mg/kg.

Approximately 90 subjects have been treated with ddI in phase I studies. Decreasing serum p24 antigen levels were noted in about 50 percent of evaluable subjects, and increases in the number of CD4 T-lymphocytes were noted in about one third of subjects.

The major dose-limiting toxicity appears to be a painful sensory-motor peripheral neuropathy. The occurrence of peripheral neuropathy was more common and occurred early in the course of treatment among subjects receiving higher daily doses of ddI, typically exceeding 12 mg/kg per day. Pancreatitis has also been reported in several subjects receiving higher daily doses of ddI. In addition, increases in uric acid levels have occurred in many subjects, but dose interruptions have not typically been needed. Rare cases of liver enzymes elevation, rash, thrombocytopenia, neutropenia, and diarrhea have been noted.

Clinical studies to evaluate the efficacy and safety of ddI are currently being done. In addition, the FDA has approved an open label study for subjects with advanced HIV disease who have, despite zidovudine therapy, rapidly progressive HIV disease as manifested by weight loss, neurologic deterioration, multiple AIDS-defining opportunistic infections, a CD4 T-lymphocyte count $<50/mm^3$, and a performance status of 40 percent or less. A compassionate plea protocol has also been approved for patients with advanced HIV disease who are intolerant of zidovudine therapy because of anemia, gastrointestinal symptoms, neurologic toxicities, or neutropenia.

COMBINATION THERAPIES

Combination microbial therapy and cancer chemotherapy have been used successfully to treat bacterial infections, fungal infections, viral infections and a variety of malignancies. Although zidovudine is effective in the treatment of HIV infection, limitations in its use have occurred due to disease progression, toxicity, and potential adverse consequences of the emergence of resistant mutants. The use of combination therapies in HIV infection, therefore, appears logical and may allow for reduced doses of individual drugs, delays in the development of reduced sensitivity, and enhanced effectiveness of anti-HIV activity. Several drug combinations in vitro have been shown to have synergistic inhibitory activity against HIV, including zidovudine and α-interferon, rsCD4 and zidovudine, castanospermine/n-butyl DNJ (glycosylation inhibitors) and zidovudine, and ddC and zidovudine. Possible synergistic or additive inhibitory activity in vitro has also been shown for combination therapies with acyclovir and zidovudine and ddI and zidovudine. In contrast, antagonistic inhibitory activity against HIV has been seen with ribavirin and zidovudine.[11]

Several studies have found that combined daily doses of 1200 mg of zidovudine and up to 5 g of acyclovir do not result in a substantial alteration of the pharmacokinetics of zidovudine. Short courses of combined therapy appear to be tolerated without additive toxicities. However, no definitive data are available that demonstrate an advantage for combination therapy over high doses of monotherapy with zidovudine. With the demonstration that lower daily doses of zidovudine may be more effective than higher doses, combination studies of acyclovir and lower daily doses of zidovudine will be needed.

The combination of 4 to 18 million units of α-interferon and 600 mg per day of zidovudine in patients with HIV-associated Kaposi's sarcoma has been found to be relatively well tolerated. The major adverse reactions seen to date include anemia, neutropenia, and hepatotoxicity. Increases in the number of CD4 T-lymphocytes, suppression of serum p24 antigen, and antitumor responses have been noted. Antitumor responses appear to be greater with the combination than with high dose α-interferon monotherapy. Low daily doses of α-interferon (1 to 9 million units) and zidovudine in combination are being evaluated in the treatment of patients with AIDS and ARC.

Studies evaluating the combination of other nucleoside anti-HIV drugs, including ddC and ddI and zidovudine, are also being done. The possibility that lower daily doses of each drug will be as effective as single drug therapy could limit the toxicities seen with either drug alone.

REFERENCES

1. Chaisson RE, Leuther MD, Allain JP, et al: Effect of zidovudine on serum human immunodeficiency virus core antigen levels. Arch Intern Med 148:2151-2153, 1988
2. Dubin G, Braffman MN: Zidovudine-induced hepatotoxicity. Ann Intern Med 110:85-86, 1989
3. Fischl MA, Richman DD, Causey DM, et al: Prolonged zidovudine therapy in patients with AIDS and advanced AIDS-related complex. JAMA 262:2405-2410, 1989
4. Fischl MA, Richman DD, Grieco MH, et al: The efficacy of azidothymidine (AZT) in the treatment of patients with AIDS and AIDS-related complex: A double-blind, placebo-controlled trial. N Engl J Med 317:185-191, 1987
5. Hirschel B, Glauser MP, Chave DR, Tauber M: Zidovudine for the treatment of thrombocytopenia associated with human immunodeficiency virus (HIV). Ann Intern Med 109:718-721, 1988
6. Larder BA, Darby G, Richman DO: HIV with reduced sensitivity to zidovudine (AZT) isolated during prolonged therapy. Science 243:1731-1734, 1989
7. Oksenhendler E, Bierling P, Ferchal F, Clauvel JP, Seligmann M: Zidovudine for thrombocytopenic purpura related to human immunodeficiency virus (HIV) infection. Ann Intern Med 110:365-368, 1989
8. Pinching AJ, Helbert M, Peddle B, et al: Clinical experience with zidovudine for patients with acquired immunodeficiency syndrome and acquired immunodeficiency syndrome-complex. J Infect Dis 18:33-40, 1989
9. Pottage JC, Benson CA, Spear JB, Landay AL, Kessier HA: Treatment of human immunodeficiency virus-related thrombocytopenia with zidovudine. JAMA 82:3045-3048, 1989
10. Richman DD, Fischl MA, Grieco MH, et al: The toxicity of azidothymidine (AZT) in the treatment of patients with AIDS and AIDS-related complex: A double-blind, placebo-controlled trial. N Engl J Med 317:192-197, 1987
11. Spector SA, Kennedy C, McCutchan JA, et al: The antiviral effect of zidovudine and ribavirin in clinical trials and the use of p24 antigen levels as a virologic marker. J Infect Dis 159:822-828, 1989

12. Stambuck D, Hawkins D, Gazzard BG: Zidovudine treatment of patients with acquired immunodeficiency syndrome and acquired immunodeficiency syndrome-complex: St. Stephen's Hospital experience. J Infect Dis 18:41-51, 1989
13. Walker RE, Parker RL, Kovacs JA, et al: Anemia and erythropoiesis in patients with the acquired immunodeficiency syndrome (AIDS) and Kaposi's sarcoma treated with zidovudine. Ann Intern Med 108:372-376, 1988
14. Yarchoan R, Thomas R, Grafman J, et al: Long-term administration of 3'-azdio-2',3'-dideoxythymidine to patients with AIDS-related neurologic disease. Ann Neurol 23(suppl):S82-S87, 1988

9

DERMATOLOGIC CARE IN THE AIDS PATIENT:

A 1990 Update

TIMOTHY G. BERGER, MD

Skin disease is an extremely common complication of HIV infection, occurring in up to 90 percent of cases.[5] Some of the skin conditions are common also in uninfected persons (e.g., seborrheic dermatitis) but are more severe with HIV infection. Other skin diseases are particularly associated with HIV infection (e.g., bacillary angiomatosis). The average HIV-infected patient has at least two and often more skin conditions simultaneously. It is useful to classify the cutaneous disorders seen with HIV disease as infectious disorders, hypersensitivity disorders and drug reactions, or neoplasms. The treatment of these conditions is summarized in Table 9–1 on pp 116-117.

INFECTIOUS CUTANEOUS DISORDERS

Bacterial Infections

Staphylococcus aureus is the most common cutaneous bacterial pathogen.[7] The following patterns of staphylococcal infection are seen: folliculitis, bullous impetigo, ecthyma, abscesses, hidradenitis suppurativa–like plaques, and cellulitis. Folliculitis is the most common form of staphylococcal infection seen in HIV-infected persons (Fig. 9–1). The central trunk, groin, and face are the most common sites of infection. The primary lesion is a follicular pustule, but lesions may be almost urticarial. Many HIV-infected patients have staphylococcal folliculitis of the trunk with severe pruritus, one of the more treatable pruritic eruptions seen in HIV disease.[7]

114

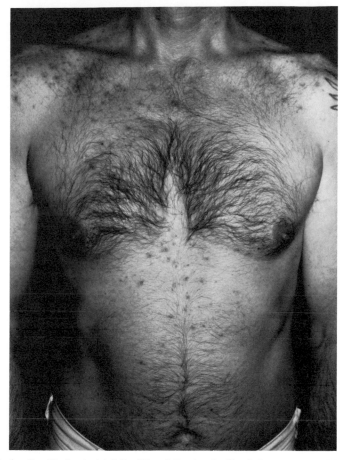

FIGURE 9–1. Pruritic bacterial folliculitis of the trunk. *Staphylococcus aureus* was cultured from a lesion, and the condition cleared with oral antibiotics.

Often many of the lesions have been excoriated, and the patient must be carefully examined for a primary lesion adequate for culture. Bullous impetigo is common in the groin and axillae, presenting as flaccid blisters which quickly rupture, leaving small, superficial erosions with a peripheral scale. The lesions are usually asymptomatic and occur more commonly during hot, humid weather. Ecthyma is a punched-out ulcer with a sharp border (Fig. 9–2). The base may be purulent or may be covered with a thick, adherent crust. Lesions are most common on the lower legs, commonly overlying a preexisting dermatitis. Violaceous, tender, cystic plaques and nodules in the axillae and groin may be due to *S. aureus* alone, as are virtually all suppurative abscesses. All of the above patterns may be accompanied by an associated cellulitis. The treatment of cutaneous staphylo-

TABLE 9–1.   DIAGNOSIS AND TREATMENT OF SKIN CONDITIONS COMMONLY SEEN WITH HIV INFECTION

CONDITION	MORPHOLOGY	LOCATION	TREATMENT	DURATION
Staphylococcal folliculitis	Erythematous follicular pustules or papules; may be pruritic	Face, trunk, groin	Dicloxacillin 500 mg p.o. q.i.d. or other penicillinase-resistant antistaphylococcal antibiotic	7-10 d
			Refractory: Add rifampin 600 mg q.d. to above	First 5 d of antibiotic therapy with above
Bacillary angiomatosis	Friable, vascular papules, cellulitic plaques, subcutaneous nodules	Skin, bone, liver, spleen, lymph node	Erythromycin 500 mg q.i.d. *or* Rifampin 600 mg q.d.	Skin, only 14–21 d Bone, unknown but at least 6 wk
Herpes zoster (shingles)	Grouped vesicles on erythematous bases	Dermatomal distribution; may spill onto adjacent dermatomes	Acute: acyclovir 800 mg p.o. 5 times per day	7-10 d
			Dissemination, severe immunosuppression, or involvement of ophthalmic branch of trigeminal nerve: acyclovir 10 mg/kg i.v. q. 8 h. (corrected for creatinine clearance)	10 d Give i.v. until no new blisters for 72 h, then finish with oral as above
Herpes simplex	Grouped vesicles on erythematous bases rapidly evolving into superficial mucocutaneous ulcerations or fissures; necrotizing ulcers may be seen when chronic	Face, hand, or anogenital	Acute: acyclovir 200-400 mg p.o. 5 times per day	7-10 d
			Oral acyclovir failure or dissemination: acyclovir 5 mg/kg i.v. q. 8 h. (corrected for creatinine clearance)	7-10 d or until ulcers healed and no new lesions for 3 d
			Maintenance: acyclovir 200 mg p.o. t.i.d. or 400 mg p.o. b.i.d.	Indefinitely
			Acyclovir resistance: foscarnet (investigational)	
Molluscum contagiosum	2-5 mm pearly flesh-colored papules often with central umbilication	Face, anogenital	Cryotherapy *or* Topical cantharidin sparingly applied for 4-6 h to nonanogenital lesions and then washed off *or* Electrosurgery *or* Curettage	For all treatments, repeat at 2- to 3-wk intervals until resolved

Condition	Clinical features	Location	Treatment	Duration
Insect bite reactions	Erythematous, urticarial papules	Scabies: axillae, groin, fingerwebs	Electrosurgery *or* Curettage. Scabies: lindane 1% lotion for 12 h	Twice, 1 wk apart
		Fleas: lower legs. Mosquitoes: upper and lower extremities	Fleas, mosquitoes: 1. Insect repellants 2. Antihistamines 3. Insecticide spray environment (fleas)	Constant regular use
Photosensitivity	Eczematous eruption	Face (tip of nose), extensor forearms, neck	1. Sun protection, sunscreens 2. Discontinue photosensitizing medications 3. Topical steroids	Continuous for 1 and 2; As needed for 3
Eosinophilic folliculitis	Urticarial follicular papules	Trunk and face	Oral antihistamines *and* Topical steroids *or* Ultraviolet light	Constant treatment
Seborrheic dermatitis	Fine white scaling without erythema (dandruff) to patches and plaques of erythema with indistinct margins and yellowish, greasy scale	Scalp, central face, eyebrows, nasolabial and retroauricular folds, chest, upper back, axillae, groin	Hydrocortisone 2.5% cream and ketoconazole 2% cream applied b.i.d. Severe: ketoconazole 200-400 mg p.o. q.d. Maintenance: Hydrocortisone 1% cream and ketoconazole 2% cream applied b.i.d.	Until lesions resolve; 3-4 wk; Indefinitely
Psoriasis/Reiter's syndrome	Sharply marginated plaques with a silvery scale	Elbows, knees, lumbosacral	Triamcinolone acetonide 0.1% cream t.i.d.	Indefinitely

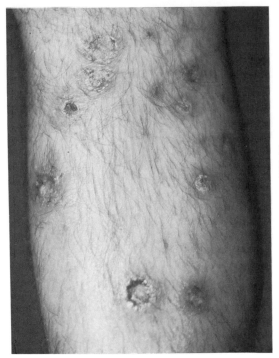

FIGURE 9–2. Ecthyma, showing punched-out staphylococcal ulcers of the lower leg.

coccal infections is determined by the severity of the infection and the presence of systemic symptoms. Patients with chills, fever, large abscesses, or cellulitis are usually admitted for intravenous therapy. Abscesses should be incised and drained. Localized infection may be treated on an outpatient basis with oral agents once cultures are taken. Patients are reexamined after 3 to 5 days to check for improvement to be sure that the appropriate antibiotic was chosen. A penicillinase-resistant penicillin or first-generation cephalosporin is the first choice for therapy. Since nasal carriage approaches 50 percent in these patients, rifampin 600 mg in a single daily dose may be added in refractory or relapsing cases. Washing with benzoyl peroxide or antibacterial soaps may be beneficial to prevent relapse but should be accompanied by vigorous lubrication since dry skin is so common.

Bacillary angiomatosis is an uncommon chronic bacterial infection seen mostly in immune suppression, especially symptomatic HIV disease.[10] The causative organism is felt to be closely related or identical to the bacterium causing cat-scratch disease. It is extremely difficult to culture, so the diagnosis is established by identifying histopathologically the causative agent in affected tissue. This disease should be suspected in patients with lesions of the skin or bone. The skin lesions have been most commonly recognized and are subcutaneous nodules, friable vascular papules (like granulation tissue), or cellulitic plaques (Fig. 9–3). They may occur anywhere on the

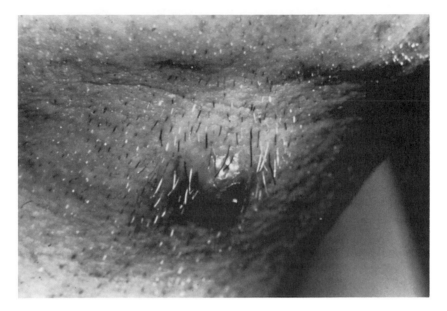

FIGURE 9–3. Smooth, 4-mm angiomatous papule on the chin at the site of a cat scratch. Biopsy revealed numerous bacteria, confirming the diagnosis of bacillary angiomatosis.

skin or mucosal surfaces, especially the respiratory tract and conjunctiva.[4] Erosive bone lesions are common and may appear up to a year before the skin lesions. Other internal organs may also be involved, especially liver, spleen, and lymph nodes.[1] Before the recognition of bacillary angiomatosis as an infectious disease, several affected persons died,[4] and there have been recent reports of deaths associated with visceral disease as well.[14] Indicators of chronic infection such as fever, night sweats, anemia, or an elevated sedimentation rate may occur. Since these symptoms also occur in HIV disease, their importance may be overlooked. The diagnosis of bacillary angiomatosis should be entertained in any HIV-infected person with vascular lesions of the skin or subcutaneous tissue, and a skin biopsy should be performed. The pathology of the skin lesions is that of vascular proliferation with marked edema and infiltration with many polymorphonuclear leukocytes. The lesion may be initially mistaken for Kaposi's sarcoma or a pyogenic granuloma (Fig. 9–4).[11] Since Kaposi's sarcoma rarely if ever involves the bone, a patient with vascular skin lesions and bone lesions most likely has bacillary angiomatosis. To confirm the diagnosis, the skin biopsy may be examined with silver stains or by electron microscopy. Since this disease has been reported from only a few centers, often the most direct approach to establishing the diagnosis is to seek consultation from a pathologist who has experience with this disease.

It is critically important to establish this diagnosis, since bacillary an-

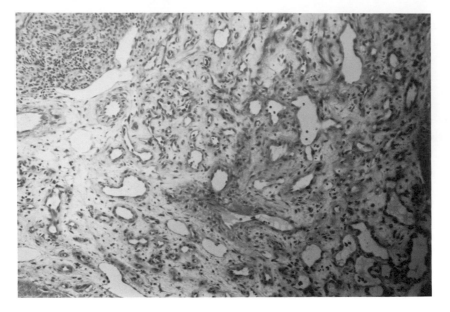

FIGURE 9—4. Biopsy from a lesion of bacillary angiomatosis showing a proliferation of vessels lined with plump (epithelioid) endothelial cells. The background stroma is edematous, and there are multiple fragments of polymorphonuclear leukocyte nuclei scattered throughout. These latter two features are not seen in Kaposi's sarcoma.

giomatosis may be fatal if untreated and in our hands has been an easily treatable disease. The treatment of choice is erythromycin orally at a dose of 500 mg four times daily. Rifampin at a dose of 600 mg daily has also been effective. The penicillins, cephalosporins, and ciprofloxacin have not been effective in our experience. Skin lesions usually resolve with 2 to 3 weeks of treatment. Visceral disease should probably be treated longer, but the duration of treatment has yet to be established due to the small number of reported patients.

Viral Infections

The herpes viruses are the most common cutaneous viral pathogens, with herpes simplex (HSV) varicella zoster viruses causing the majority of infections. The reader is referred to Chapter 21 in this text for a more complete discussion, but several important points must be emphasized. Herpes zoster commonly occurs during the asymptomatic period of HIV disease.[12] Any person, especially anyone under 65, who develops shingles should be queried about risk factors for HIV infection. Usually, the course of herpes zoster is uneventful, although occasionally persistent postherpetic neuralgia may occur. In patients with more advanced HIV

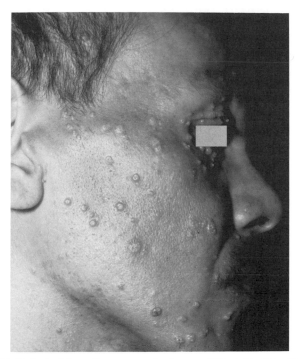

FIGURE 9—5. Multiple facial molluscum contagiosum. This extensive disease usually is associated with advanced HIV disease (OI's, CD4 <200, and standard symptoms). Lesions are largely refractory to all but surgical destruction when the patient is severely immune-suppressed.

disease, herpes zoster may be very painful, severe, and prolonged. Dissemination may occur but is usually limited to skin. In my experience, disseminated herpetic lesions are almost always due to varicella zoster virus, not HSV.

Herpes simplex infections occur in the genital, digital, and orofacial areas. Any persistent, nonhealing ulcer in an HIV-infected person must be suspected of being HSV-related. It is not unusual for lesions to be secondarily infected, so cultures may yield *S. aureus* or other pathogens. A viral culture or fluorescent antibody examination should be performed. If this is negative, consider a biopsy of the edge of the ulcer. It is impossible to clinically diagnose chronic ulcerations in this setting, and multiple cultures and often skin biopsy are required to establish the diagnosis.

Molluscum contagiosum is extremely common in patients with symptomatic HIV disease. Lesions present as umbilicated, pearly, 2- to 5-mm papules on the face, genital area, and scattered on the trunk (Fig. 9–5). There is a particular predilection for lesions to occur on the eyelids. Lesions may number from one to hundreds. Occasional lesions may exceed 1 cm (giant molluscum). Their pearly border and telangiectasias may lead to the misdiagnosis of basal cell carcinoma. Complete eradication is extremely difficult. Lesions are usually treated with destructive modalities (cryotherapy with liquid nitrogen, light electrocautery, or curettage). Topical retinoic acid (Retin A) applied once nightly to the face may slow down the rate of appearance, but, unless applied to the point of severe irritation, does little for established lesions. It cannot be used on the eyelids or genitalia. We and others have seen disseminated cryptococcosis mimic molluscum contagiosum.[6]

HYPERSENSITIVITY DISORDERS

Many of the disorders that cause the pruritic eruptions so common in HIV disease are poorly characterized, their pathogenesis not understood, and the optimal treatments unknown.[2] Excluding drug reactions, diagnosing even half the pruritic eruptions seen in HIV disease is quite good for the current state of knowledge.

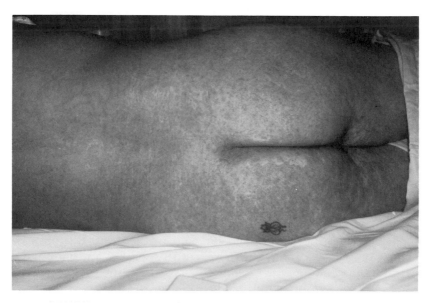

FIGURE 9–6. Widespread maculopapular eruption typical of rashes seen with SMT/TMP and other antibiotics.

Drug Reactions

It has long been recognized that approximately 50 percent of persons treated with trimethoprim-sulfamethoxazole (TMP-SMT) for *Pneumocystis carinii* pneumonia develop a widespread maculopapular eruption.[8] The rash may resolve with continued treatment but often persists or progresses with continuation. Similar reactions are seen with almost all other medications given to HIV-infected persons. Reactions seem to be most common to antibiotics, especially the penicillins and sulfa drugs (Fig. 9–6). Cutaneous reactions are rare to certain frequently used medications, especially acyclovir and zidovudine. Whether HIV-infected persons have a higher rate of reaction to drugs other than TMP-SMT is unknown. In addition to maculopapular reactions, urticaria, erythema multiforme, and fixed drug eruptions may be seen. In some patients the erythema multiforme may be severe. Stevens-Johnson syndrome or toxic epidermal necrolysis (Fig. 9–7). Any HIV-infected person with a widespread eruption should be carefully evaluated for the possibility that it is induced by medication.

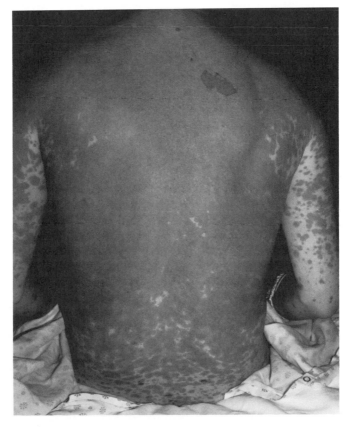

FIGURE 9–7. Drug-induced erythema multiforme major.

Insect Bite Reactions

Scabies, flea bites, and mosquito bites may all be extremely florid in the setting of HIV disease. These eruptions present as nonfollicular papules to cellulitic plaques with marked pruritus. The offending arthropod is identified by the distribution of the eruption or simply by discovering which biting insects are present in the patient's environment. In San Francisco, fleas are a common cause of lower leg pruritic papules, nodules, and blisters. In Miami, mosquitoes are apparently the most important cause of pruritic papules of the extremities.[13] In all patients, the fingerwebs, genitalia, axillae, and feet should be carefully examined for lesions. When lesions are found in these areas, they should be scraped to search for scabetic mites. Scabies is spread by close personal contact, so the affected person must also be examined for sexually transmitted diseases. Treatment of scabies is by standard methods. Other insect bite reactions are treated in three steps: (1) eliminate the biting insects from the patient's environment with insecticides; (2) make the patient less attractive to the insect with insect repellents (Avon Skin So Soft, products containing diethyl toluamide [DEET]); and (3) block the patient's reaction to the bite with potent antihistamines taken regularly, rather than as needed. At least a generous nightly dose should be given (e.g., hydroxyzine 50 to 75 mg), with additional doses during the day if this is inadequate. Longer-acting antihistamines may be more beneficial (e.g., terfenadine, astemizole, or doxepin). Persistent pruritic papules are treated with medium- to high-potency topical steroids until they resolve.

Photosensitivity

HIV disease alone or the medications HIV-infected patients take may lead to photodermatitis, cutaneous eruptions solely in sun-exposed areas (Fig. 9–8).[15] These eruptions initially may appear as pruritic scaly patches or like an enhanced sunburn, which may progress. They are frequently excoriated and become thickened and often hypopigmented. With time the eruptions may extend to unexposed skin. Shortwave ultraviolet irradiation is the usual precipitating spectrum. Photodermatitis is managed by (1) discontinuation of potential photosensitizers (sulfa and nonsteroidal antiinflammatory drugs [NSAIDs]), (2) sun avoidance and protecting the patient from the sun with sunscreens, hats, and clothing, and (3) applying a medium- to high-potency topical steroid to the lesions. In my experience this is relatively easy to manage if the pattern is recognized. If the condition is allowed to persist, the patient may progress to a state of enhanced photosensitivity which will not respond to these simple measures.

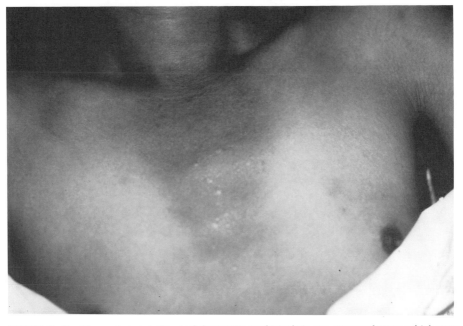

FIGURE 9—8. Hyperpigmentation and dermatitis exclusively in sun-exposed areas, which may be induced by certain medications (sulfa drugs, NSAIDs) or may be due to HIV infection alone.

Pruritic Folliculitis

Only about one third to one half of HIV-infected persons with pruritic folliculitis have *S. aureus* infection.[7] The cause of the folliculitis in the rest is unknown. Usually a skin biopsy is required to rule out other infectious processes (systemic fungal infections) or to determine the composition of the inflammatory infiltrate. Eosinophilic folliculitis is a chronic, waxing and waning follicular eruption.[3] The primary lesion is an up to 1 cm edematous papule with a tiny central pustule. The lesions are scattered on the trunk, head, and neck. Cultures for bacteria are uniformly negative, and the patients do not respond to antibiotics effective against *S. aureus*. Skin biopsy reveals inflammation containing significant numbers of eosinophils surrounding and involving the hair follicle. No organisms are seen in most cases, although occasionally *Demodex* may be found. This mite is commonly found in skin biopsy specimens, so its significance is unknown. Therapy with crotamiton or lindane, which kill *Demodex,* may rarely improve these patients. In my experience antihistamines on a long-term basis (astemizole, doxepin, or temaril) and potent topical steroids are partially effective. Phototherapy with ultraviolet irradiation may be beneficial.[3]

Papulosquamous Disorders

Three dermatologic disorders characterized by scaling patches and plaques are seen more commonly in HIV-infected persons—seborrheic dermatitis, psoriasis, and Reiter's syndrome.[5] Seborrheic dermatitis is extremely common, affecting to varying degrees a high percentage of persons with symptomatic HIV disease (Fig. 9–9). Lesions are usually located in the hairy areas of the central face, scalp, chest, back, and groin. The lesions are mildly erythematous with a yellowish, greasy scale. When limited to the face, lesions are usually asymptomatic, but scalp and trunk lesions are often

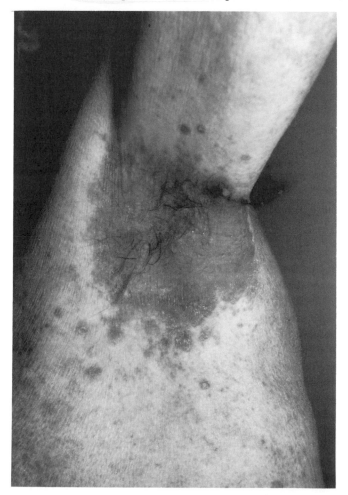

FIGURE 9–9. Seborrheic dermatitis of the axilla in a patient with AIDS. Seborrheic dermatitis is commonly accentuated in the axillae and groin in HIV-infected persons and is distinguished from cutaneous candidiasis by a negative potassium hydroxide scraping. The patient was treated successfully with a mild topical steroid and an imidazole cream mixed together and applied twice daily.

pruritic (Fig. 9–10). Therapy for the scalp includes the regular use of a dandruff shampoo containing selenium sulfide (Selsun), zinc pyrithione (Head & Shoulders, Danex, Zincon), or sulfur and salicylic acid (Vanseb, Sebulex). In addition, a medium-potency steroid solution (triamcinolone 0.1 percent) may be applied. For facial, trunk, and groin lesions, a topical imidazole cream (ketoconazole 2% or clotrimazole 1 percent), plus a low potency topical steroid (hydrocortisone 1 to 2.5 percent or desonide 0.05 percent) is applied twice daily. For refractory trunk lesions, the strength of the topical steroid may be increased. For severe cases, a 2- to 4-week course of oral ketoconazole, 200 to 400 mg daily, may lead to improvement.

Psoriasis often begins after HIV infection, and preexisting psoriasis may flare following infection. The initial lesions frequently begin like seborrheic dermatitis but extend to the axillae and groin and finally involve the elbows, knees, and lumbosacral areas (Fig. 9–11). The lesions of psoriasis and seborrheic dermatitis in the axillae and groin are identical. When psoriasis involves the trunk, it tends to form more fixed, less easily treatable lesions

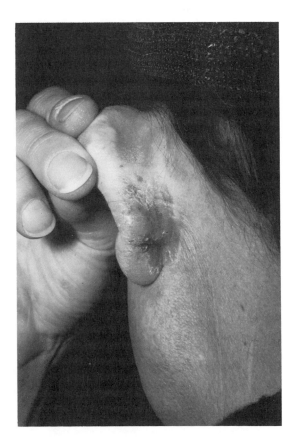

FIGURE 9–10. Seborrheic d matitis in the retroauricular ar Erosion, weeping, and second staphylococcal infection are co mon in this location.

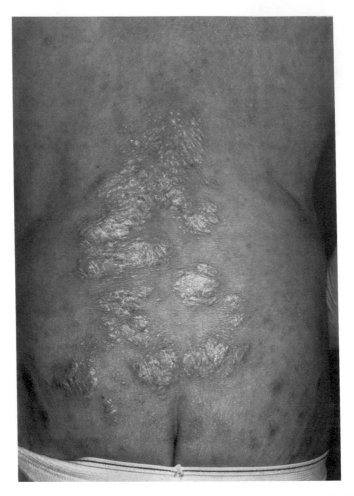

FIGURE 9–11. Typical plaquelike psoriasis that began in the sixth decade in this HIV-infected man. Pruritus was severe.

with a thicker scale. Psoriasis of the palms and soles often begins as superficial pustules which evolve into hyperkeratotic papules identical to the keratoderma blenorrhagia of Reiter's syndrome (Fig. 9–12). Arthritis may be present with psoriasis alone or as a part of Reiter's syndrome. Mild to moderate psoriasis is managed with topical steroids and tar. Patients with severe psoriasis and HIV disease may note a significant improvement of their skin lesions with zidovudine therapy.[9] Methotrexate has been associated with rapid immune suppression and death in HIV-infected persons with psoriasis and Reiter's syndrome and should be considered an agent of last resort.[16]

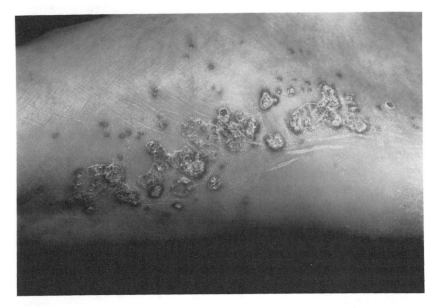

FIGURE 9–12. Pustules evolving into keratotic plaques on the sole. This was the initial manifestation of psoriasis in this HIV-infected person. While identical to the lesions seen in Reiter's syndrome, this patient had no other characteristic stigmata.

REFERENCES

1. Angritt P: Case for diagnosis. Milit Med 153:M26-M32, 1988
2. Berger TG: Evaluation and treatment of pruritus in the HIV-infected patient. In Volberding P, Jacobson MA (eds): AIDS Clinical Review 1989. New York, Marcel Dekker, 1989, pp 205-220
3. Buchness MR, Lim HW, Hatcher VA, et al: Eosinophilic pustular folliculitis in the acquired immunodeficiency syndrome: Treatment with ultraviolet B phototherapy. N Engl J Med 318:1183-1186, 1988
4. Cockrell CJ, Whitlow MA, Webster GF, et al: Epithelioid angiomatosis: A distinct vascular disorder in patients with the acquired immunodeficiency syndrome or AIDS-related complex. Lancet 2:654-656, 1987
5. Coldiron BM, Bergstresser PR: Prevalence and clinical spectrum of skin disease in patients infected with human immunodeficiency virus. Arch Dermatol 125:357-361, 1989
6. Concus AP, Helfand RF, Imber MJ, et al: Cutaneous cryptococcosis mimicking molluscum contagiosum in a patient with AIDS. J Infect Dis 158:897-898, 1988
7. Duvic M: Staphylococcal infections and the pruritus of AIDS-related complex. Arch Dermatol 123:1599, 1987
8. Gordin FM, Simon GL, Wofsy CB, et al: Adverse reactions to trimethoprim-sulfamethoxazole in patients with the acquired immunodeficiency syndrome. Ann Intern Med 100:495-498, 1984
9. Kaplan MH, Sadick NS, Wieder J, et al: Antipsoriatic effects of zidovudine in human immunodeficiency virus-associated psoriasis. J Am Acad Dermatol 20:76-82, 1989
10. Koehler JE, LeBoit PE, Egbert BM, et al: Cutaneous vascular lesions and disseminated cat-scratch disease in patients with the acquired immunodeficiency syndrome (AIDS) and AIDS-related complex. Ann Intern Med 109:449-455, 1988

11. LeBoit PE, Berger TG, Egbert BM, et al: Bacillary (epithelioid) angiomatosis: The histopathology and differential diagnosis of a pseudoneoplastic infection in patients with human immunodeficiency virus disease. Am J Surg Pathol 13:909-920, 1989

12. Melbye M, Grossman RJ, Goedert JJ: Risk of AIDS after herpes zoster. Lancet 1:728-730, 1987

13. Penneys NS, Nayar JK, Bernstein H, et al: Chronic pruritic eruption in patients with acquired immunodeficiency syndrome associated with increased antibody titers to mosquito salivary gland antigens. J Am Acad Dermatol 21:421-425, 1989

14. Simon DM, Benson CA, Loew J, et al: Fatal disseminated cat-scratch disease in HIV-infected patients. In Program and Abstracts of the 29th Interscience Conference on Antimicrobial Agents and Chemotherapy (Abstract #382), American Society for Microbiology, Houston, 1989

15. Toback AC, Longley J, Cardullo AC, et al: Severe chronic photosensitivity in association with acquired immunodeficiency syndrome. J Am Acad Dermatol 15:1056–1057, 1986

16. Winchester R, Bernstein DH, Fischer HD, et al: The co-occurrence of Reiter's syndrome and acquired immunodeficiency. Ann Intern Med 106:19-26, 1987

10

DIAGNOSIS AND MANAGEMENT OF THE ORAL MANIFESTATIONS OF HIV INFECTION AND AIDS

JOHN S. GREENSPAN, BSc, BDS, PhD, FRCPath
DEBORAH GREENSPAN, BDS
JAMES R. WINKLER, DMD

Oral lesions have been recognized as prominent features of AIDS and HIV infection since the beginning of the epidemic.[16] Some of these changes are reflections of reduced immune function, manifested as oral opportunistic conditions, and these are often the earliest clinical features of HIV infection. Some, in the presence of known HIV infection, are highly predictive of the ultimate development of the full syndrome, whereas others represent the oral features of AIDS itself. The particular susceptibility of the mouth to HIV disease is a reflection of a wider phenomenon. Oral opportunistic infections can be seen in a variety of conditions in which the teeming and varied microflora of the mouth take advantage of local and systemic immunologic and metabolic imbalances. These include oral infections in primary immunodeficiency,[34] leukemia,[3] and diabetes,[14] and those resulting from radiation therapy, cancer chemotherapy, and bone marrow suppression.[2,8,10]

Oral lesions seen in association with HIV infection are classified in Table 10-1, and our general approach to the diagnosis and management of oral HIV disease is summarized in Table 10-2.

131

TABLE 10–1.   ORAL LESIONS IN HIV INFECTION

Fungal
  Candidiasis
    Pseudomembranous
    Atrophic
    Angular cheilitis
    Hyperplastic
  Histoplasmosis
  Geotrichosis
  Cryptococcosis
Bacterial
  Atypical gingivitis
  HIV-associated periodontitis
  Necrotizing stomatitis
  Mycobacterium avium intracellulare complex
  Klebsiella stomatitis

Viral
  Herpes simplex
  Herpes zoster
  Hairy leukoplakia
  Warts
Neoplastic
  Kaposi's sarcoma
  Non-Hodgkin's lymphoma
  Squamous cell carcinoma (?)
Other
  Recurrent aphthous ulcers
  Idiopathic thrombocytopenic purpura
  Xerostomia
  Salivary gland enlargement

CANDIDIASIS

Pseudomembranous candidiasis (thrush) was described in the first group of AIDS patients[16] and has been shown to be a harbinger of the full-blown syndrome in HIV-seropositive individuals.[32,39] However, it is not well recognized that this oral fungal condition can take several forms, some of them with subtle clinical appearances.[25,46] The most common form, pseudomembranous candidiasis, presents as removable white plaques on any oral mucosal surface (Fig. 10–1). These plaques may be as small as 1 to 2 mm or may be extensive and widespread. They can be wiped off, leaving an erythematous, or even bleeding, mucosal surface.

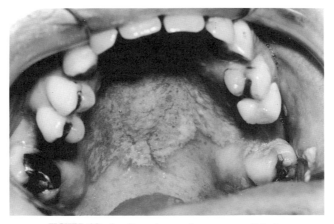

FIGURE 10–1. Pseudomembranous candidiasis.

**TABLE 10–2.   DIAGNOSIS AND MANAGEMENT OF ORAL
HIV DISEASE**

CONDITION	DIAGNOSIS	MANAGEMENT
Fungal		
Candidiasis	Clinical appearance KOH preparation Culture	Antifungals
Histoplasmosis	Biopsy	Systemic therapy
Geotrichosis	KOH preparation Culture	Polyene antifungals
Cryptococcosis	Culture Biopsy	Systemic therapy
Bacterial		
HIV-associated gingivitis	Clinical appearance	Plaque removal Chlorhexidine
HIV-associated periodon- titis	Clinical appearance	Plaque removal, debride- ment Povidone-iodine; metronida- zole Chlorhexidine
Necrotizing stomatitis	Clinical appearance Culture and biopsy (to ex- clude other causes)	Debridement Povidone-iodine; metronida- zole Chlorhexidine
Mycobacterium avium intra- cellulare complex	Culture Biopsy	Systemic therapy
Klebsiella stomatitis	Culture	Systemic therapy (based on antibiotic sensitivity test- ing)
Viral		
Herpes simplex	Clinical appearance Immunofluorescence on smears	Most cases are self-limiting Oral acyclovir for prolonged cases (over 10 days)
Herpes zoster	Clinical appearance	Oral or intravenous acy- clovir
Hairy leukoplakia	Clinical appearance Biopsy; in situ hybridization for Epstein-Barr virus	Not routinely treated Oral acyclovir for severe cases
Warts	Clinical appearance Biopsy	Excision
Neoplastic		
Kaposi's sarcoma	Clinical appearance Biopsy	Palliative surgical or laser excision for some bulky or unsightly lesions; ra- diation therapy; chemo- therapy
Non-Hodgkin's lymphoma	Biopsy	Chemotherapy
Squamous cell carcinoma	Biopsy	Excision or radiation ther- apy, or both

KOH = Potassium hydroxide.   *Continued.*

TABLE 10–2. DIAGNOSIS AND MANAGEMENT OF ORAL HIV DISEASE—continued

CONDITION	DIAGNOSIS	MANAGEMENT
Other		
Recurrent aphthous ulcers	History Clinical appearance Biopsy (to exclude other causes)	Topical steroids
Idiopathic thrombocytopenic purpura	Clinical appearance Hematologic work-up	
Xerostomia	History; clinical appearance; salivary flow measurements	Salivary stimulants or change in systemic medication, or both Topical fluorides
Salivary gland enlargement	Clinical appearance Biopsy (to exclude other causes—needle or labial salivary gland biopsy)	

The atrophic form (Fig. 10–2) is seen as smooth red patches on the hard or soft palate, buccal mucosa, or dorsal surface of the tongue. These lesions may seem insignificant and may be missed unless a thorough oral mucosal examination is performed in good light. Occasionally, *Candida* causes hyperkeratosis (candidal leukoplakia). Such white lesions cannot be wiped off but regress with prolonged antifungal therapy. Candidal leukoplakia may be seen on the buccal mucosa, tongue, and hard palate. It can be confused with hairy leukoplakia and other forms of leukoplakia. Distinguishing between them involves smears, histopathologic study, and therapeutic response (see later discussion on hairy leukoplakia). Angular cheilitis owing to *Candida* infection produces erythema, cracks, and fissures at the corner of the mouth.

Diagnosis of oral candidiasis involves potassium hydroxide preparation of a smear from the lesion (Fig. 10–3). Culture provides information on the species involved. Biopsy is of use for the diagnosis of candidal leukoplakia and to aid in distinguishing it from other forms of leukoplakia.

Oral candidiasis in HIV infection usually responds to topical antifungal agents. These include nystatin vaginal tablets, 100,000 units three times daily, dissolved slowly in the mouth; nystatin oral pastilles, 200,000 units, one pastille five times daily, or clotrimazole oral tablets, 10 mg, one tablet five times daily. Oral ketoconazole in tablet form, 200 mg once daily, is a systemic antifungal agent that can be used as an alternative. It is effective if absorbed. Antifungal therapy should be maintained for 1 to 2 weeks, and some patients may need maintenance therapy because of frequent

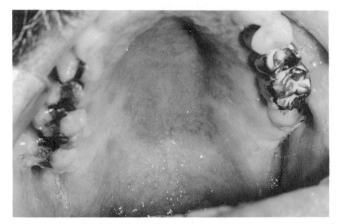

FIGURE 10-2. Atrophic candidiasis.

relapse. Angular cheilitis usually responds to topical antifungal creams, including triamcinalone, and nystatin (Mycolog) or clotrimazole.

Occasionally, other and unusual oral fungal lesions are seen. These include histoplasmosis,[25] geotrichosis (D. Greenspan and J. S. Greenspan, unpublished observations), and cryptococcosis.[15,35]

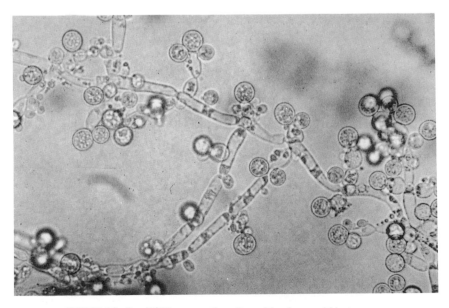

FIGURE 10-3. KOH preparation. Fungal hyphae and blastospores.

GINGIVITIS AND PERIODONTITIS

Unusual forms of gingivitis and periodontal disease are seen in association with HIV infection. The gingiva may show a fiery red marginal line (Fig. 10–4), even in clean mouths showing absence of significant accumulations of plaque.[30,51,52] The periodontal disease resembles, in some respects, acute necrotizing ulcerative gingivitis (ANUG) superimposed on rapidly progressive periodontitis (Fig. 10–5). Thus, there may be halitosis and a history of rapid onset. There is necrosis of the tips of interdental papillae with the formation of cratered ulcers. However, in contrast to

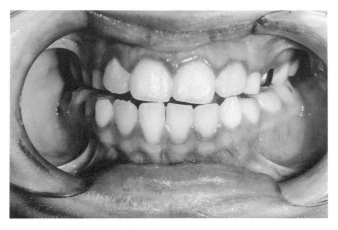

FIGURE 10–4. HIV-associated gingivitis.

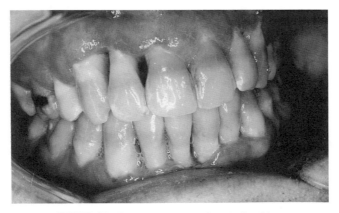

FIGURE 10–5. HIV-associated periodontitis.

ANUG, these patients complain of spontaneous bleeding and severe, deep-seated pain, which is not readily relieved by analgesics. There may be rapid progressive loss of gingival and periodontal soft tissues and extraordinarily rapid destruction of supporting bone. Teeth may therefore loosen and even exfoliate. The periodontal disease often demonstrates a severity and a rapid rate of progression that have not been seen by the majority of currently practicing dentists and periodontists. Exposure and even sequestration of bone may occur, producing necrotizing stomatitis lesions similar to the noma seen in severely malnourished persons in World War II and more recently in the developing countries in association with malnutrition and chronic infections such as malaria. The pathologic and microbiologic features of these remarkable periodontal lesions are under investigation. Current standard therapy for gingivitis and periodontitis is ineffectual. Instead, the therapeutic regimen that is emerging involves thorough debridement curettage followed by a combination of topical antiseptics, notably povidone-iodine irrigation (Betadine) with chlorhexidine (Peridex) mouthrinses, sometimes supplemented with short-course metronidazole (Flagyl) in extremely severe cases.[53] Treatment will fail if thorough local removal of bacteria and diseased hard and soft tissue is not achieved.

OTHER BACTERIAL LESIONS

A few cases have been seen of oral mucosal lesions associated with unusual bacteria, including *Klebsiella pneumoniae* and *Enterobacter cloacae*. These have been diagnosed using aerobic and anaerobic cultures and have responded to antibiotic therapy based on in vitro sensitivity assays.[25] Oral ulcers due to *Mycobacterium avium* have also been described.[50]

HERPES SIMPLEX

Oral lesions due to herpes simplex virus (HSV) are a common feature of HIV infection. The condition usually presents as recurrent intraoral lesions with crops of small, painful vesicles that ulcerate. These lesions commonly appear on the palate or gingiva. Smears from the lesions may reveal giant cells, and HSV can be identified using monoclonal antibodies and immunofluorescence.[13] The lesions usually heal, although they may recur. In patients with a history of prolonged bouts (more than 10 days) of such lesions it may be considered appropriate to treat with oral acyclovir as soon as symptoms are reported. Usually, one 200-mg capsule taken five times a day is effective. Acyclovir-resistant herpes of the lips and perioral structures has been described.[37] The lesions responded to Foscarnet.

HERPES ZOSTER

Both chickenpox and herpes zoster (shingles)[38,47] have been seen in association with HIV infection. In orofacial zoster, the vesicles and ulcers follow the distribution of one or more branches of the trigeminal nerve on one side. Facial nerve involvement with facial palsy (Ramsay Hunt syndrome) may also occur. Prodromal symptoms may include pain referred to one or more teeth, which often prove to be vital and noncarious. The ulcers usually heal in 2 to 3 weeks, but pain may persist. Oral acyclovir in doses up to 4 g/d may be used in severe cases, but occasionally patients may need to be hospitalized for intravenous acyclovir therapy.

HAIRY LEUKOPLAKIA

First seen on the tongue in homosexual men,[19,20] hairy leukoplakia has now been described in several oral mucosal locations and in all risk groups for AIDS.[7,26,33,42,43,44,54] Hairy leukoplakia produces white thickening of the oral mucosa, often with vertical folds or corrugations (Fig. 10–6 and Color Plate IB). The lesions range from a few millimeters to involvement of the entire dorsal surface of the tongue. The differential diagnosis includes candidal leukoplakia, smokers' leukoplakia, epithelial dysplasia or oral cancer, white sponge nevus, and the plaque form of lichen planus. Biopsy reveals epithelial hyperplasia with a thickened parakeratin layer showing surface irregularities, projections or "hairs," vacuolated prickle cells, and very little inflammation.[11,20] Epstein-Barr virus can be identified in vacuolated and other prickle cells as well as in the superficial layers of the epithelium using cytochemistry, electron microscopy, Southern blot, and

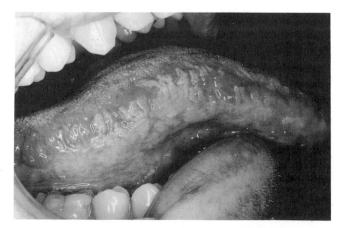

FIGURE 10–6. Hairy leukoplakia.

in situ hybridization.[4,9,29,40] For cases in which biopsy is not considered appropriate (hemophiliacs, children, large-scale epidemiologic studies), we have developed cytospin and filter in situ hybridization techniques.[28] The possibility exists that a second virus is also involved.[29] Langerhans cells are sparse or absent from the lesion.[6]

Almost all patients with hairy leukoplakia are HIV-seropositive, about 75 percent have HIV viremia, and many subsequently develop AIDS (about 33 percent at 12 months and 66 percent at 21 months).[5,24] Cases with tiny or extensive lesions show no difference in this tendency.[45] Rare cases have been described in HIV-negative individuals.[22]

Hairy leukoplakia appears to be an EBV-induced benign epithelial hyperplasia. High doses of oral acyclovir appear to reduce the lesion clinically,[12] and we have shown that the acyclovir prodrug desciclovir can eliminate both the lesion and the EBV infection present in the epithelial cells.[21] However, these effects are soon reversed after cessation of acyclovir or desciclovir therapy. Hairy leukoplakia has not been seen on other than oral mucosal surfaces.[31]

WARTS

Oral lesions due to human papillomavirus (HPV) can present as single or multiple papilliferous warts with multiple white and spikelike projections, as pink cauliflowerlike masses (Fig. 10–7), as single projections, or as flat lesions resembling focal epithelial hyperplasia.[25,49] In HIV infection, we have seen numerous examples of each type. Southern blot hybridization

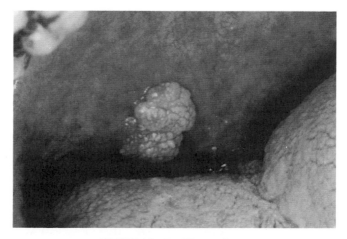

FIGURE 10–7. Wart, palate.

has revealed not (as would be expected) HPV types 6, 11, 16, and 18, which are usually associated with anogenital warts, but HPV type 7, which is usually associated with butcher's warts of skin, or HPV types 13 and 32, previously associated with focal epithelial hyperplasia.[23] Venereal transmission thus seems not to be involved in these warts. Instead, they may be attributable to activation of latent HPV infection or perhaps autoinfection from skin and face lesions.

If large, extensive, or otherwise troublesome, these oral warts can be removed using surgical or laser excision. In some cases, we have seen recurrence after therapy and even extensive spread throughout the mouth.

NEOPLASTIC DISEASE

Kaposi's Sarcoma

Kaposi's sarcoma in AIDS produces oral lesions in many cases.[35] The lesions occur as red or purple macules, papules, or nodules. Occasionally, the lesions may be of the same color as the adjoining normal mucosa. Although frequently asymptomatic, pain may occur because of traumatic ulceration with inflammation and infection. Bulky lesions may be visible or may interfere with speech and mastication. Diagnosis involves biopsy.[18]

Lesions at the gingival margin frequently become inflamed and painful because of plaque accumulation. Excision, by surgical means or by laser, is readily performed and can be repeated if the lesion again produces problems. Local radiation therapy has also been used to reduce the size of such lesions. Oral lesions usually regress when patients receive chemotherapy for aggressive Kaposi's sarcoma.

Lymphoma

Although not as frequent as oral Kaposi's sarcoma, oral lesions are a common feature of HIV-associated lymphoma.[55] Poorly defined alveolar swellings or discrete oral masses in individuals who are HIV-seropositive may prove on biopsy to be non-Hodgkin's lymphoma. No treatment is provided for the oral lesions separate from the systemic chemotherapy regimen that is usually used in such cases.

Carcinoma

Several cases have been seen of oral squamous cell carcinoma, particularly of the tongue, in young male homosexuals. It is not clear whether these lesions are related to HIV infection.[49]

OTHER LESIONS

Recurrent aphthous ulcers (RAU) are a common finding in the normal population. There is an impression, not as yet substantiated by prospective studies of incidence, that RAU is more common among HIV-seropositive individuals.[25] These lesions present as recurrent crops of small (1 to 2 mm) to large (1 cm) ulcers on the nonkeratinized oral and oropharyngeal mucosa. These can interfere significantly with speech and swallowing and may present considerable problems in diagnosis. When large and persistent, biopsy may be indicated to exclude lymphoma. The histopathologic features of RAU are those of nonspecific inflammation. Treatment with topical steroids is often effective in reducing pain and accelerating healing. A valuable agent is fluocinonide (Lidex), 0.05 percent ointment, mixed with equal quantities of Orabase applied to the lesion up to six times daily. This regimen is particularly effective for early lesions. Decadron elixir, 0.5 mg/ml used as a rinse and expectorated, is also helpful, particularly when the location of the lesion makes it difficult for the patient to apply Lidex.

Idiopathic thrombocytopenic purpura may produce oral mucosal ecchymoses or small blood-filled lesions.[25] Spontaneous gingival bleeding may occur. Diagnosis by hematologic evaluation is usually straightforward, but, as with any systemic condition presenting as oral lesions, full work-up is indicated.

We have seen several cases of parotid enlargement in pediatric AIDS cases (Fig. 10–8) and more recently among adults who are HIV-seropos-

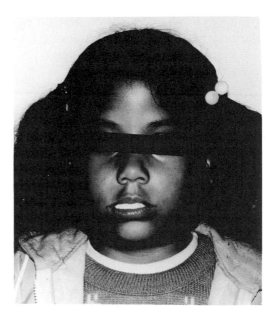

FIGURE 10–8. Parotid enlargement.

itive. No specific cause has been determined, although viral causes are suspected.[1,41,48] Diagnosis, to exclude lymphoma, leukemia, and other causes of salivary gland enlargement, may involve labial salivary gland biopsy and major salivary gland needle biopsy. Some of these cases show xerostomia. Furthermore, the latter condition may be seen in association with HIV infection in the absence of salivary gland enlargement. The patient may complain of oral dryness, and there may be signs of xerostomia, such as lack of pooled saliva, failure to elicit saliva expression from Stensen's or Wharton's ducts, and obvious mucosal dryness. Tests of salivary function, notably stimulated parotid flow-rate determination, show reduced salivary flow. Some of these cases are attributable to side effects of medications that reduce salivation. In such cases it may be possible to arrange to change the medications or their doses. In other cases, stimulation of salivary flow by use of sugarless candy may alleviate some of the discomfort. Topical fluorides and other preventive dentistry approaches are used to reduce the frequency of caries.

SUMMARY

The oral manifestations of HIV infection present as a variety of opportunistic infections, neoplasms, and other lesions. Some of these are common, perhaps the most common, features of HIV disease and are highly predictive of the development of AIDS. Clinicians caring for HIV-infected persons should become familiar with the diagnosis and management of this group of conditions.

The oral lesions of HIV infection present challenges of diagnosis and therapy. As the epidemic progresses, it can be expected that further lesions will be observed and that additional rational and effective therapeutic approaches will be developed.

REFERENCES

1. Ammann AJ: The acquired immunodeficiency syndrome in infants and children. Ann Intern Med 103:734, 1985
2. Barrett AP: Clinical characteristics and mechanisms involved in chemotherapy-induced oral ulceration. Oral Surg 63:424, 1983
3. Barrett AP: Oral changes as initial diagnostic indicators in acute leukemia. J Oral Med 41:234, 1986
4. Belton CM, Eversole LR: Oral hairy leukoplakia: Ultrastructural features. J Oral Pathol 15:493, 1986
5. Centers for Disease Control: Oral viral lesion (hairy leukoplakia) associated with acquired immunodeficiency syndrome. MMWR 34:549, 1985
6. Daniels TE, Greenspan D, Greenspan JS, et al: Absence of Langerhans cells in oral hairy leukoplakia, an AIDS-associated lesion. J Invest Dermatol 89:178, 1987
7. De Maubeuge J, Ledoux M, Feremans W, et al: Oral "hairy" leukoplakia in an African AIDS patient. J Cutan Pathol 13:235, 1986

8. DePaola LG, Peterson DE, Overholser CJ Jr, et al: Dental care for patients receiving chemotherapy. J Am Dent Assoc 112:198, 1986
9. DeSouza YG, Greenspan D, Felton JR, Hartzog GA, Hammer M, Greenspan JS: Localization of Epstein-Barr virus DNA in the epithelial cells of oral hairy leukoplakia by in situ hybridization of tissue sections [Letter]. N Engl J Med 320:1559-1560, 1989
10. Dreizen S, McCredie KB, Bodey GP, et al: Quantitative analysis of the oral complications of antileukemia chemotherapy. Oral Surg 62:650, 1986
11. Eversole LR, Jacobsen P, Stone CE, et al: Oral condyloma planus (hairy leukoplakia) among homosexual men: A clinicopathologic study of thirty-six cases. Oral Surg 61:249, 1986
12. Friedman-Kien AE: Viral origin of hairy leukoplakia (Letter). Lancet 2:694, 1986
13. Fung JC, Shanley J, Tilton RC: Comparison of herpes-simplex virus-specific DNA probes and monoclonal antibodies. J Clin Microbiol 22:48, 1985
14. Glavind L, Lund B, Loe H: The relationship between peridontal state and diabetes duration, insulin dosage and retinal changes. J Periodontol 39:341, 1968
15. Glick M, Cohen SG, Cheney RT, et al: Oral manifestations of disseminated *Cryptococcus neoformans* in a patient with acquired immunodeficiency syndrome. Oral Surg 64:454, 1987
16. Gottlieb MS, Schroff R, Schantez HM, et al: *P. pneumoniae* and mucosal candidiasis in previously healthy homosexual men: Evidence of a new acquired cellular immunodeficiency. N Engl J Med 305:1435, 1981
17. Winkler JR, Murray PA, Grassi M, et al: Diagnosis and management of HIV-associated periodontal lesions. J Am Dent Assoc 119(suppl):255-345, 1989
18. Green TL, Beckstead JH, Lozada-Nur F, et al: Histopathologic spectrum of oral Kaposi's sarcoma. Oral Surg 58:306, 1984
19. Greenspan D: Oral viral leukoplakia ("hairy" leukoplakia): A new oral lesion in association with AIDS. Compend Contin Educ Dent 6:204, 1985
20. Greenspan D, Greenspan JS, Conant M, et al: Oral "hairy" leukoplakia in male homosexuals: Evidence of association with both papillomavirus and a herpes-group virus. Lancet 2:831, 1984
21. Greenspan D, Greenspan JS, DeSouza Y, et al: Efficacy of BWA515U in treatment of EBV infection in hairy leukoplakia. (Submitted for publication)
22. Greenspan D, Greenspan JS, DeSouza Y, Levy JA, Unger AM: Oral hairy leukoplakia in an HIV-negative renal transplant recipient. J Oral Pathol Med 18:32-34, 1989
23. Greenspan D, de Villiers EM, DeSouza Y, Greenspan JS: Unusual HPV types in oral warts in association with HIV infection. J Oral Pathol 17:482-487, 1989
24. Greenspan D, Greenspan JS, Hearst NG, et al: Relation of oral hairy leukoplakia to infection with the human immunodeficiency virus and the risk of developing AIDS. J Infect Dis 155:475, 1987
25. Greenspan D, Greenspan JS, Pindborg JJ, et al: AIDS and the Dental Team. Copenhagen, Munksgaard, 1986
26. Greenspan D, Hollander H, Friedman-Kien A, et al: Oral hairy leukoplakia in two women, a haemophiliac and a transfusion recipient (Letter). Lancet 2:978, 1986
27. Greenspan JS, Greenspan D: Diagnosis and management of oral hairy leukoplakia. Oral Surg Oral Med Oral Pathol 67:396-403, 1989
28. Greenspan JS, Greenspan D, DeSouza Y, et al: Diagnosis and investigation of hairy leukoplakia using non-invasive techniques (Abstract). Presented at III International Conference on Acquired Immunodeficiency Syndrome (AIDS), Washington, DC, 1987
29. Greenspan JS, Greenspan D, Lennette ET, et al: Replication of Epstein-Barr virus within the epithelial cells of oral "hairy" leukoplakia, an AIDS-associated lesion. N Engl J Med 313:1564, 1985
30. Greenspan JS, Greenspan D, Winkler JR, et al: AIDS—oral and periodontal changes. In Genco RJ, et al (eds): Contemporary periodontics, St Louis, CV Mosby Co, 1990
31. Hollander H, Greenspan D, Stringari S, et al: Hairy leukoplakia and the acquired immunodeficiency syndrome. Ann Intern Med 104:892, 1986
32. Klein RS, Harris CA, Small CB: Oral candidiasis in high-risk patients as the initial manifestation of the acquired immunodeficiency syndrome. N Engl J Med 311:354, 1984
33. Konrad K: Orale "haarige" Leukoplakie—klinische Fruehmanifestation der HTLV-III-Infektion. Wien Klin Wochenschr 3(Suppl):702, 1986

34. Leggott PJ, Robertson PB, Greenspan D, et al: Oral manifestation of primary and acquired immunodeficiency diseases in children. Pediatr Dent 9:98, 1987
35. Lozada F, Silverman S, Migliorati CA, et al: Oral manifestations of tumor and opportunistic infections in the acquired immunodeficiency syndrome (AIDS): Findings in 53 homosexual men with Kaposi's sarcoma. Oral Surg 56:491, 1983
36. Lynch DP, Naftolin LZ: Oral *Cryptococcus neoformans* infection in AIDS. Oral Surg 64:449, 1987
37. MacPhail LA, Greenspan D, Schiødt M, Drennan D, Mills J: Acyclovir-resistant, foscarnet-sensitive oral herpes simplex type 2 lesion in a patient with AIDS. Oral Surg Oral Med Oral Pathol 67:427-432, 1989
38. Melbye M, Grossman RJ, Goeder JJ, et al: Risk of AIDS after herpes zoster. Lancet 1:728, 1987
39. Murray HW, Hillman JK, Rubin BY, et al: Patients at risk for AIDS-related opportunistic infections. N Engl J Med 313:1504, 1985
40. Nasemann T, Kimmig W, Schaeg G, et al: Orale "hairy" Leukoplakie-electronenoptische Schnelldiagnostik durch Negative-Staining-Verfahren. Hautarzt 37:571, 1986
41. Pahwa S, Kaplan M, Fikrig S, et al: Spectrum of human T-cell lymphotropic virus type III infection in children. JAMA 255:2299, 1986
42. Phelan JA, Saltzman BR, Friedland GH, et al: Oral findings in patients with acquired immunodeficiency syndrome. Oral Surg 64:50, 1987
43. Reichart P, Pohle HD, Gelderblom H, et al: Orale Manifestationen bei AIDS. Dtsch Z Mund Kiefer Geschichtschr 9:167, 1985
44. Rindum JL, Schiødt M, Pindborg JJ, et al: Oral hairy leukoplakia in three hemophiliacs with human immunodeficiency virus infection. Oral Surg 63:437, 1987
45. Schiødt M, Greenspan D, Daniels TE, Greenspan JS: Clinical and histologic spectrum of oral hairy leukoplakia. Oral Surg Oral Med Oral Pathol 64(6):716-720, 1987
46. Schiødt M, Pindborg JJ: Aids and the oral cavity. Epidemiology and clinical oral manifestations of human immune deficiency virus infection: A review. Int J Oral Maxillofac Surg 16:1, 1987
47. Schiødt M, Rindum JL, Bygbjerg I: Chickenpox with oral manifestations in an AIDS patient. Tandlaegebladet 91:316, 1987
48. Schiødt M, Greenspan D, Daniels TE, Nelson J, Leggott PJ, Wara DW, Greenspan JS: Parotid gland enlargement and xerostomia associated with labial sialadenitis in HIV-infected patients. In 2nd International Symposium on Sjogren's Syndrome. J Autoimmunity 2(4):415, 1989
49. Silverman S, Migliorati CA, Lozada-Nur F, et al: Oral findings in people with or at high risk for AIDS: A study of 375 homosexual males. J Am Dent Assoc 112:187, 1986
50. Volpe F, Schimmer A, Barr C: Oral manifestations of disseminated *Mycobacterium avium intracellulare* in a patient with AIDS. Oral Surg 60:567, 1985
51. Winkler JR, Murray PA: Periodontal disease. J Calif Dent Assoc 15:20, 1987
52. Winkler JR, Murray PA, Grassi M: Clinical evaluation and management of HIV-associated periodontal lesions. J Periodontol, 1990 (in press)
53. Winkler JR, Murray PA, Grassi M, et al: Diagnosis and management of HIV-associated periodontal lesions. J Am Dent Assoc 119(suppl):255-345, 1989
54. Wray D, Moody GH, McMillan A: Oral "hairy" leukoplakia associated with human immunodeficiency virus infection: Report of two cases. Br Dent J 161:338, 1986
55. Ziegler JL, Miner RC, Rosenbaum E, et al: Outbreak of Burkitt's-like lymphoma in homosexual men. Lancet 2:631, 1982

11

AIDS-ASSOCIATED GASTROINTESTINAL DISEASE

JOHN P. CELLO, MD

Gastrointestinal (GI) tract abnormalities are commonly encountered in the evaluation and treatment of patients with AIDS.[7] Although some of these GI manifestations, such as weight loss, anorexia, and large-volume diarrhea, can be difficult to diagnose and treat specifically, many other manifestations of HIV infection, particularly those in the esophagus, liver, biliary tract, and rectosigmoid colon, can be expeditiously evaluated, definitively diagnosed, and specifically treated. In this chapter the most common GI manifestations of HIV infection are reviewed in relation to specific organs.

ESOPHAGEAL DISEASES

Dysphagia, odynophagia, and retrosternal esophageal pain (esophagospasm), are common among patients with acute and chronic HIV infection. An acute AIDS esophagitis has been reported in eight patients during the initial illness from HIV infection.[17] These patients had dysphagia, odynophagia, and retrosternal pain lasting 2 to 14 days. Endoscopic examination showed focal, discrete esophageal ulcerations 0.2 to 1.5 cm in diameter. The esophageal symptoms disappeared spontaneously over a 10-day to 20-week period without any definitive therapy as symptoms of acute HIV infection resolved.[17]

Dysphagia (difficulty swallowing with a sensation of food sticking) is the most common esophageal complaint in AIDS patients. By far the most common organism associated with dysphagia is *Candida albicans;* the majority of patients have both oral thrush and esophageal candidiasis (Table 11–1). In patients with oral thrush and esophageal complaints, a course

TABLE 11-1. CLINICAL FEATURES OF AIDS-ASSOCIATED ESOPHAGITIS

PARAMETER	*CANDIDA*	CYTOMEGALOVIRUS	HERPES VIRUS
Thrush	Usual	Occasional	Occasional
Dysphagia	Severe	Moderate	Moderate
Odynophagia	Rare	Moderate	Severe
Esophagospasm	Rare	Moderate	Severe
Localization	Poor	Good	Excellent
Endoscopic features	Diffuse plaques	Giant shallow ulcers	Deep ulcers
Diagnostic tests	Histology, cytology	Histology	Histology, culture
Therapy	Ketoconazole	Ganciclovir	Acyclovir
Response to therapy	Good	Poor	Good

of antifungal therapy including ketoconazole, 200 mg/day, is indicated. Barium contrast radiography may support the diagnosis of esophageal candidiasis (Fig. 11-1). Endoscopy to document esophageal involvement in AIDS patients with oral thrush and dysphagia is unnecessary unless treatment with ketoconazole fails to relieve symptoms significantly.[22,23] Large, yellow-white plaques throughout the esophagus are usually noted in *Candida* esophagitis, and biopsies or direct cytology brushings should be performed to look for tissue-invasive pseudomycelia (Fig. 11-2). Even when symptoms respond favorably to antifungal therapy, esophageal lesions may not resolve completely despite months of therapy.[22]

Pain on swallowing (odynophagia), retrosternal episodic pain without swallowing (esophagospasm), and dysphagia occur more commonly in patients whose esophagitis is caused by herpes simplex virus (HSV) or cytomegalovirus (CMV) than in those with *Candida* esophagitis. Although discrete, single ulcers have been reported in CMV esophagitis, usually esophageal lesions caused by CMV are large (2 to 10 cm in length), shallow, superficial ulcerations extending through much of the esophagus (Fig. 11-2).[19] The ulcerations may be so extensive and circumferential that virtually no normal mucosa is encountered, only infected granulation tissue. Biopsy specimens should be obtained from these large, shallow ulcerations for histologic and viral culture studies. Many patients with CMV esophagitis have CMV-infected endothelial cells, which suggests vasculitis as a possible pathophysiologic mechanism.[5,19] Although patients with CMV esophagitis may have an initially favorable response to ganciclovir (DHPG), relapses are common[10] and maintenance therapy is usually indicated.

Although sometimes indistinguishable from CMV ulcerations, HSV ulcerations are generally fewer, smaller, and deeper. Patients with acute herpetic esophagitis may have aphthoid ulcerations (shallow ulcerations overlying edematous, erythematous mucosa) a few millimeters in diameter; however, chronic herpetic esophageal ulcerations tend to be deeper, clean based, and 1 to 2 cm in diameter. These larger, deeper chronic herpetic

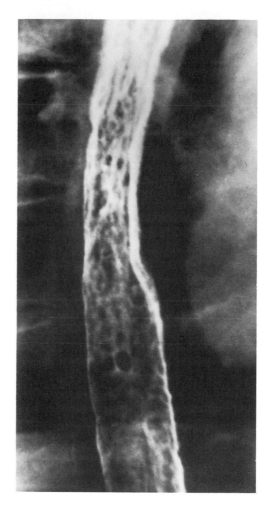

FIGURE 11–1. Upper gastrointestinal barium radiograph in patient with severe *Candida* esophagitis. Mucosa is covered diffusely with plaques and shallow ulcerations.

ulcerations also tend to be associated clinically with intense esophagospasm, odynophagia, and dysphagia. Biopsy specimens should always be obtained from these ulcerations for histologic evaluation and viral cultures. Fortunately, the clinical response to acyclovir has been gratifying among patients with HSV esophagitis.

Rarely, primary lymphoma, Kaposi's sarcoma, and esophageal squamous cell carcinoma have been noted in patients with AIDS. In addition to these AIDS-related esophageal diseases, severe esophageal acid peptic reflux with esophagitis and esophageal ulcerations may occur in bedridden AIDS and ARC patients. Furthermore, nonsteroidal anti-inflammatory agents, tetracycline, and potassium chloride pills may produce discrete esophageal ulcerations, particularly in bedridden patients or patients with diabetes

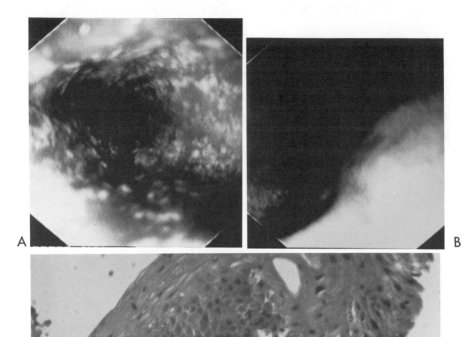

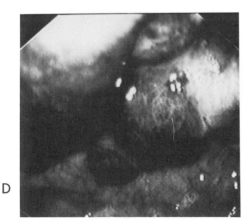

FIGURE 11–2. *A, Candida* esophagitis at endoscopy. Multiple yellow-white plaques (1 to 4 mm in diameter) coat entire esophagus. Shallow erosions are also visible. *B,* Cytomegalovirus (CMV) esophagitis at endoscopy. Large, flat, superficial ulceration is visible in midesophagus. Little exudate is present in ulcer base, which is composed largely of granulation tissue. *C,* Hematoxylin and eosin stain of esophageal biopsy material from patient with CMV esophagitis. Large cells with giant nuclei are clearly visible in lamina propria *(arrow). D,* Kaposi's sarcoma of stomach. Endoscopy demonstrates submucosal reddish nodules with intact overlying mucosa.

**TABLE 11–2.   CAUSE OF UPPER GASTROINTESTINAL TRACT
BLEEDING IN 13 AIDS PATIENTS**

Lesion	Number of Patients
Kaposi's sarcoma	
Gastric	3
Duodenal	1
Gastric lymphoma	2
Cytomegalovirus	
Esophagitis	1
Gastritis	1
Gastric ulcer	1
Duodenal ulcer	1
Duodenitis	1
Mallory-Weiss tear	1
Variceal bleeding	1

mellitus. Given the many causes of esophagitis and the good possibility of providing specific therapy, I strongly recommend endoscopy for AIDS patients with esophageal complaints (except those with oral thrush).

GASTRIC DISEASES

Nausea, vomiting, hematemesis, melena, and early satiety are occasionally encountered in patients with AIDS or ARC. A thorough investigation is indicated because many of these patients have non-AIDS-related gastrointestinal diseases. In patients with AIDS or ARC, I have encountered the full range of non-HIV-associated upper gastrointestinal disorders, including severe peptic esophagitis, gastric and duodenal peptic ulcers, pancreatitis, cholangitis, hemorrhagic gastritis, variceal hemorrhage, and Mallory-Weiss tears (Table 11–2).

Kaposi's sarcoma in the GI tract is commonly noted on endoscopy of patients with documented cutaneous or nodal Kaposi's sarcoma. In the limited published series the stomach is the most commonly involved organ in visceral Kaposi's sarcoma, followed by the colon, the duodenum, and rarely the esophagus.[6,18] In one prospective survey of 50 patients with cutaneous or nodal Kaposi's sarcoma, or both, 20 (40 percent) had GI lesions noted on endoscopy or flexible sigmoidoscopy.[6] However, only seven (23 percent) of 30 lesions seen by endoscopy or sigmoidoscopy could be confirmed histologically, probably because of the submucosal location of most Kaposi's sarcoma lesions and the limited depth of biopsy sampling.[6] Patients with GI Kaposi's sarcoma lesions may well have significantly shorter survival than those without lesions.[6] However, these lesions are themselves rarely associated with significant GI complications, although occasionally

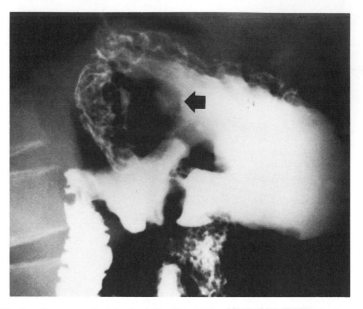

FIGURE 11–3. Upper gastrointestinal double-contrast barium radiography in patient with diffuse visceral Kaposi's sarcoma. "Target lesion" *(arrow)* consists of submucosal nodule with central umbilicated ulceration. Such lesions are also seen in patients with early gastric lymphoma or metastases to stomach (usually from lung, breast, or melanoma).

they become large and bulky, leading to GI tract bleeding, obstruction, or perforation (Fig. 11–2).

B cell non-Hodgkin's lymphomas involving the antrum are often associated with gastric outlet obstruction. Although non-AIDS-related gastric lymphomas are commonly confined to the stomach initially, AIDS-related lymphomas are more commonly multifocal with extensive disease throughout the abdomen in addition to gastric involvement. As with esophageal symptoms, nausea, vomiting, early satiety, and hematemesis indicative of gastric disease should be rapidly evaluated in patients with AIDS or ARC by early investigation, including barium double-contrast radiography. Although smaller lymphomas and Kaposi's sarcoma lesions may go undetected by radiographic techniques and require endoscopy for detection, larger masses are commonly noted radiographically as "target lesions" with central umbilicated ulcerations (Fig. 11–3). Biopsy of these lesions should be performed under endoscopic guidance. I recommend using an endoscope with a large suction channel (model No. GIF-1T10, Olympus Corp., Lake Success, N.Y., or equivalent) and large-diameter biopsy forceps (FB-13K, Olympus, or equivalent) to sample deeper into the gastric wall. Occasionally a loop cautery snare technique, similar to that employed to remove polyps, should be used to extract larger samples for histologic and immunohistochemical studies. For histologic studies of lymphomas, plastic-embedded sections should be used. For preparation of these, adequate tissue specimens must be fixed in cold paraformaldehyde in addition to the formalin fixation used for routine paraffin-imbedded sections.

HEPATOBILIARY DISEASE

Abnormal results of biochemical liver function tests, right upper quadrant abdominal discomfort, and hepatomegaly are seen with increasing frequency in patients with AIDS and ARC.[2,4,8,9,12,13,15,20,21] In addition, jaundice, severe right upper quadrant pain, and spiking fevers are encountered in patients with HIV infection. Early and *complete* invasive and noninvasive evaluation of these patients should be undertaken with particular attention to treatable non-HIV-associated biliary tract disease, such as calculous and acalculous cholecystitis, biliary strictures resulting from surgery for choledocholithiasis or from chronic pancreatitis, and hepatic abscesses. The evaluation should include prompt abdominal evaluation by ultrasonography, computed tomography (CT), or both.

Acalculous cholecystitis, including gangrenous cholecystitis (an entity rarely encountered in young, healthy, ambulatory patients), has been reported in AIDS patients, many of whom have CMV or *Cryptosporidium* noted on histologic sections.[1,9] However, the pathophysiologic features of this disease are uncertain; several patients have had CMV-infected endothelial cells, together with mucosal necrosis and ulceration, suggesting, as with esophagitis, a necrotizing vasculitis. Ultrasonography may demonstrate thickening of the gallbladder wall, air in the wall, narrowing of the lumen, pericholecystic fluid, and localized gallbladder tenderness to the palpating transducer. Nuclear scintigraphy may help substantiate the diagnosis of cholecystitis by the absence of gallbladder visualization despite adequate excretion of radionuclide into the duodenum. Appropriate surgical intervention is indicated in patients with acute acalculous cholecystitis.

Hepatic parenchymal disease is common in patients with HIV infection.[12,15,20] In our retrospective review of hepatic histologic findings, clinical features, and laboratory data in 85 AIDS patients, only one (3.8 percent) of 26 had normal percutaneous liver biopsy specimens and nine (15 percent) of 58 had normal livers at postmortem examination (Table 11–3).[20] Steatosis, portal inflammation, and poorly formed, noncaseating granulomas were the most common histologic abnormalities. AIDS-specific infections or malignancies were detected in 40 percent of both biopsy and autopsy groups. *Mycobacterium avium-intracellulare* was the most common AIDS-related pathogen in our series (Table 11–4). On postmortem evaluation, Kaposi's sarcoma was the most common AIDS-related hepatic finding in our study.[20] Intrahepatic lymphomas and CMV hepatitis were less frequently encountered.

TABLE 11-3.   HEPATIC HISTOLOGIC FINDINGS IN 85 AIDS PATIENTS

FINDING	BIOPSY (% OF TOTAL) (NO. = 26)	AUTOPSY (% OF TOTAL) (NO. = 59)	COMBINED (% OF TOTAL) (NO. = 85)
Normal	1 (3.8)	9 (15.3)	10 (11.8)
Steatosis	10 (38.5)	26 (44.1)	36 (42.4)
Portal inflammation	14 (53.8)	16 (27.1)	30 (35.3)
Congestion	1 (3.8)	18 (30.5)	19 (22.4)
Granulomas	10 (38.5)	2 (3.4)	12 (14.1)
Focal necrosis	5 (19.2)	5 (8.5)	10 (11.8)
Fibrosis or cirrhosis	4 (15.4)	4 (6.8)	8 (4.7)
Bile stasis	2 (7.7)	3 (5.1)	5 (5.9)
Kupffer cell hyperplasia	3 (11.5)	3 (5.1)	6 (7.1)
Piecemeal necrosis	2 (7.7)	1 (1.7)	3 (1.2)

From Schneiderman DJ, Arenson DM, Cello JP, et al: Hepatic disease in patients with acquired immune deficiency syndrome (AIDS). Hepatology 7:927, 1987.

TABLE 11-4.   AIDS-SPECIFIC HEPATIC HISTOLOGICAL FEATURES IN 85 PATIENTS

FINDING	BIOPSY (% OF TOTAL) (N = 26)	AUTOPSY (% OF TOTAL) (N = 59)	COMBINED (% OF TOTAL) (N = 85)
No pathogens	15 (57.7)	34 (57.6)	49 (57.6)
Mycobacterium avium-intracellulare	8 (30.8)	6 (10.2)	14 (16.5)
Kaposi's sarcoma	0 (0.0)	11 (18.6)	11 (12.9)
Cytomegalovirus	2 (7.7)	6 (10.2)	8 (9.4)
Lymphoma	2 (7.7)	2 (3.4)	4 (4.7)
Cryptococcus	0 (0.0)	2 (3.4)	2 (2.4)
Histoplasma	0 (0.0)	1 (1.7)	1 (1.2)
Coccidioides	0 (0.0)	1 (1.7)	1 (1.2)

From Schneiderman DJ, Arenson DM, Cello JP, et al: Hepatic disease in patients with acquired immune deficiency syndrome (AIDS). Hepatology 7:927, 1987.

In addition to a high frequency of Kaposi's sarcoma (10 of 26 patients), CMV (10 of 26 patients), and *M. avium-intracellulare* (5 of 26 patients), marked depletion of portal tract lymphocytes in livers of AIDS patients was found by Nakanuma et al.[15]

Although biochemical laboratory test profiles vary widely in patients with AIDS, the most common abnormalities are substantially elevated serum alkaline phosphatase levels (2 to 15 times upper limit of normal) and more modestly elevated serum transaminase concentrations (usually 2 to 10 times normal). The highest serum alkaline phosphatase levels are encountered in patients with hepatic lymphoma, granulomas, and sclerosing cholangitis.[2,20,21]

Evidence of past hepatitis B viral (HBV) infection also is nearly universal, with between 85 and 95 percent of AIDS patients demonstrating positive serologic markers for HBV. However, only infrequently (5 to 15 percent) are these patients hepatitis B surface antigen positive.[12,20]

In most instances, therefore, parenchymal liver disease in AIDS patients is a manifestation of a previously diagnosed, widely disseminated disease process, and liver biopsy infrequently documents new AIDS-specific diagnoses. Thus a percutaneous liver biopsy is not needed in the majority of patients with hepatomegaly and abnormal results of liver function tests. However, specific diagnosis of an unsuspected disorder (such as *Mycobacterium tuberculosis* infection or lymphoma) may be made on the basis of liver histologic studies, and in patients with substantial abnormal results of hepatic biochemical tests, hepatomegaly, and no documented disseminated disease (such as Kaposi's sarcoma, *M. avium-intracellulare* infection, or lymphoma), a liver biopsy and mycobacterial, fungal, and viral culture studies should be performed.

Obstructive biliary tract disease should be thoroughly and expeditiously evaluated in AIDS patients. I and others have noted profound abnormalities when ultrasonography, CT, and endoscopic cholangiography were performed in patients with HIV infection, and the full spectrum of HIV disease manifested in the biliary tree has yet to be elucidated.[1,4,9,13,16,21] Patients with AIDS-associated biliary tract disease have fever, pain, and tenderness in the right upper quadrant and dramatic increases in serum alkaline phosphatase levels (2 to 20 times more than the upper limits of normal).[13,21] Occasionally jaundice has been noted. In the majority of the patients with AIDS-associated biliary tract disease, ultrasonography and CT of the abdomen show prominent intrahepatic and extrahepatic bile ducts with dilation down to the periampullary area and marked thickening of the ductal walls.[4,13,21] Patients with these findings should be more thoroughly investigated with direct cholangiography, particularly endoscopic retrograde cholangiopancreatography (ERCP), which is clearly more sensitive than either ultrasonography or CT scanning. Of 35 AIDS patients undergoing ERCP at San Francisco General Hospital over the past 4 years, 14 had intrahepatic and extrahepatic sclerosing cholangitis changes (including irregular ductal mucosa) and papillary stenosis (Fig. 11–4, *A*), six had intrahepatic ductal sclerotic changes alone, three had papillary stenosis alone (Fig. 11–4, *B*), and four had high-grade extrahepatic bile duct obstruction (Fig. 11–4, *C*). Only eight of 35 AIDS patients studied by ERCP because of pain and markedly elevated serum alkaline phosphatase levels had normal cholangiograms (Table 11–5). All 12 patients with papillary stenosis *and* abdominal pain underwent ERCP sphincterotomy with multiple biopsies of the ampulla of Vater. Although the right upper quadrant abdominal pain and spiking fevers responded significantly to sphincterotomy, serum alkaline phosphatase levels rose despite establishment of adequate distal duct drainage, which probably reflects ongoing intrahepatic ductal disease. Twelve (44 percent) of 27 patients with abnormal cholangiograms were found to have specific AIDS-related pathogens or malig-

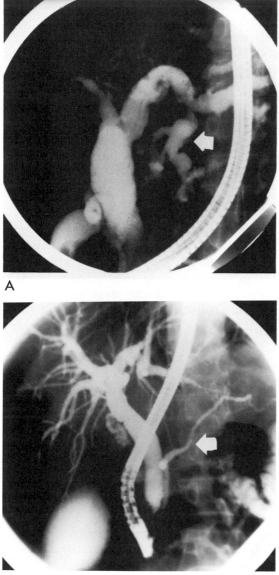

FIGURE 11–4. Endoscopic retrograde cholangiopancreatography (ERCP) in AIDS patients with "AIDS cholangiopathy." *A,* Sclerosing cholangitis and papillary stenosis. Beading, focal stricturing, and dilation of intrahepatic ducts *(arrow)* are present, as well as dilation and irregular mucosa in extrahepatic duct. Distal common bile duct is narrowed. *B,* Papillary stenosis alone. ERCP demonstrated normal pancreatic duct *(large arrow)* and dilated but smooth-walled extrahepatic bile duct. Little drainage occurred for 2 hours after ERCP.

nancies in the regions of ductal disease demonstrated by cholangiography (four with CMV, four with *Cryptosporidium,* one with CMV and *Cryptosporidium,* one with Kaposi's sarcoma, one with *M. avium-intracellulare,* and one with lymphoma).

The pathophysiology of AIDS-associated sclerosing cholangitis and papillary stenosis is uncertain, although CMV and cryptosporidial ulceration and subsequent fibrotic stricturing of the bile duct have been suggested by

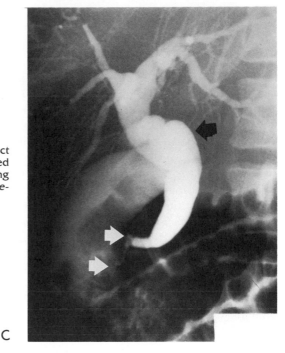

FIGURE 11–4, cont'd. *C,* Bile duct stricture. Extrahepatic duct is dilated *(black arrow).* There is 1.4 cm long distal common bile duct stricture *(between white arrows).*

C

our studies and by the limited additional reports. As suggested by our cholangiographic findings in a few patients without jaundice or ductal dilation detected by CT or ultrasonography, biliary sclerotic changes among AIDS patients may be far more common than is widely appreciated.

TABLE 11–5. CLINICAL FEATURES OF AIDS CHOLANGIOPATHY*

FEATURE	ABNORMAL ERCP FINDINGS (N = 27)	NORMAL ERCP FINDINGS (N = 8)	P VALUE
Age (yr)	37 ± 2	36 ± 4	NS
AIDS duration (mo)	6.9 ± 1.0	7.4 ± 3.0	NS
Right upper quadrant pain	21/27 (78%)	6/8 (75%)	NS
Abnormal ultrasound	18/25 (72%)	1/7 (14%)	0.02
Abnormal CT scan	7/8 (88%)	0/6 (0)	0.01
Alkaline phosphatase (IU/L)	763 ± 131	777 ± 163	NS
Alanine aminotransferase (IU/L)	100 ± 21	111 ± 39	NS
Bilirubin (mg/dl)	1.4 ± 0.6	1.0 ± 0.3	NS

NS, Not significant.
*In 35 patients studied at San Francisco General Hospital. Data are expressed as mean ± standard deviation or as number and percentage of patients examined.

SMALL BOWEL DISEASES

Cramping paraumbilical abdominal pain, weight loss, and large-volume diarrhea are common in patients with HIV disease (Slim's disease). Indeed, the AIDS wasting syndrome (HIV infection and profound diarrhea for 30 days or more without superimposed opportunistic enteric infections) has been accepted as a CDC case definition for AIDS. However, the majority of AIDS patients with cramping paraumbilical pain and associated large-volume diarrhea and weight loss have specific small bowel infections (Table 11–6). Certainly, infections caused by routine colonic bacterial pathogens, such as *Salmonella, Shigella,* and *Campylobacter,* which may be persistent and mimic chronic small bowel disease, should be excluded by adequate culture techniques. Routine and atypical parasitic infestations, including *Giardia lamblia, Entamoeba histolytica, Cryptosporidium,* and *Isospora belli,* likewise must be excluded.[3,16,24,31] In most cases these parasites can be easily isolated from the stools of patients with weight loss and severe diarrhea (Plate IE). Recently a microsporidium, *Encephalitozoon cunicule,* was recognized as a new AIDS-associated pathogen; electron microscopy of small bowel mucosa is required to make this diagnosis. In one third of AIDS patients with infectious diarrhea whose stools contain no enteric pathogens according to culture studies and ova and parasites examination, CMV or *M. avium-intracellulare* is the cause of diarrhea (Table 11–6). The clinical spectrum of disease among patients with CMV and *M. avium-intracellulare* is highly variable. Many patients remain minimally symptomatic whereas others have profound dehydrating diarrhea, malabsorption, and severe abdominal pains. Small bowel vasculitis and ulceration caused by CMV may even

TABLE 11–6.   INFECTIOUS DIARRHEA IN AIDS PATIENTS*

CAUSE	NUMBER	PERCENTAGE
Cytomegalovirus	15	20
Mycobacterium avium-intracellulare	10	14
Salmonella	10	14
Cryptosporidium	8	11
Entamoeba histolytica	6	8
Giardia lamblia	4	5
Herpes simplex virus	4	5
Campylobacter jejuni	3	4
Isospora belli	2	3
Clostridium difficile	2	3
Candida	2	3
Strongyloides	2	3
Kaposi's sarcoma	1	1
Other pathogens	5	7
	74	

Data from Smith PD, Lane C, Vee J, et al: Ann Intern Med 108:328, 1988; and Antony MA, Brandt LJ, Klein RS, et al: Dig Dis Sci 33:1141, 1988.
*In 43 patients, some with multiple pathogens.

progress to perforation of the small bowel. *M. avium-intracellulare* is easily noted on histologic sections of small and large bowel mucosa, since the macrophages are filled with acid-fast-staining mycobacteria.

In addition to AIDS-associated pathogens, HIV infection of the enterocytes or lamina propria may cause abnormalities of the small bowel mucosa.[11] Limited studies to date have demonstrated the gamut of pathologic findings, from normal small bowel mucosa to subtotal villous atrophy (decreased villous height) and associated crypt changes consisting largely of decreased mitoses (hypoplasia).[11,30] Moreover, decreased epithelial cell heights, increased numbers of intraepithelial lymphocytes and plasma cells, spherical intracellular viruslike particles, and decreased brush border enzyme activity have been reported in histologic evaluation of small bowel biopsy specimens.[11,30] These changes may represent viral infection of the enterocytes by HIV itself or an unidentified opportunistic viral agent. If a patient's stool evaluations show no specific pathogens, a series of small bowel biopsies may be indicated. Multiple biopsy specimens should be taken from the small bowel to look for the previously indicated pathogens (specifically CMV, *M. avium-intracellulare,* and *Cryptosporidium*) and additional histologic abnormalities. Although biopsy of small bowel mucosa is traditionally performed with "per oral capsule" techniques, others and I prefer to use long, flexible fiberoptic endoscopes for this procedure. Since many patients have nausea, vomiting, and abdominal pain in addition to weight loss and diarrhea, endoscopy can be used to inspect the esophagus and stomach at the same time biopsies are taken from the proximal small bowel.

COLORECTAL DISEASES

As mentioned previously in the section dealing with diseases of the small intestine, diarrhea is common in patients with HIV infection. Among patients with predominantly colorectal disease, as distinct from small bowel disease, colitic diarrhea tends to be associated with frequent small-volume stools, left lower quadrant or suprapubic cramping, rectal urgency (tenesmus), and often proctalgia and dyskesia (painful defecation). On occasion a small amount of bright red blood may be noted. In the majority of these patients with colitic diarrhea, specific bacterial and parasitic pathogens can be easily isolated by careful analysis of the stools, including routine bacterial culture studies and microscopy for intestinal parasites. Some patients have classic herpetic perianal ulcerations, which can be diagnosed by specific viral culture of swabs taken directly from the perianal area.

In AIDS patients with symptoms of proctitis and no abnormalities on stool evaluation, examination with a flexible sigmoidoscope (usually employing a 60 cm long, fully immersible instrument) is indicated. I and others have described CMV proctocolitis with sigmoidoscopic features suggestive of focal ischemic colitis, consisting of submucosal hemorrhages and discrete but shallow ulcerations of distal colonic mucosa.[10,14] CT scans of patients with CMV colitis may demonstrate diffuse colonic wall thickening indicative of a transmural inflammatory or infiltrative process. Barium contrast radiography of the colon commonly shows edematous haustral folds, shallow ulcerations, and diffuse granularity of the mucosa. The spectrum of CMV infection in the colon is broad, ranging from asymptomatic infection to severe ulceration and perforation. In addition to perianal disease, herpetic ulcerations of the distal colon may be encountered in patients with HSV-1 or HSV-2. Specifically directed biopsies for histologic studies and viral culture are indicated. In patients with persistent diarrhea, *Chlamydia* should also be sought by specific stool culture. Even in the absence of focal or diffuse colonic mucosal changes, biopsy specimens should be obtained for histologic evaluation to look for the occasional patient with *Cryptosporidium* not detected in the stool. In rare instances, Kaposi's sarcoma lesions may become large, bulky, and ulcerative in patients with visceral involvement and may lead to obstruction and substantial hemorrhage.[5]

In addition to HIV-associated pathologic processes, idiopathic inflammatory bowel disease and colorectal neoplasms (including anal cancer) must be carefully excluded from the diagnosis, particularly in middle-aged patients with recently diagnosed AIDS or ARC.

PERITONEAL DISEASES

Patients with AIDS or ARC occasionally have a sudden onset of ascites. Some HIV-infected patients have underlying cirrhosis (resulting from alcoholism or viral hepatitis), and a sizable percentage of these patients have transudative ascites related to their chronic liver disease. However, exudative ascites (ascites protein concentration greater than 1.5 to 2 g/dl) should be thoroughly evaluated in patients with HIV infection. Careful evaluation of the ascitic fluid, including cytologic studies (sampling large volumes) and acid-fast stains, should be employed early to exclude malignancy and tuberculous peritonitis from the diagnosis. In addition to paracentesis, CT scanning may be helpful in evaluating patients with ascites, particularly those with large, bulky peritoneal, omental, mesenteric, or retroperitoneal masses that can be easily approached by CT-guided aspiration cytology. In several patients with recent onset of exudative ascites and no abnormalities or equivocal evaluations by paracentesis or fine needle aspiration biopsy, I have performed laparoscopic evaluations with directed biopsy of peritoneal lymphomatous implants. Such implants usually appear as pink, fleshy nodules 2 to 10 mm in diameter. Tuberculous peritonitis is easily recognizable as 1 to 2 mm whitish tubercles diffusely studding the visceral and parietal peritoneum. In addition to finding tuberculous and lymphomatous peritonitis, I have encountered two patients who had peritonitis symptoms and exudative ascites and whose periotoneal biopsy specimens contained CMV.

REFERENCES

1. Antony MA, Brandt LJ, Klein RS, et al: Infectious diarrhea in patients with AIDS. Dig Dis Sci 33:1141, 1988
2. Blumberg RS, Kelsey P, Perrone T, et al: Cytomegalovirus- and *Cryptosporidium*-associated acalculous gangrenous cholecystitis. Am J Med 76:1118, 1984
3. Caccamo D, Perez NK, Marchevsky A: Primary lymphoma of the liver in the acquired immunodeficiency syndrome. Arch Pathol Lab Med 110:553, 1986
4. Cello JP: Gastrointestinal manifestations of HIV infection. In Sande MA, Volberding PA (eds): The Medical Management of Aids. Philadelphia, WB Saunders Co, 1988, pp 141-152
5. Cello JP, Wilcox CM: Evaluation and treatment of gastrointestinal tract hemorrhage in patients with AIDS. In Friedman SL (guest ed): Gastrointestinal Manifestations of AIDS. Philadelphia, WB Saunders Co, 1988, pp 639-648
6. DeHovitz JA, Pape JW, Boney M, et al: Clinical manifestations and therapy of *Isospora belli* infection in patients with the acquired immunodeficiency syndrome. N Engl J Med 315:87, 1986
7. Dolmatch BL, Laing FC, Federle MP, et al: AIDS-related cholangitis: Radiographic findings in nine patients. Radiology 163:313, 1987
8. Freedman PG, Weiner BC, Balthazar EJ: Cytomegalovirus esophagogastritis in a patient with acquired immunodeficiency syndrome. Am J Gastroenterol 80:434, 1985
9. Friedman SL, Wright TL, Altman DF: Gastrointestinal Kaposi's sarcoma in patients with acquired immunodeficiency syndrome: Endoscopic and autopsy findings. Gastroenterology 89:102, 1985
10. Gelb A, Miller S: AIDS and gastroenterology. Am J Gastroenterol 81:619, 1986
11. Glasgow BJ, Anders K, Layfield LJ, et al: Clinical and pathologic finding of the liver in the acquired immune deficiency syndrome. Am J Clin Pathol 83:582, 1985
12. Kavin H, Jonas RB, Chowdhury L, et al: Acalculous cholecystitis and cytomegalovirus infection in the acquired immunodeficiency syndrome. Ann Intern Med 104:53, 1986
13. Koretz SH, Collaborative DHPG Treatment Study Group: Treatment of serious cytomegalovirus infections with 9-(1,3-dihydroxy-2-propoxymethyl) guanine in patients with AIDS and other immunodeficiencies. N Engl J Med 314:801, 1986
14. Kotler DP, Gaetz HP, Lange M, et al: Enteropathy associated with the acquired immunodeficiency syndrome. Ann Intern Med 101:421, 1984
15. Lake-Bakaar G, Tom W, Lake-Bakaar D, et al: Gastropathy and ketoconazole malabsorption in the acquired immune deficiency syndrome (AIDS). Ann Intern Med 109:471, 1988
16. Lebovics E, Thung SN, Schaffner F, et al: The liver in the acquired immunodeficiency syndrome: A clinical and histologic study. Hepatology 5:293, 1985
17. Margulis SJ, Honig CL, Soave R, et al: Biliary tract obstruction in the acquired immunodeficiency syndrome. Ann Intern Med 105:207, 1986
18. Meilselman MS, Miller-Catchpole R, Christ M, et al: *Campylobacter pylori* gastritis in the acquired immunodeficiency syndrome. Gastroenterology 95:209, 1988
19. Meiselman MS, Cello JP, Margaretten W: Cytomegalovirus colitis: Report of the clinical, endoscopic and pathologic findings in two patients with the acquired immune deficiency syndrome. Gastroenterology 88:171, 1985
20. Nakanuma Y, Liew CT, Peters RL, et al: Pathologic features of the liver in acquired immune deficiency syndrome (AIDS). Liver 6:158, 1986
21. Pitlik S, Fainstein V, Garza D, et al: Human cryptosporidiosis: Spectrum of disease; Report of six cases and review of the literature. Arch Intern Med 143:2269, 1983
22. Rabeneck L, Boyko WJ, McLean DM, et al: Unusual esophageal ulcers containing enveloped virus-like particles in homosexual men. Gastroenterology 90:1882, 1986

23. St. Onge G, Bezahler GH: Giant esophageal ulcer associated with cytomegalovirus. Gastroenterology 83:127, 1982
24. Saltz RK, Kurtz RC, Lightdale CJ, et al: Kaposi's sarcoma: Gastrointestinal involvement correlation with skin findings and immunologic function. Dig Dis Sci 29:817, 1984
25. Schneiderman DJ, Arenson DM, Cello JP, et al: Hepatic disease in patients with acquired immune deficiency syndrome (AIDS). Hepatology 7:925, 1987
26. Schneiderman DJ, Cello JP, Laing FC: Papillary stenosis and sclerosing cholangitis in the acquired immunodeficiency syndrome. Ann Intern Med 106:546, 1987
27. Smith PD, Lane C, Vee J, et al: Intestinal infections in patients with the acquired immunodeficiency syndrome (AIDS). Ann Intern Med 108:328, 1988
28. Tavitian A, Raufman JP, Rosenthal LE, et al: Ketoconazole-resistant *Candida* esophagitis in patients with acquired immunodeficiency syndrome. Gastroenterology 90:443, 1986
29. Tavitian A, Raufman JP, Rosenthal LE: Oral candidiasis as a marker for esophageal candidiasis in the acquired immunodeficiency syndrome. Ann Intern Med 104:54, 1986
30. Ullrich R, Zeitz M, Heise W, et al: Small intestinal structure and function in patients infected with human immunodeficiency virus (HIV): Evidence for HIV-induced enteropathy. Ann Intern Med 111:15, 1989
31. Wolfson JS, Richter JM, Waldron MA, et al: Cryptosporidiosis in immunocompetent patients. N Engl J Med 312:1278, 1985

12

MANAGEMENT OF THE NEUROLOGIC COMPLICATIONS OF HIV-1 INFECTION AND AIDS

RICHARD W. PRICE, MD
BRUCE BREW, MB, BS

HIV-1 infection and particularly its late phase, AIDS, are complicated by a variety of central nervous system (CNS) and peripheral nervous system (PNS) disorders (for general reviews, see references 11, 12, 49, and 87). Classification of these disorders according to their underlying pathophysiologic or pathogenetic process provides a framework for comprehending the conditions to which these patients are susceptible (Table 12–1) and makes it possible to deal systematically with new or unusual conditions.

In practice, however, a neurologist confronted with a sick patient begins with neuroanatomic localization. Therefore in this chapter we discuss the major neurologic disorders according to their predominant pathologic anatomy. Another important consideration for differential diagnosis is the stage of systemic HIV-1 infection and degree of underlying immunosuppression at the time of presentation. The immune status strongly affects vulnerability to disease and hence strongly influences the probabilities of differential diagnosis. Because of this, we discuss the neurologic aspects of early HIV-1 infection separately before dealing with the more common conditions that occur in the AIDS phase of infection.

Our studies of the neurologic complications of AIDS are supported by Public Health Service Grant No. NS-21703 from the National Institutes of Health.

TABLE 12–1.   CLASSIFICATION OF THE NEUROLOGIC COMPLICATIONS OF HIV-1 INFECTION ACCORDING TO UNDERLYING PATHOPHYSIOLOGIC AND PATHOGENETIC CATEGORIES

UNDERLYING PROCESS	EXAMPLES
Opportunistic infections	Cerebral toxoplasmosis
	Cryptococcal meningitis
	Progressive multifocal leukoencephalopathy
Opportunistic neoplasms	Primary central nervous system lymphoma
	Metastatic lymphoma
Metabolic, toxic, and other complications of systemic disease	Hypoxic encephalopathy
	Sepsis
	Stroke
Functional (psychiatric) disorders	Anxiety disorder
	Psychotic depression
Unique conditions that may be related to a primary effect of HIV-1 itself	AIDS dementia complex
	Predominantly sensory polyneuropathy
Autoimmune disorders	Guillain-Barré syndrome
	Chronic idiopathic demyelinating polyneuropathy

NERVOUS SYSTEM INVOLVEMENT EARLY IN HIV-1 INFECTION

Although major clinical attention has focused on the late neurologic sequelae of infection, HIV-1 infection may be accompanied by clinically significant neurologic disorders earlier, even at the time of initial systemic HIV-1 infection. A number of observations also suggest that the CNS is commonly infected by HIV-1 early in the course of systemic infection.

Early Neurologic Complications of HIV-1 Infection

A variety of CNS disorders have been described in association with seroconversion or, less commonly, somewhat later during the asymptomatic phase of systemic disease.[9,13,25,39] These may occur from days to weeks after the seroconversion-related illness that resembles mononucleosis, evolve acutely or subacutely, and take the form of focal or diffuse encephalitis, meningitis, ataxia, or myelopathy, either alone or with PNS abnormalities, including brachial plexopathy or neuropathy. These disorders are monophasic, and most patients recover within a number of weeks, although cognitive deficits may persist in some. The cerebrospinal fluid (CSF) usually shows a minor lymphocyte-predominant pleocytosis with a modest rise in protein concentration. The computed tomography (CT) brain scan is normal, but the electroencephalogram may show focal or diffuse slowing. These early syndromes are apparently uncommon, but their incidence may be underappreciated because they are clinically indistinguishable from other acute viral or postinfectious encephalitides, most of which are never specifically diagnosed. The patient may not have a background systemic illness that leads the clinician to suspect HIV-1 infection, and even when such an illness is present, the acute systemic manifestations of HIV-1 may not be recognized when neurologic disease is prominent. Even in patients serotested in the acute phase, HIV-1 antibodies may not be detected. Immunologic assessment also is usually unrewarding because T-lymphocyte subsets are often normal or include only transient elevation of the CD8+ subset with or without depression of the CD4+ subset. Consequently, serologic studies are needed in the acute period and convalescence (which lasts 6 to 10 weeks or longer), and in some patients virus isolation or antigen detection may be required for diagnosis.

More common than the later seroconversion-related deficits is the development of demyelinating neuropathies during the asymptomatic, or latent, phase of HIV-1 infection. These resemble Guillain-Barré syndrome or the chronic inflammatory demyelinating polyneuropathy seen in other contexts, except with HIV-1 the CSF often exhibits uncharacteristic, albeit mild, pleocytosis.[20] The pathophysiologic pattern of these neuropathies probably parallels that of these disorders in other settings and has an autoimmune basis. Patients appear to respond favorably to plasmapheresis (currently the recommended treatment) or corticosteroids, although their prognosis may not be as good as that of non-HIV-1-infected patients.[19]

Asymptomatic HIV-1 Infection of the Central Nervous System

Although clinically overt nervous system involvement may occur early in the course of HIV-1 infection, neurologically asymptomatic infection is more common. Studies of CSF in HIV-infected patients have shown (1) abnormalities in "routine" studies such as cell counts and protein and immunoglobulin measurements; (2) local, intra-blood-brain barrier synthesis of anti-HIV-1 antibody; and (3) isolation of virus.[1,30,36,37,55,78,79] These abnormalities have been noted in fully functional, asymptomatic patients who have remained well on follow-up for a year or more; they have a practical bearing on the interpretation of CSF findings in neurologic diagnosis. Physicians must take into account such "incidental" abnormalities in cell counts, protein and immunoglobulin levels, oligoclonal bands, and HIV-1 recovery when interpreting results of CSF studies performed for other diagnostic purposes or in monitoring therapy.

With respect to the biology of HIV-1, the CSF findings imply that nervous system involvement is a part of the ecology of the virus in the human host.

They indicate that HIV-1 can be relatively nonpathogenic for the CNS, which leads to the critical question of what causes the conversion of this asymptomatic state to aseptic meningitis or parenchymal encephalitis in some patients.[71,72,75]

LATE NERVOUS SYSTEM INVOLVEMENT BY HIV-1

In the late stages of HIV-1 infection, when immune defenses have been severely compromised and systemic complications have begun to appear, the nervous system becomes highly susceptible to a wide array of disorders involving all levels of the neuraxis: meninges, brain, spinal cord, peripheral nerve, and muscle.

Meningitis

Several disorders may involve the leptomeninges in patients with advanced HIV-1 disease (Table 12–2), with symptoms ranging from mild headache to severe disability with hydrocephalus and cranial nerve palsies. In addition, a number of conditions can mimic meningitis; for example, headache may initially be an important symptom in parenchymal brain diseases, such as toxoplasmosis and primary CNS lymphoma, or in non-neurologic disorders. We have been struck by the number of patients who were referred for evaluation of headache and soon showed signs of overt *Pneumocystis carinii* pneumonia, specific treatment of which ended the headache.

Among the true meningitides, a syndrome of aseptic meningitis may occur acutely at the time of seroconversion as described previously but is more common in advanced HIV-1 infection.[41,42,87] Hollander has divided the disorder into two types: an acute and a chronic form.[42] Both occur in the late phase of HIV-1 infection, usually in the setting of ARC or, less frequently, AIDS. Both are accompanied by meningeal symptoms, including headache, but meningeal signs are more characteristic of the acute form. Palsies affecting cranial nerves V, VII, and VIII may also complicate the course. Bell's palsy sometimes recurs. The CSF shows a mild mononuclear pleocytosis, usually with normal glucose and slightly elevated protein levels. The meningitis is presumed to result from direct HIV-1 infection of the meninges because the virus can be readily isolated from the CSF and because no other cause has been identified. Whether HIV-1 infection is the sole or even major cause of the disorder can be questioned, however, since other causes of aseptic meningitis might provoke an influx of HIV-1-infected lymphocytes and monocytes into the CSF, increasing the

TABLE 12–2. MENINGITIDES COMPLICATING HIV-1 INFECTION

Aseptic meningitis (HIV-1)
Cryptococcal meningitis
Tuberculous meningitis *(Mycobacterium tuberculosis)*
Syphilitic meningitis
Lymphomatous meningitis (metastatic)

likelihood of virus isolation. In addition, because of the high prevalence of mild abnormalities in the CSF of HIV-1-infected patients described earlier, this aseptic meningitis may be difficult to distinguish from another cause of headache that coexists with the asymptomatic CSF abnormalities discussed previously. Although the degree of pleocytosis might be used as a guide, presuming that the cellular reaction is involved in the genesis of symptoms, how should 5 to 20 cells/mm^3 in the CSF be interpreted? Further study is needed to clarify this issue. The syndrome is benign but may imply a poor prognosis because it signals impending progression to AIDS in some patients. Use of antiretroviral therapy for this disorder has not been reported.

The most important meningeal infection in AIDS patients is caused by *Cryptococcus neoformans.*[18,47] This usually presents as subacute meningitis or meningoencephalitis with headache, nausea, vomiting, and confusion, just as in non-AIDS patients. In some patients symptoms are remarkably mild and the CSF is close to normal, with few or no cells and little or no perturbation in glucose or protein levels (see Chapter 17).

Whether tuberculous meningitis in HIV-1-infected patients differs in clinical presentation, course, and response to therapy from the classic form in which subacute or chronic meningitis is manifest as headache, stiff neck, cranial nerve palsies, hydrocephalus, and vascular occlusions is not yet certain (see Chapter 19).

The extent to which underlying HIV-1 infection alters the presentation, clinical course, or response to therapy of CNS syphilis has not been defined precisely.[43] The previously discussed CSF abnormalities common in asymptomatic HIV-seropositive persons, including elevated protein levels and cell counts, make it harder to interpret such findings in patients with positive serologic tests for syphilis or those undergoing treatment. Given this state of knowledge, most clinicians favor overtreatment of newly diagnosed or previously untreated syphilis seropositivity (see Chapter 7).[53,60]

Systemic lymphoma complicating HIV-1 infection may secondarily spread to the CNS and primarily involve the meninges.[88] Clinical manifestations, if any are present, usually include cranial nerve palsies, headaches, or increased intracranial pressure (see Chapter 22).

TABLE 12–3. DIFFUSE BRAIN DISEASE COMPLICATING HIV-1 INFECTION

With Concomitant Depression of Alertness
    Metabolic encephalopathies (alone or as an exacerbating influence)
    Toxoplasmosis ("encephalitic" form)
    Cytomegalovirus encephalitis
    Herpes encephalitis
    Acute HIV-1 encephalitis
With Preservation of Consciousness
    AIDS dementia complex

Dementia and Diffuse Brain Disease

Involvement of the brain parenchyma in AIDS can be divided into conditions that cause predominantly focal symptoms and signs and those that cause more diffuse dysfunction (Table 12–3). Some of these disorders may overlap. For example, cerebral toxoplasmosis may have an "encephalitic," as well as the more common focal, presentation. However, this division is valuable as a first step in differential diagnosis. The nonfocal disorders can be subdivided into those causing parallel impairment of alertness and cognition, those with diffuse encephalopathy or delirium, and a disorder in which alertness is characteristically spared while cognition, motor function, and behavior are impaired, is the AIDS dementia complex.

Diffuse Encephalopathies

The diffuse encephalopathies include the metabolic or toxic encephalopathies developing in AIDS patients as sequelae of the systemic nonneurologic diseases, such as pneumonias with hypoxia and generalized sepsis. Similarly, various CNS-active drugs may cloud mentation or alertness just as in non-AIDS patients. These effects can occur alone but commonly exacerbate or unmask the AIDS dementia complex, resulting in a mixture of the two conditions. HIV-1-infected patients may also be more sensitive to neuroleptic agents, resulting in parkinsonian or other movement disorders as side effects at seemingly low doses.[40]

Certain brain infections may also produce diffuse brain dysfunction. CNS toxoplasmosis characteristically causes focal neurologic symptoms and signs but in some patients may appear as a generalized encephalopathy with clouding of consciousness and bilateral cerebral dysfunction.[63] This may be a particularly fulminating illness that is related to the presence of abundant *Toxoplasma* microabscesses, which may be poorly imaged by CT scan (see Chapter 16). CNS lymphoma may infiltrate deep structures and impair cognition and motor function without prominent focal symptoms or signs.

The clinical importance of CNS cytomegalovirus (CMV) infection has not been determined. Systemic CMV infection is of course common in

AIDS patients, and pathologic evidence of mild brain infection, marked by scattered microglial nodules with occasional characteristic intranuclear inclusion bodies, can be detected in the brains of perhaps one fourth of patients dying of AIDS (see Chapter 21).[61,67] However, clinicopathologic correlation suggests that CMV usually plays only a minor role in causing overt CNS dysfunction.[61] On the other hand, a small number of patients have more severe CMV encephalitis with subacute clouding of consciousness and in some cases seizures. The clinical diagnosis in such patients is difficult. In some the presence of ventricular ependymitis with local contrast enhancement detected by CT or magnetic resonance imaging may be helpful. CSF cultures are usually negative except in patients with radiculomyelitis (see later discussion).[59] The effect of ganciclovir or other anti-CMV therapy on the course of CMV encephalitis has not been adequately assessed. Encephalitis related to HSV-1 and HSV-2 also occurs in AIDS patients and may manifest itself as a subacute nonfocal encephalopathy.[49]

AIDS Dementia Complex

The AIDS dementia complex, characterized by a triad of cognitive, motor, and behavioral dysfunctions,[62,73,76] is probably the most common CNS complication of HIV-1 infection and will probably develop eventually in most AIDS patients to some extent. Characteristically it appears after the development of the major opportunistic infections or neoplasms that define systemic AIDS, although it sometimes occurs before major systemic complications.[14,64] However, results of recent larger cohort studies indicate that this syndrome is uncommon in patients who are systemically well.[45,56,85] On the other hand, once ARC develops, as many as one third of patients have equivocal or mild abnormalities on history or neuropsychologic testing.[45] Our clinical experience suggests that early in the course of systemic AIDS perhaps one third of patients exhibit mild dementia and another one fourth have a subclinical cognitive loss that can be documented by careful neurologic history and examination or neuropsychologic examination. In late AIDS as many as two thirds of patients exhibit mild to severe dementia and an additional one fourth have subclinical AIDS dementia complex.

Clinical Features.   Despite the presence of several terms for this syndrome, we prefer "AIDS dementia complex" because of the prominence of cognitive dysfunction in the disorder along with the frequency of motor and behavioral signs, which may predominate in some cases.[73,85] The clinical features of the AIDS dementia complex are briefly summarized in Table 12–4. Patients' earliest symptoms are usually difficulty with concentration and memory. Affected patients begin to lose their train of thought or conversations. Many complain of slowness in thinking. Complex tasks become more difficult and take longer to complete, and memory impairment or difficulty in concentration leads to missed appointments and the need to keep lists.

**TABLE 12–4. MAJOR CLINICAL MANIFESTATIONS
OF AIDS DEMENTIA COMPLEX**

	EARLY	LATE
Cognition	Inattention, reduced concentration, forgetfulness	Global dementia
Motor performance	Slowed movements, clumsiness, ataxia	Paraplegia
Behavior	Apathy, altered personality (agitation)	Mutism

Despite the complaints, results of bedside mental status tests may be within normal limits early in the evolution of the illness, although responses are characteristically slow. As the disease progresses, patients perform poorly on tasks requiring concentration and attention, such as word and digit reversals and serial 7's. With increasing severity, a larger array of mental status tests show abnormalities. Slowness of response remains prominent, and affected individuals may appear apathetic, with poor insight and indifference to their illness.

Symptoms of motor dysfunction usually lag behind intellectual impairment. Complaints include poor balance or coordination. Patients may drop things more frequently or become slower and less precise with normal hand activities, such as eating or writing. Gait incoordination may result in more frequent tripping or falling or a perceived need to walk more carefully. Even when other symptoms are lacking, motor abnormalities can almost always be detected on examination early in the course of the disease. These include slowing of rapid successive and alternating movements of the extremities and eyes. Abnormal reflexes may also be present, with generalized hyperreflexia and development of release signs such as snout, glabellar, and, less commonly, grasp responses. As the disease evolves, ataxia and subsequently leg weakness limit walking. Pathologic examination of patients with early or predominating spastic-ataxic gait usually shows vacuolar myelopathy (see the following discussion). Bladder and bowel incontinence is common in the late stages of the disease.

Psychologic depression is surprisingly uncommon in these patients, despite the prominence of psychomotor slowing. Patients appear uninterested and lack initiative, but without dysphoria. In a minority a more agitated organic psychosis is the initial or predominant aspect of the illness. Such patients are irritable and hyperactive and may become overtly manic.

In the end stage of the AIDS dementia complex, patients are nearly vegetative, lying in bed with a vacant stare, unable to ambulate, and incontinent. However, unless intercurrent illness develops, alertness is usually preserved.

In children the disorder has the same general features, although the course may vary somewhat and has either a progressive or a static form.[4,15,33]

The progressive form is characterized by the gradual loss of previously acquired motor skills in conjunction with the evolution of motor abnormalities ranging from spastic paraparesis to quadriplegia with pseudobulbar palsy and rigidity. Acquired microcephaly is almost universal.

AIDS Dementia Complex Staging.   For adult patients we have adopted a method of staging the severity of the AIDS dementia complex based on functional cognitive and motor status (Table 12–5).[72–74] We have found this to be useful in providing a common descriptive vocabulary for both clinical and investigative purposes.

Neuropsychologic Test Profile.   Formal neuropsychologic studies quantitatively support the clinical findings described previously and are helpful in establishing impairment and in serially following the course of disease or response to therapy. In general, the neuropsychologic tests most sensitive to AIDS dementia complex require some or all of the following: performance under time pressure, problem solving, visual scanning, visual-motor integration, motor speed, and alternation between two performance rules or stimulus sets.[90]

Neurodiagnostic Studies.   Neuroimaging procedures and CSF examination are essential to the evaluation of AIDS patients with CNS dysfunction. Although most often nonspecific, imaging results are useful as an adjunct to diagnosis of the AIDS dementia complex and, perhaps more important, are particularly helpful in excluding other neurologic conditions complicating AIDS. Neuroradiologic findings in the AIDS dementia com-

TABLE 12–5.   CLINICAL STAGING OF AIDS DEMENTIA COMPLEX

STAGE	CHARACTERISTICS
0 (normal)	Normal mental and motor function
0.5 (subclinical or equivocal)	Either minimal or equivocal *symptoms* or motor dysfunction characteristic of AIDS dementia complex (ADC), or mild signs (snout response, slowed extremity movements) but *without impairment of work or capacity to perform activities of daily living* (ADLs); gait and strength are normal
1 (mild)	Unequivocal evidence (symptoms, signs, neuropsychologic test performance) of functional intellectual or motor impairment characteristic of ADC but able to perform *all but the more demanding aspects of work or ADLs;* can walk without assistance
2 (moderate)	Cannot work or maintain the more demanding aspects of daily life, but able to perform *basic activities of self-care*; ambulatory but may require a single prop
3 (severe)	*Major intellectual incapacity* (cannot follow news or personal events, cannot sustain complex conversation, considerable slowing of all output) or *motor disability* (cannot walk unassisted but requires walker or personal support, usually with slowing and clumsiness of arms as well)
4 (end stage)	*Nearly vegetative*; intellectual and social comprehension and responses are at rudimentary level; nearly or absolutely mute; paraparetic or paraplegic with double incontinence

plex include the nearly universal finding of cerebral atrophy. Widened cortical sulci and enlarged ventricles are usually clearly evident by CT scanning or MRI.[62] Also, in some patients MRI shows patchy or diffuse T2-weighted abnormalities in the hemispheric white matter and, less commonly, the basal ganglia or thalamus. Children with AIDS-related dementia often have basal ganglia calcification and atrophy.[3]

Examination of the CSF in AIDS dementia complex reveals abnormalities in both routine and more specialized tests. However, routine analysis is confounded by the CSF abnormalities described earlier in patients with asymptomatic HIV-1 infection. This includes HIV-1 isolation from CSF.[38,50,66] On the other hand, the likelihood of detecting HIV-1 p24 core antigen in the CSF increases with AIDS dementia complex severity, although free antigen is still a relatively infrequent finding and thus of low sensitivity diagnostically.[66,70] More recently, we have found that the CSF concentrations of beta$_2$-microglobulin and neopterin correlate with both the severity of the AIDS dementia complex and its response to antiretroviral therapy.[7,8] Although these are nonspecific markers of immune activation, they may prove to have an ancillary role in diagnosis and assessment of therapeutic response.

Neuropathology. Histologic abnormalities in demented AIDS patients are most prominent in the subcortical structures and can be segregated into three seemingly discontinuous, but frequently overlapping, sets: gliosis and diffuse white matter pallor, multinucleated cell encephalitis, and vacuolar myelopathy; a less common additional finding is diffuse or focal spongiform change of the cerebral white matter.[61,72] The most common of these is the central astrocytosis and accompanying diffuse white matter pallor, which in isolation correlates with milder AIDS dementia complex. Inflammation is characteristically scant, consisting of a few perivascular lymphocytes and brown-pigmented macrophages accompanying the astrocytosis.

Multinucleated cells are characteristically found in patients with more severe clinical disease.[22,61] The multinucleated cells usually resemble macrophages and, indeed, are accompanied by neighboring macrophage and microglial reaction along with local edema and white matter rarefaction. They are most often concentrated in the white matter and deep gray structures.

Although inflammation with multinucleated cells may also be present in the spinal cord, in our experience a vacuolar myelopathy is more common.[61,68] The pathologic features of the latter resemble subacute combined degeneration resulting from vitamin B$_{12}$ deficiency, but levels of this vitamin are generally normal in serum. Although the incidence of vacuolar myelopathy is generally correlated with the other pathologic abnormalities found in the brain, the myelopathy can occur in the absence of the multinucleated cells. Our studies suggest that vacuolar myelopathy is independent of productive HIV-1 infection,[83] although others have suggested findings to the contrary.[29]

Etiology and Pathogenesis. Evidence from a growing number of studies supports a primary role for HIV-1 in the AIDS dementia complex, at least in a subset of patients.[24,32,35,38,72,82,84] There is also a growing consensus that macrophages and microglia, along with multinucleated cells derived from these two cell types, are the principal participants in productive infection.[34,35,46,57,77,89,92,93] Whether other cell types in the brain, including the native astrocytes, oligodendrocytes, or neurons, are also infected is less clear and requires further investigation. Cell culture studies have demonstrated low-level infection of astrocytic cells, perhaps involving a non-CD4 virus-cell interaction (see Chapter 2).[16]

Having said that HIV-1 can be found in the brains of demented individuals, we should emphasize that this is not an invariable finding. Our studies have shown that, in patients with subclinical or mild AIDS dementia complex (stage 0.5 or 1), the chief pathologic findings are astrocytosis and white matter pallor.[21] Even in some patients with more severe (stage 2 or 3) AIDS dementia complex, these are the sole histologic findings. As a rule, multinucleated cell encephalitis with histologically demonstrable HIV-1 infection is found only in the more severely affected patients (stage 2 or greater). Since HIV-1 infection is confined almost exclusively to brains with multinucleated cells, only this group of patients can justifiably be referred to as exhibiting HIV-1 encephalitis. As a consequence of the discrepancy between clinical deficit and both the pathologic and virologic features, indirect pathogenetic processes relating infection and brain injury have been proposed.[72,75] These processes may involve virus-coded toxins, such as gp120, or cell-coded toxins, particularly cytokines.

Treatment. Several studies have indicated that the AIDS dementia complex may respond to zidovudine.[69,83,94] Optimal dosages have not yet been established. More recently, preliminary reports suggest that the newer nucleoside analog, dideoxyinosine, may also have a salutary effect on this condition (see Chapter 8).[95]

Focal Brain Diseases

A number of focal brain disorders may affect AIDS patients (Table 12–6). Evaluation of these conditions begins with the recognition of their focal nature along with associated background systemic symptoms and signs (such as fever and headache). Investigations include neuroradiologic characterization and, often, a strategy involving therapeutic trial, followed in some patients by brain biopsy.

The temporal profile of the focal brain disorders is an important aspect of their clinical presentation. Abrupt onset suggests either a vascular cause

TABLE 12–6. FOCAL BRAIN DISEASE COMPLICATING HIV-1 INFECTION

Acute
   Vascular disorders
Subacute
   Cerebral toxoplasmosis
   Primary central nervous system lymphoma
   Progressive multifocal leukoencephalopathy
   Tuberculous brain abscess *(Mycobacterium tuberculosis)*
   Cryptococcoma
   Varicella-zoster virus encephalitis
   Herpes encephalitis

or seizure. AIDS patients may suffer transient ischemic attacks or even strokes leaving residual brain injury.[17,31] The pathogenesis is often unclear, but fortunately most have a benign outcome.

The most common focal disorders, however, characteristically have a subacute onset and evolve over days or sometimes weeks. Of these, cerebral toxoplasmosis characteristically progresses the most rapidly (days) and progressive multifocal leukoencephalopathy (PML) the most slowly (weeks). Primary CNS lymphoma lies somewhere between. All cause similar neurologic deficits, although there are usually differences in the associated findings. Thus the initial symptoms of toxoplasmosis are commonly a combination of focal deficit and generalized encephalopathy with confusion or clouding of consciousness.[63] This contrasts at least at onset, with PML, in which focal neurologic deficits are unaccompanied by either diffuse brain dysfunction or evidence of a systemic toxic state.[5,48] The CNS lymphomas, when accompanied by significant mass effect or when deep in the frontal or periventricular region, may cause more global mental dysfunction. Varicella-zoster virus (VZV) encephalitis may be focal and mimic PML[44] but has not yet been recognized ante mortem. HSV-1 or HSV-2 encephalitis, if focal, also tends to be associated with additional generalized impairment. Cryptococcoma is usually a complication of cryptococcal meningitis, but when it occurs alone, cryptococcal antigen may be absent from the CSF, making diagnosis difficult.[47]

In patients with focal disease, cerebral toxoplasmosis is the first diagnosis considered because of its frequency (5 to 15 percent of AIDS patients) and response to therapy (see Chapter 16). In evaluation of these patients neuroimaging techniques, particularly CT and more recently MRI, are critical both to confirm the presence of macroscopic focal disease and to determine the nature of the abnormalities. Multiple lesions involving the cortex or deep brain nuclei (thalamus, basal ganglia) surrounded by edema strongly favor cerebral toxoplasmosis. In most cases toxoplasmosis abscesses exhibit ringlike contrast enhancement on the CT scan, but homogeneous contrast enhancement or nonenhancing hypodense lesions may be noted. Double-dose contrast CT studies, or preferably MRI, may more clearly define the lesions or show additional spherical lesions characteristic of the disease. Only rarely is the CT scan normal.[63,65]

Cerebral lymphoma may produce a similar CT appearance, although the lesions of lymphoma commonly exhibit more diffuse or less clear-cut contrast enhancement, tend to be less numerous when seen radiologically, and are more often located in the white matter adjacent to the lateral ventricles. Primary CNS lymphomas of B cell origin are opportunistic neoplasms that complicate the course of AIDS in approximately 5 percent of patients, although this estimate includes lymphomas noted incidentally at autopsy.[67,88] If present, symptoms of primary brain lymphomas are progressive focal or multifocal neurologic deficits similar to those in toxoplasmosis, although the tempo of disease evolution is usually slower. Neuroradiologic studies are usually sensitive in detecting primary brain lymphomas but do not establish a definitive diagnosis. Characteristically these tumors are multicentric but usually only one or two lesions appear on the CT or MRI scan. Their location is characteristically deep in the brain surrounding the ventricles and most often in the white rather than gray matter. On CT scan they may be enhanced by contrast administration, but often such enhancement is weak or absent. MRI scanning is more sensitive. However, final diagnosis relies on brain biopsy.

In treatment of cerebral toxoplasmosis, and indeed in all AIDS patients, use of corticosteroids should be avoided when possible. This is particularly important when a therapeutic trial to differentiate between toxoplasmosis and CNS lymphoma is being considered. Since symptoms of the latter may respond to corticosteroids alone, clinical or CT improvement from a combination of antibiotic and steroid treatment is difficult to interpret. In addition, corticosteroids further impair immune defenses in AIDS patients, which could worsen not only toxoplasmosis but also other systemic opportunistic infections. However, if cerebral edema threatens to cause brain herniation, judicious short-term use of corticosteroids may be instituted along with appropriate specific therapy and subsequently tapered rapidly once the patient improves.

PML is an opportunistic infection caused by JC virus, a human papovavirus. The disease is characterized by selective white matter destruction.[5,48,80] Clinical evolution is usually more protracted than that of either toxoplasmosis or CNS lymphoma, and altered consciousness related to brain swelling is not a feature. Definitive diagnosis is made only on the basis of brain biopsy or autopsy, although suspicion is aroused by the clinical history and an examination suggesting more than one cerebral focus, along with a CT or MRI scan demonstrating white matter lesions, without mass effect and usually without contrast enhancement. No therapy has been proven effective for the disease. Spontaneous sustained remission of PML has recently been reported in two AIDS patients.[6]

VZV and, to a lesser extent, HSV-1 and HSV-2 have been reported to cause CNS disease in AIDS patients, although this is unusual. VZV infections are of three types: (1) multifocal direct brain infection affecting principally the white matter and partially mimicking PML,[44] (2) cerebral vasculitis that characteristically occurs in the setting of ophthalmic herpes zoster and causes contralateral hemiplegia,[27] and (3) myelopathy complicating herpes zoster.[26] Both HSV-1 and HSV-2 have been identified in the brains of some AIDS patients,[49] but the clinical correlates of these infections in AIDS patients have not yet been wholly delineated.

Myelopathies

Acute or subacute myelopathies are unusual complications of AIDS but include transverse myelitis related to herpes zoster [26] and spinal lymphomas (Table 12–7). In addition, severe CMV-related polyradiculopathy that progresses over a number of weeks may involve the spinal cord[58] (see the following discussion). Combined CMV and HSV infection of the spinal cord has also been described,[91] although antemortem recognition may be exceptionally difficult.

In our experience the more slowly progressive vacuolar myelopathy is far more common.[61,68] Usually it is accompanied by dementia, and it has therefore been included under the clinical term "AIDS dementia complex" discussed previously. It may occur in relative isolation or with marked preponderance. Patients exhibit progressive, painless gait disturbance with ataxia and spasticity. Bladder and bowel difficulty usually becomes significant only after considerable gait symptoms, whereas sensory disturbance is less conspicuous unless the patient has concomitant neuropathy. Patients do not have a distinct demarcation in the spinal cord level of sensory or motor impairment as in transverse myelopathy. Even in patients with seemingly isolated lower extremity symptoms, examination usually reveals some evidence of disturbance higher in the neuraxis. In typical instances we do not recommend myelography. Spinal MRI is useful in evaluating AIDS myelopathies, but thus far our attempts to detect vacuolar change by this method have been disappointing.

TABLE 12–7. MYELOPATHIES COMPLICATING HIV-1 INFECTION

Acute or Subacute
    Transverse myelitis
        Varicella-zoster virus (herpes zoster)
        Spinal epidural or intradural lymphoma
    With polyradiculopathy
        Cytomegalovirus
Subacute or Chronic, Progressive
    Vacuolar myelopathy
    HTLV-I-associated myelopathy

An additional cause of myelopathy in HIV-1-infected patients is coinfection with a second retrovirus, human T lymphotropic virus type I (HTLV-1).[10,81] This relates principally to the convergent epidemiologic pattern of these infections rather than to increased disease susceptibility resulting from immunosuppression. HTLV-I-associated myelopathy occurs principally in intravenous drug abusers.[10] The disorder is similar clinically to vacuolar myelopathy but can be distinguished by pathologic studies. Clinical diagnosis is suspected when the patient is HTLV-I seropositive. Specific diagnosis may prove to be important, since HTLV-I-associated myelopathy, at least in a patient without AIDS, may respond to immunosuppressive therapies, including plasmapheresis.[54]

Peripheral Neuropathies

Peripheral neuropathies of several types may complicate the various stages of HIV-1 infection (Table 12–8). Those occurring early in infection were discussed previously. Late neuropathies include herpes zoster and the ascending polyradiculopathy caused by CMV.[28,58] Diagnosis of the latter is aided by finding polymorphonuclear pleocytosis in the CSF. Thickened spinal roots viewed by myelography or MRI scanning have also been reported. Although CMV can be cultured from CSF of patients with these neuropathies, viral replication and the appearance of cytopathologic changes in culture take too long to rely on as a guide for the rapid institution of specific antiviral therapy.

Mononeuritis multiplex is unusual but has been described in ARC and AIDS; biopsy has shown axonal degeneration, sometimes with an accompanying segmental demyelination.[52] Inflammatory cells are present, but

TABLE 12–8. PERIPHERAL NEUROPATHIES COMPLICATING HIV-1 INFECTION

Early
    Mononeuritides, brachial plexopathy
    Acute demyelinating polyneuropathy
Latent Period
    Acute demyelinating polyneuropathy (Guillain-Barré)
    Chronic idiopathic demyelinating polyneuropathy
Late
    Mononeuritis multiplex
    Predominantly sensory polyneuropathy
    Autonomic neuropathy
    Cytomegalovirus-associated polyradiculopathy
    Herpes zoster
    Mononeuropathies associated with aseptic meningitis
    Mononeuropathies secondary to lymphomatous meningitis
    Toxic neuropathies (dideoxycytidine, dideoxyinosine)

evidence of a vasculitis in the form of vasonecrosis with or without fibrosis has thus far not been documented despite the suspicion that vascular involvement probably underlies the patchy distribution and abrupt onset of nerve dysfunction.

The most common neuropathy in AIDS patients is a distal, predominantly sensory and axonal neuropathy.[87] Characteristically, the sensory symptoms far exceed either sensory or motor dysfunction. The prevalence of this disorder has not been determined, but in mild form it is probably common. In some patients sensory symptoms such as "burning feet" resemble those in severe alcoholic or diabetic neuropathy. Even in patients with the severe form, sensory loss and motor weakness are usually mild, although the painful paresthesias and burning may prevent walking. The pathogenesis of this neuropathy is uncertain; the suspicion that it may be related to direct HIV-1 infection of nerve or dorsal root ganglion has not been confirmed. Anecdotal experience suggests that it does not generally respond to zidovudine. Treatment therefore relies on symptom management with tricyclic and analgesic agents.

The toxic axonal neuropathies caused by some of the newer antiretroviral nucleoside drugs, including dideoxyinosine and dideoxycytidine, are likely to be increasingly important in the next several years.[95] Their clinical features are similar to those of AIDS-related sensory polyneuropathy, with distal pain or paresthesias as the initial and predominant clinical feature. Patients with underlying neuropathies of other types may be particularly vulnerable to this complication.

Autonomic neuropathy has also been reported in AIDS patients.[21,51] Clinical features range from severe positional hypotension to cardiovascular collapse in patients undergoing invasive procedures such as lung biopsy.

Myopathies

Myopathies may also occur at several stages of HIV-1 infection but are less common and less well characterized than the neuropathies. A wide range of presentation is possible, from asymptomatic elevation of creatine kinase levels to progressive proximal weakness.[23,86] A polymyositis- or dermatomyositis-like illness has been described in AIDS patients, but as with the other myopathies, the pathogenesis is not clear. Viral antigens have been found in the inflammatory lymphoid cells but not in myocytes, and one report has identified multinucleated giant cells in the inflammatory infiltrate.[2]

Recent reports suggest that zidovudine may also cause myopathy. The clinical features have not been well delineated, but proximal muscles, especially of the legs, seem to be most affected, and the term "saggy butt syndrome" has caught the fancy of clinicians familiar with the condition.

SUMMARY

   The approach to diagnosis and management of the neurologic complications of HIV-1 infection and AIDS follows that used in general neurologic
practice. The differences are related to the altered disease probabilities in
a group of patients whose vulnerabilities to opportunistic and HIV-1-
related neurologic disease far overshadow the background incidence of
"ordinary" neurologic diseases. With the diagnosis of underlying HIV-1
infection and an understanding of its systemic stage, the neurologic history
establishes the temporal profile of the disease and usually makes a tentative
anatomic localization possible. The neurologic examination refines this localization and uncovers additional, including asymptomatic, abnormalities.
Neuroimaging studies using CT or MRI, and less commonly myelography
or angiography, add further precision to localization and narrow the range
of possible underlying pathologic processes. Electrodiagnosis using electroencephalography or evoked potentials may also be helpful in delineating
and localizing physiologic dysfunction. Nerve conduction studies and elec-
tromyography can similarly refine diagnosis of neuromuscular disease. CSF
examination provides a direct view of inflammatory reactions in the meninges and can be used to diagnose certain invading organisms or neoplasms. Therapeutic trial and brain biopsy may be needed for exact diagnosis in some instances. These evaluations, pursued with a background
understanding of the spectrum of neurologic disorders affecting HIV-1-
infected patients, allows accurate neurologic diagnosis in the great majority
of patients. As with other aspects of AIDS, this is an important exercise,
since an increasing number of these neurologic disorders can be treated
with gratifying relief of morbidity or prevention of death.

REFERENCES

   1. Appleman ME, Marshall DW, Brey RL, et al: Cerebrospinal fluid abnormalities in pa-
       tients without AIDS who are seropositive for the human immunodeficiency virus.
       J Infect Dis 158:193-199, 1988
   2. Bailey RO, Turok DI, Jaufmann BP, et al: Myositis and acquired immunodeficiency
       syndrome. Hum Pathol 18:749, 1987
   3. Belman AL, Lantos G, Horoupian D, et al: Calcification of the basal ganglia in infants
       and children. Neurology 36:1192, 1986
   4. Belman AL, Ultmann MH, Horoupian D, et al: Neurological complications in infants
       and children with acquired immune deficiency syndrome. Ann Neurol 18:560, 1985
   5. Berger JR, Kaszovitz B, Post JD, et al: Progressive multifocal leukoencephalopathy as-
       sociated with human immunodeficiency virus infection. Ann Intern Med 107:78, 1987
   6. Berger JR, Mucke L: Prolonged survival and partial recovery in AIDS-associated PML.
       Neurology 38:1060-1065, 1988
   7. Brew BJ, Bhalla RB, Fleischer M, et al: Cerebrospinal fluid beta-2 microglobulin in
       patients infected with human immunodeficiency virus type 1. Neurology 39:830-834,
       1989
   8. Brew BJ, Bhalla R, Schwartz M, et al: CSF neopterin in HIV-1 infection and as a function
       of AIDS dementia complex (ADC) severity (Abstract). Presented at the Fifth Inter-
       national Conference on AIDS, Montreal, Canada, June 5-9, 1989

9. Brew BJ, Cooper DA, Perdices MJ, et al: The neurological complications of HIV infection in the absence of significant immunodeficiency. Aust NZ J Med (in press)
10. Brew BJ, Hardy W, Zuckerman E, et al: AIDS-related vacuolar myelopathy is not associated with coinfection by HTLV-1. Ann Neurol 26:679-681, 1989
11. Brew BJ, Sidtis J, Petito CK, et al: The neurological complications of AIDS and human immunodeficiency virus infection. In Plum F (ed): Advances in Contemporary Neurology. Philadelphia, FA Davis Co, 1988, pp 1-49
12. Britton CB, Miller JR: Neurologic complications in acquired immunodeficiency syndrome (AIDS). Neurol Clin 2:315, 1984
13. Carne CA, Smith A, Elkington SG, et al: Acute encephalopathy coincident with seroconversion for anti-HTLV-III. Lancet 2:1206, 1985
14. Centers for Disease Control: Revision of the CDC surveillance case definition for acquired immunodeficiency syndrome. MMWR 36:1S-14S, 1987
15. Centers for Disease Control: Classification system for human immunodeficiency virus (HIV) infection in children under 13 years of age. MMWR 36:225-236, 1987
16. Cheng-Mayer C, Rutka JT, Rosenblum ML, et al: Human immunodeficiency virus can productively infect cultured human glial cells. Proc Natl Acad Sci USA 84:3526, 1987
17. Cho ES, Sharer LR, Peress NS, et al: Intimal proliferation of leptomeningeal arteries and brain infarcts in subjects with AIDS. J Neuropathol Exp Neurol 46:385, 1987
18. Chuck SL, Sande MA: Infections with *Cryptococcus neoformans* in the acquired immunodeficiency syndrome. N Engl J Med 321:794-799, 1989
19. Cornblath DR: Treatment of the neuromuscular complications of human immunodeficiency virus infection. Ann Neurol 23:588-591, 1988
20. Cornblath DR, McArthur JC, Kennedy PGE, et al: Inflammatory demyelinating peripheral neuropathies associated with human T-cell lymphotropic virus type III infection. Ann Neurol 21:32, 1986
21. Craddock C, Pasvol G, Bull R, et al: Cardiorespiratory arrest and autonomic neuropathy in AIDS. Lancet 2:16, 1987
22. Cronin KC, Rosenblum M, Brew BJ, et al: HIV-1 brain infection: Distribution of infection and clinical correlates (Abstract). Presented at the Fifth International Conference on AIDS, Montreal, Canada, June 5-9, 1989
23. Dalakas MC, Pezeshkpour GH, Gravell M, et al: Polymyositis associated with AIDS retrovirus. JAMA 256:2381, 1986
24. De La Monte SM, Ho DD, Schooley RT, et al: Subacute encephalomyelitis of AIDS and its relation to HTLV-III infection. Neurology 37:562-569, 1987
25. Denning DA, Anderson J, Rudge P, et al: Acute myelopathy associated with primary infection with human immunodeficiency virus. Br Med J 294:143, 1987
26. Devinsky O, Cho ES, Petito CK, et al: Herpes zoster myelitis (Abstract). Neurology 37(suppl 1):319, 1987
27. Eidelberg D, Sotrel A, Horoupian DS, et al: Thrombotic cerebral vasculopathy associated with herpes zoster. Ann Neurol 19:7-14, 1986
28. Eidelberg D, Sotrel A, Vogel H, et al: Progressive polyradiculopathy in acquired immune deficiency syndrome. Neurology 36:912, 1986
29. Eilbott DJ, Peress N, Burger H, et al: Human immunodeficiency virus type 1 in spinal cords of acquired immunodeficiency syndrome patients with myelopathy: Expression and replication in macrophages. Proc Natl Acad Sci USA 86:3337-3341, 1989
30. Elovaara I, Iivanainen M, Sirkka-Liisa V, et al: CSF protein and cellular profiles in various stages of HIV infection related to neurological manifestations. J Neurol Sci 78:331, 1987
31. Engstrom JW, Lowenstein DH, Bredesen DE: Cerebral infarctions and transient neurologic deficits associated with acquired immunodeficiency syndrome. Am J Med 86:528-532, 1989
32. Epstein LG, Sharer LR, Cho ES, et al: HTLV-III/LAV like retrovirus particles in the brains of patients with AIDS encephalopathy. AIDS Res 1:447, 1985
33. Epstein LG, Sharer LR, Joshi V, et al: Progressive encephalopathy in children with acquired immune deficiency syndrome. Ann Neurol 17:488, 1985
34. Gabuzda DH, Ho DD, De La Monte SM, et al: Immunohistochemical identification of HTLV-III antigen in brains of patients with AIDS. Ann Neurol 20:289, 1986

35. Gartner S, Markovits P, Markovits DM, et al: Virus isolation from an identification of HTLV-III/LAV producing cells in brain tissue from a patient with AIDS. JAMA 256:2365, 1986
36. Goudsmit J, deWolf F, Paul DA, et al: Expression of human immunodeficiency virus antigen (HIV-Ag) in serum and cerebrospinal fluid during acute and chronic infection. Lancet 2:177, 1986
37. Goudsmit J, Wolters EC, Bakker M, et al: Intrathecal synthesis of antibodies to HTLV-III in patients without AIDS or AIDS related complex. Br Med J 292:1231, 1986
38. Ho DD, Rota TR, Schooley RT, et al: Isolation of HTLV-III from cerebrospinal fluid and neural tissues of patients with neurologic syndromes related to the acquired immunodeficiency syndrome. N Engl J Med 313:1493, 1985
39. Ho DD, Sarngadharan MG, Resnick L, et al: Primary human T-lymphotropic virus type III infection. Ann Intern Med 103:880, 1985
40. Hollander H, Golden J, Mendelson T, et al: Extrapyramidal symptoms in AIDS patients given low dose metoclopromide or chlorpromazine. Lancet 2:1186, 1985
41. Hollander H, Levy JA: Neurologic abnormalities and recovery of human immunodeficiency virus from cerebrospinal fluid. Ann Intern Med 106:692-695,1987
42. Hollander H, Stringari S: Human immunodeficiency virus-associated meningitis: Clinical course and correlations. Am J Med 83:813, 1987
43. Hook EW III: AIDS commentary: Syphilis and HIV infection. J Infect Dis 160:530-534, 1989
44. Horten B, Price RW, Jimenez D: Multifocal varicella-zoster virus leukoencephalitis temporarily remote from herpes zoster. Ann Neurol 9:251-266, 1981
45. Janssen RS, Saykin AJ, Cannon L, et al: Neurological and neuropsychological manifestations of HIV-1 infection: Association with AIDS-related complex but not asymptomatic HIV-1 infection. Ann Neurol 26:592-600, 1989
46. Koenig S, Gendelman HE, Orenstein JM, et al: Detection of AIDS virus in macrophages in brain tissue from AIDS patients with encephalopathy. Science 233:1089, 1986
47. Kovacs JA, Kovacs AA, Polis M, et al: Cryptococcosis in the acquired immunodeficiency syndrome. Ann Intern Med 103:533-538, 1985
48. Krupp LB, Lipton RB, Swerdlow ML, et al: Progressive multifocal leukoencephalopathy: Clinical and radiographic features. Ann Neurol 17:344, 1985
49. Levy RL, Bredesen DE, Rosenblum ML: Neurological manifestations of the acquired immunodeficiency syndrome (AIDS): Experience at UCSF and review of the literature. J Neurosurg 62:475, 1985
50. Levy JA, Shimabukuro J, Hollander H, et al: Isolation of AIDS associated retroviruses from cerebrospinal fluid and brain of patients with neurological symptoms. Lancet 2:586, 1985
51. Lin-Greenberg A, Taneja-Uppal N: Dysautonomia and infection with the human immunodeficiency virus. Ann Intern Med 106:167, 1987
52. Lipkin WI, Parry G, Kiprov D, et al: Inflammatory neuropathy in homosexual men with lymphadenopathy. Neurology 35:1479, 1985
53. Lukehart S, Hook E, Baker-Znder S, et al: Invasion of the central nervous system by *Treponema pallidum:* Implications for diagnosis and treatment. Ann Intern Med 109:855-862, 1988
54. Matsuo H, Nakamura T, Tsujihata M, et al: Plasmapheresis in treatment of human T-lymphotropic virus type-I associated myelopathy. Lancet 2:1109-1113, 1989
55. McArthur JC, Cohen BA, Farzadegan H, et/al: Cerebrospinal fluid abnormalities in homosexual men with and without neuropsychiatric findings. Ann Neurol 23:534-537, 1988
56. McArthur JC, Cohen BA, Selnes OA, et al: Low prevalence of neurological and neuropsychological abnormalities in otherwise healthy HIV-1 infected individuals: Results from the multicenter AIDS cohort study. Ann Neurol 26:601-611, 1989
57. Michaels J, Price RW, Rosenblum MK: Microglia in the human immunodeficiency virus encephalitis of acquired immune deficiency syndrome: Proliferation, infection and fusion. Acta Neuropathol 76:373-379, 1988
58. Miller RG, Storey J, Greco C: Successful treatment of progressive polyradiculopathy in AIDS patients (Abstract). Neurology 39(suppl):271, 1989

59. Morgello S, Cho ES, Nielsen S, et al: Cytomegalovirus encephalitis in patients with acquired immunodeficiency syndrome. Hum Pathol 18:289, 1987
60. Musher DM: Editorial on syphilis in HIV: How much penicillin cures early syphilis? Ann Intern Med 109:849-851, 1988
61. Navia BA, Cho ES, Petito CK, et al: The AIDS dementia complex. II. Neuropathology. Ann Neurol 19:525, 1986
62. Navia BA, Jordan BD, Price RW: The AIDS dementia complex. I. Clinical features. Ann Neurol 19:517, 1986
63. Navia BA, Petito CK, Gold JWM, et al: Cerebral toxoplasmosis complicating the acquired immune deficiency syndrome: Clinical and neuropathological findings in 27 patients. Ann Neurol 19:224, 1986
64. Navia BA, Price RW: The acquired immunodeficiency syndrome dementia complex as the presenting or sole manifestation of human immunodeficiency virus infection. Arch Neurol 44:65, 1987
65. Nolla-Salas J, Ricart C, D'Olhaberriague L, et al: Hydrocephalus: An unusual CT presentation of cerebral toxoplasmosis in a patient with acquired immunodeficiency syndrome. Eur Neurol 27:130-132, 1987
66. Paul MO, Brew BJ, Khan A, et al: Detection of HIV-1 in cerebrospinal fluid (CSF): Correlation with presence and severity of the AIDS dementia complex (Abstract). Presented at the Fifth International Conference on AIDS, Montreal, Canada, June 5-9, 1989
67. Petito CK, Cho ES, Lemann W, et al: Neuropathology of acquired immunodeficiency syndrome (AIDS): An autopsy review. J Neuropathol Exp Neurol 45:635, 1986
68. Petito CK, Navia BA, Cho ES, et al: Vacuolar myelopathy pathologically resembling subacute combined degeneration in patients with acquired immunodeficiency syndrome (AIDS). N Engl J Med 312:874, 1985
69. Pizzo PA, Eddy J, Falloon J, et al: Effect of continuous intravenous infusion of zidovine (AZT) in children with symptomatic HIV infection. N Engl J Med 319:889-896, 1988
70. Portegies P, Epstein LG, Hung ST, et al: Human immunodeficiency virus type 1 antigen in cerebrospinal fluid: Correlation with clinical neurological status. Arch Neurol 46:261-264, 1989
71. Price RW, Brew B: Infection of the central nervous system by human immunodeficiency virus: Role of the immune system in pathogenesis. Ann NY Acad Sci 540:162-175, 1988
72. Price RW, Brew B, Sidtis J, et al: The brain in AIDS: Central nervous system HIV-1 infection and the AIDS dementia complex. Science 239:586-592, 1988
73. Price RW, Brew BJ: The AIDS dementia complex. J Infect Dis 158:1079-1083, 1988
74. Price RW, Brew BJ, Sidtis JJ, et al: A system for staging the AIDS dementia complex: Correlations with neurological and neuropsychological assessments (Abstract). Presented at the Fifth International Conference on AIDS, Montreal, Canada, June 5-9, 1989
75. Price RW, Brew BJ, Rosenblum M: The AIDS dementia complex and HIV-1 brain infection: A pathogenetic model of virus-immune interaction. In Waksman BH (ed): Immunologic Mechanisms in Neurologic and Psychiatric Disease. New York, Raven Press, 1990
76. Price RW, Sidtis JJ, Navia BA: AIDS dementia complex. In Rosenblum ML, Levy RM, Bredesen DE (eds): AIDS and the Nervous System, New York, Raven Press, 1988
77. Pumarola-Sune T, Navia BA, Cordon-Cardo C, et al: HIV antigen in the brains of patients with the AIDS dementia complex. Ann Neurol 21:490, 1987
78. Resnick L, Berger JR, Shapshak P, et al: Early penetration of the blood-brain-barrier by HIV. Neurology 38:9-14, 1988
79. Resnick L, DiMarzo-Veronese F, Schupbach J, et al: Intra-blood-brain-barrier synthesis of HTLV-III specific IgG in patients with neurologic symptoms associated with AIDS or AIDS-related complex. N Engl J Med 313:1498, 1985
80. Richardson EP: Progressive multifocal leukoencephalopathy. In Vinken PJ, Bruyn GW (eds): Handbook of Clinical Neurology, vol 9. Amsterdam, Elsevier, 1970, pp 485-499
81. Rosenblum MR, Brew BJ, Aronow HA, et al: Clinical-pathological features of HTLV-I associated myelopathy (HAM) in AIDS (Abstract). Presented at the Fifth International Conference on AIDS, Montreal, Canada, June 5-9, 1989

82. Rosenblum M, Scheck A, Cronin K, et al: Dissociation of AIDS related vacuolar myelopathy and productive HIV-1 infection of the spinal cord. Neurology 39:892-896, 1989
83. Schmitt FA, Bigleg JW, McKinnis R, et al: Neuropsychological outcome of azidothymidine (AZT) in the treatment of AIDS and AIDS-related complex: A double blind, placebo-controlled trial. N Engl J Med 319:1573-1578, 1988
84. Shaw GM, Harper ME, Hahn BH, et al: HTLV-III infection in brains of children and adults with AIDS encephalopathy. Science 227:177, 1985
85. Sidtis J, Price RW: Early HIV-1 infection and the AIDS dementia complex. Neurology (in press)
86. Simpson DM, Bender AN: Human immunodeficiency virus-associated myopathy: Analysis of 11 patients. Ann Neurol 24:79-84, 1988
87. Snider WD, Simpson DM, Nielsen S, et al: Neurological complications of acquired immune deficiency syndrome: Analysis of 50 patients. Ann Neurol 14:403, 1983
88. So YT, Beckstead JH, Davis RL: Primary central nervous system lymphoma in acquired immune deficiency syndrome: A clinical and pathological study. Ann Neurol 20:566, 1986
89. Stoler MH, Eskin TA, Benn S, et al: Human T cell lymphotropic virus type III infection of the central nervous system: A preliminary in situ analysis. JAMA 256:2360, 1986
90. Tross S, Price RW, Navia BA, et al: Neuropsychological characterization of the AIDS dementia complex: A preliminary report. AIDS 2:81-88, 1988
91. Tucker T, Dix RD, Katzen C, et al: Cytomegalovirus and herpes simplex virus ascending myelitis in a patient with acquired immune deficiency syndrome. Ann Neurol 18:74-79, 1985
92. Vazeux R, Brousse N, Jarry A, et al: AIDS subacute encephalitis: Identification of HIV-infected cells. Am J Pathol 126:403, 1987
93. Wiley CA, Schrier RD, Nelson JA, et al: Cellular localization of human immunodeficiency virus infection within the brains of acquired immune deficiency syndrome patients. Proc Natl Acad Sci USA 83:7089, 1986
94. Yarchoan R, Berg G, Brouwers P, et al: Response of human immunodeficiency virus associated neurological disease to 3'-azido-3'-deoxythymidine. Lancet 1:132, 1987
95. Yarchoan R, Mitsuya H, Thomas RV, et al: In vivo activity against HIV and favorable toxicity profile of 2',3'dideoxyinosine. Science 245:412-415, 1989

13

HEMATOLOGIC MANIFESTATIONS OF HIV INFECTION

JULIE HAMBLETON, MD
DONALD I. ABRAMS, MD

HIV infection is associated with a wide spectrum of hematologic abnormalities. Abnormalities may be found in all stages of HIV disease and involve the bone marrow, cellular elements of the peripheral blood, and coagulation pathways. The origin of these abnormalities involves many factors. A direct suppressive effect of HIV infection, ineffective hematopoiesis, infiltrative disease of the bone marrow, nutritional deficiencies, peripheral consumption secondary to splenomegaly or immune dysregulation, and drug effect all contribute to the variety of hematologic findings. Many of these abnormalities are clinically significant, whereas others may be more of academic interest. Specific abnormalities in the bone marrow, peripheral blood cell lines, and coagulation complex are reviewed here in turn.

BONE MARROW

Hematologic abnormalities are common in patients with HIV infection. Ineffective hematopoiesis has been described as resulting from direct suppression by HIV infection, infiltrative disease (whether of infectious or neoplastic origin), nutritional deficiencies, and drug effect.

HIV infection alone has been shown to suppress normal hematopoiesis.[6,23] Donahue et al isolated bone marrow progenitors from patients with AIDS and ARC.[6] They found that the progenitor cells responded to recombinant human granulocyte-macrophage colony–stimulating factor and recombinant erythropoietin. However, sera taken from patients with antibody to HIV suppressed the in vivo growth of these progenitor cells,

182

while not suppressing the in vivo growth of progenitor cells taken from HIV-seronegative control subjects.[6] These findings suggest that antibodies to an HIV-associated envelope glycoprotein actually contribute to the myelosuppression of HIV-infected cells. Moreover, in this study, the sera from patients with HIV infection and cytopenias did not reveal elevated levels of in vitro colony-stimulating factors or interleukin-1. This suggests that HIV-infected T lymphocyte and monocytes do not produce adequate amounts of cytokines, thus contributing to the cytopenias characteristic of HIV infection.

Morphologic Features

The morphologic features of bone marrow findings in patients with AIDS have been described.[1,5] Bone marrow biopsies are frequently performed to evaluate peripheral cytopenias or persistent fevers in AIDS patients. The majority of the patients demonstrate normocellular marrow elements. Investigators have reported an increased proportion of plasma cells, as well as lymphoid aggregates composed of benign-appearing, well-differentiated lymphoctyes.[1,5,23] These findings suggest B cell proliferation related to chronic antigenic stimulation or dysregulation secondary to HIV infection. Increased immunoglobulin production is also often noted.

The myeloid/erythroid cell ratio is generally normal in patients undergoing bone marrow biopsy. Reticulin fiber staining commonly reveals increased reticulin fibrosis. Abnormalities in maturation with dysmyelopoiesis, megaloblastosis, and hemophagocytosis have also been described, and myeloproliferative syndromes and leukemia have not been found to be more prevalent in AIDS patients.[1,23]

Infiltrative disease of the bone marrow commonly contributes to the hematologic abnormalities seen in AIDS patients. Infectious causes of infiltrative diseases include mycobacterial disease (both *Mycobacterium avium-intracellulare* and *M. tuberculosis*), fungal disease (*Histoplasma, Cryptococcus,* and *Coccidioides*), and rarely parasitic disease (*Pneumocystis* and *Leishmania*). Neoplastic infiltration is due primarily to lymphoma. Infiltration of the bone marrow by *M. avium-intracellulare* usually results in isolated anemia; infiltrative disease of other causes is typically manifest as pancytopenia.

Nutritional Effects

Nutritional deficiency has not been well documented as a direct cause of hematologic abnormalities. Disorders of iron metabolism or iron deficiency and occult vitamin B_{12} deficiency have been described. Folate deficiency, on the other hand, has not been noted to be more prevalent in this patient population.

Variable iron stores from increased to absent have been reported. The overwhelming majority of patients have ineffective incorporation of iron into the erythroid cell line, the so-called anemia of chronic disease. This leads to normal or increased iron stores noted on Prussion blue iron staining of the bone marrow biopsy. On the other hand, chronic blood loss from the gastrointestinal tract secondary to neoplastic infiltration or invasive infectious enteropathies may lead to iron deficiency. In a series of 201 bone marrow biopsies reviewed at San Francisco General Hospital, 75 percent of the patients had normal iron stores regardless of their hemoglobin level at time of biopsy.

Patients with AIDS have been found to have lower than normal serum vitamin B_{12} levels, which is thought to be secondary to altered vitamin B_{12} transport proteins[23] or to abnormal absorption of the vitamin. Given the extent of gastrointestinal dysfunction with chronic diarrhea in this patient population, vitamin B_{12} deficiency from occult malabsorption may contribute to the anemia commonly seen. Harriman et al described a cohort of 11 men with AIDS or asymptomatic HIV infection.[9] Eight of the 11 patients had an abnormal Schilling test after being given intrinsic factor and pancrease. Only three patients had low serum vitamin B_{12} levels. Duodenal biopsy specimens revealed chronic inflammation with mononuclear cell infiltration of the lamina propria. Specimens from five of six patients demonstrated HIV in the mononuclear cells.

Perhaps HIV enteropathy involving the terminal ileum where vitamin B_{12} absorption takes place contributes to subclinical malabsorption and occult deficiency. This may, in turn, contribute to the neurologic and hematologic abnormalities seen in HIV-related disease. Although these issues have not been fully explored, vitamin B_{12} levels should be followed periodically in patients with AIDS. This may be particularly important in patients being treated with zidovudine, since concomitant vitamin B_{12} deficiency may potentiate the drug-induced anemia.

Diagnostic Utility of Bone Marrow Biopsy

For the most part the marrow changes in HIV-infected patients appear to be nonspecific and offer the clinician little as a diagnostic or prognostic tool. In certain conditions, however, bone marrow aspiration, culture, and biopsy are indicated.

Patients with both non-Hodgkin's and Hodgkin's lymphoma in the setting of HIV infection are frequently found to have marrow involvement. Marrow examination is useful not only for staging but also to assess the myeloid reserves before initiation of cytotoxic therapy. Patients with thrombocytopenia in the absence of anemia or leukopenia warrant bone marrow evaluation to ensure an adequate level of megakaryocytes. In rare instances diagnoses other than immune thrombocytopenic purpura, such as acute leukemia, may be established.

Occasionally a patient has increased constitutional symptoms associated with anemia or other cytopenias, or both. In the absence of a revealing workup, bone marrow examination may be indicated to rule out lymphoma or underlying opportunistic infection. Kaposi's sarcoma does not characteristically appear in the bone marrow aspirate or biopsy specimen, but lymphomatous involvement may be found. Granulomatous disease with a positive acid-fast bacillus stain suggests M. avium-intracellulare and M. tuberculosis infection, although well-formed granulomas may not be apparent. In a review of 201 bone marrow aspirates and biopsies performed at San Francisco General Hospital, a new AIDS diagnosis was confirmed in fewer than 15 patients. The majority of new diagnoses were mycobacterial disease, primarily M. avium-intracellulare.

PERIPHERAL CELL LINES

Peripheral cytopenias are common in HIV-infected individuals and are due to either decreased production in the bone marrow or accelerated destruction in the peripheral circulation. In general, the cytopenias increase in frequency as HIV disease progresses. Zon and Groopman found anemia, granulocytopenia, and thrombocytopenia in 17, 8, and 13 percent, respectively, of asymptomatic HIV-infected individuals.[31] These percentages all increase with advancing HIV disease.

Erythrocytes

Review of the peripheral blood smear in patients with HIV infection often reveals nonspecific abnormalities. Anisopoikilocytosis, often with ovalocytes and rouleau formation, is a common finding.[28] Increased vacuolization of peripheral monocytes has also been described.[28] These changes are not fully understood. Splenomegaly may cause shearing of cells, and rouleau formation may reflect the hypergammaglobulinemia seen in these patients.

Anemia has been reported to occur in 66 to 85 percent of patients with documented AIDS.[23,31] In patients with persistent lymphadenopathy the development of anemia often antedates the evolution to overt AIDS.

Most AIDS patients with anemia have the anemia of chronic disease type. In such states, the reticuloendothelial system has adequate iron stores, but the inability to use this stored iron results in ineffective hematopoiesis with a normocytic, normochromic anemia.

Iron deficiency with a microcytic, hypochromic anemia may result from chronic blood loss. This loss may be due to Kaposi's sarcoma or lympho-matous involvement of the gastrointestinal tract. Thrombocytopenia with resultant occult bleeding may occasionally lead to iron deficiency.

Infiltrative disease of the bone marrow caused by *M. avium-intracellulare* is a common cause of isolated anemia, usually without concomitant dec-rement in the other cell lines. Some of the most profound anemias, with hemotocrit values in the 15 to 20 percent range, occur in patients with mycobacterial disease. Similarly, profound anemia may develop in patients with lymphoma, but often with concomitant cytopenias of the other cell lines.

Antibody-mediated peripheral consumption of red blood cells causes anemia but is not commonly seen in AIDS patients. McGinniss et al have described the presence of red blood cell autoantibodies in a cohort of patients with AIDS, ARC, and asymptomatic HIV infection. Forty-three percent of the AIDS patients in their study had a positive direct antiglobulin test (direct Coombs' test), and other antibodies against various red cell surface antigens were detected.[16] At San Francisco General Hospital it has been estimated that 20 percent of patients with HIV infection have a pos-itive direct antiglobulin test before their first red cell transfusion.[27] Despite the documentation of erythrocyte autoantibodies, however, frank hemolysis in this patient population is rare.

Marked anemia has been observed during treatment of AIDS oppor-tunistic infections. Various antibiotics and antiviral agents have been im-plicated. Dapsone, frequently used for treatment of *Pneumocystis carinii* pneumonia, may induce methemoglobinemia or hemolysis in a glucose 6-phosphate dehydrogenase–deficient individual. Zidovudine antiretro-viral therapy results in a transfusion-dependent anemia in approximately 20 percent of patients.[22]

Transfusion of packed red blood cells is indicated in patients with symp-tomatic anemia, regardless of the cause. At present no indication exists for use of irradiated packed cells. For a general approach to HIV-infected patients with anemia, refer to Table 13–1.

Leukocytes

HIV infection affects the lymphocyte, neutrophil, and macrophage-monocyte cell lines. The hallmark of HIV infection is the progressive de-pletion of CD4 + lymphocytes. Presumably this decrement occurs through direct viral invasion of the cells. Early in HIV infection an initial increase occurs in the CD8 + cell population before a decline in the CD4 + cells is noted. Infection of macrophages and monocytes and the triggering of an autoimmune response are two other mechanisms by which lymphocyte depletion may occur. Normally, activated T lymphocytes and monocytes produce cytokines or growth factors necessary for stem cell growth and

TABLE 13–1. SPECIAL CONSIDERATIONS IN THE APPROACH TO ANEMIA IN HIV-INFECTED PATIENTS

Microcytosis
Consider involvement of the gastrointestinal tract with Kaposi's sarcoma, lymphoma, or infectious enteropathy (especially cytomegalovirus colitis) with resultant iron deficiency secondary to chronic blood loss.

Macrocytosis
Consider:
Vitamin B_{12} or folate deficiency secondary to enteropathy with malabsorption
Hemolysis with reticulocytosis
   Drugs—dapsone, sulfa
   Autoimmune
   Thrombotic thrombocytopenic purpura, hemolytic uremic syndrome, or disseminated
     intravascular coagulation
Azidothymidine (AZT) drug therapy
If patient is receiving AZT therapy:
   Check erythropoietin level
   If <500 mU/dl, consider recombinant human erythropoietin therapy
   Evaluate vitamin B_{12} level and treat if low

Normocytic anemia
If hemoglobin level >10 g/dl, the patient exhibits no unexplained constitutional symptoms, and no other cell lines are involved, the most likely diagnosis is anemia of chronic disease secondary to HIV infection. Continued observation is advised.
If hemoglobin <10 g/dl, the patient exhibits unexplained constitutional symptoms, or other cell lines are involved, consider bone marrow infiltration.

DIFFERENTIAL DIAGNOSIS
Acid-fast bacillus (AFB): *Mycobacterium avium-intracellulare* or *M. tuberculosis*
Disseminated fungal disease
   Cryptococcosis
   Histoplasmosis
   Coccidioidomycosis
Lymphoma

EVALUATION
Blood culture for *M. avium-intracellulare* and fungus
Cryptococcal antigen testing
Giemsa stain of peripheral blood for histoplasmosis
Purified protein derivative (PPD) and *Coccidioides* skin testing
Tissue biopsy if clinically indicated
   Lymph node
   Liver
Bone marrow biopsy
   Plastic sections for neoplasms
   Special stains and culture for AFB and fungi

differentiation. HIV invasion of these cells decreases production of these cytokines.

Granulocytopenia independent of drugs is noted in approximately 50 percent of patients with AIDS. The most common cause is thought to be ineffective granulopoiesis; however, various investigators have also documented the presence of antineutrophilic antibodies as one cause of peripheral neutropenia.[6,14,15,17,23]

Defects in qualitative functions of the monocyte-macrophage and granulocyte lines have also been described. Defective polymorphonuclear leukocyte chemotaxis, deficient degranulating responses, inhibition of leukocyte migration, and ineffective killing have all been reported.[18,29] Monocytes also exhibit a marked reduction in chemotaxis in response to stimuli.

Drug-induced neutropenia is common in HIV-infected patients.[22] Medications used to treat such infections as *Pneumocystis carinii* pneumonia, toxoplasmosis, and cytomegaloviral retinitis or colitis cause neutropenia. Zidovudine also may cause neutropenia, often necessitating dose reduction or cessation of therapy.

Bacteremia does not develop in many patients with HIV-related immune neutropenia; it occurs more frequently in patients with drug-induced neutropenia. In a retrospective review of community-acquired bacteremia in patients with AIDS, 10 of 14 patients with neutropenia of varying causes had gram-positive isolates.[12] These findings suggest that antimicrobial therapy for febrile neutropenic patients with AIDS should include both gram-positive and gram-negative coverage.

HIV-Related Thrombocytopenia

Thromobocytopenia is the most common platelet abnormality in HIV-infected patients. In patients with HIV-related thrombocytopenia, platelet-associated immunoglobulin is present.[11,25] The presence of a specific autoantibody against the platelet membrane has also been found in non-thrombocytopenic patients with AIDS and ARC. Some researchers have postulated that patients who become thrombocytopenic in the setting of platelet-associated immunoglobulin G have the most unencumbered reticuloendothelial system. As patients become more ill, circulating immune complexes and hypergammaglobulinemia block the spleen's ability to remove antibody-coated platelets from the circulation. In thrombocytopenic patients observed at San Francisco General Hospital, the low platelet count spontaneously resolved as the patients' disease evolved to overt AIDS, supporting this hypothesis.[2]

Circulating immune complexes that precipitate on the platelet surface and lead to destruction via clearance by the reticuloendothelial system have been described.[11] Patients with HIV-related thrombocytopenia have far higher levels of circulating immune complexes that can be eluted from their platelets than do patients with non-HIV-related thrombocytopenia.

Most patients with HIV-related immune thrombocytopenia (ITP) have only minor submucosal bleeding characterized by petechiae, ecchymoses, and occasional epistaxis. Rare patients have gastrointestinal blood loss, but most patients do not have life-threatening bleeding episodes. Unlike patients with non-AIDS-related ITP, those with HIV-associated ITP may have mild splenomegaly, especially if generalized lymphadenopathy is present.

Laboratory tests generally reveal an isolated thrombocytopenia. Anemia and leukopenia are not usual accompanying features. Review of the peripheral blood smear shows a dearth of platelets, with occasional large forms. Bone marrow biopsy shows an increased number of megakaryocytes, typical of peripheral platelet consumption. The helper/suppressor T lymphocyte ratio is reversed. This is frequently the result of increased numbers of the CD8+ suppressor/cytotoxic lymphocytes with relatively well-preserved numbers of CD4+ cells.

Patients who have HIV-related thrombocytopenia when initially examined are at risk of overt AIDS by virtue of the underlying retroviral infection regardless of the therapeutic intervention for their thrombocytopenia. In a natural history study of patients at San Francisco General Hospital, the projected 5-year rate of development of overt AIDS was 50 percent.[2] Normalization of thrombocytopenia often antedates the development of AIDS, in much the same way as the disappearance of lymphadenopathy in patients with persistent generalized lymphadenopathy may be the harbinger for life-threatening disease. A group of New York University researchers has suggested that thrombocytopenia is an epiphenomenon that imparts no further prognostic significance than the presence of HIV antibody positivity itself.[11]

Management

In patients with HIV infection, thrombocytopenia may develop secondary to a therapeutic intervention. This includes antibiotics for treatment of an AIDS opportunistic infection or cytotoxic chemotherapeutic agents for HIV-related malignancies. In these situations severe thrombocytopenia should be managed as it is in non-HIV-infected individuals. Medications causing thrombocytopenia should be discontinued, and platelet transfusions should be administered when indicated.

Steroid therapy is the mainstay of treatment of thrombocytopenia in the non-HIV-infected patients with ITP. Its efficacy in patients with HIV-related ITP, however, is variable. Most patients do not maintain an improvement in their platelet count as steroid doses are tapered. The overall response to steroid therapy (prednisone 1 mg/kg/d) is good. However, with an attempt to taper the steroids, the platelet count often returns to baseline levels. The risk of further immune suppression in HIV-infected patients with steroid therapy is real. In a series of patients treated at San Francisco General Hospital, no cases of AIDS-related opportunistic infection or malignancy occurred as a direct consequence of steroid therapy. However, reactivation of minor opportunistic infections including herpes virus infections, oral candidiasis, and a central nervous system dysphoric syndrome commonly followed treatment.

Splenectomy has been a successful therapeutic intervention for patients who fail to respond to steroid therapy. At San Francisco General Hospital, 10 of 15 patients had complete responses following splenectomy.[24] Complications following surgery in patients with HIV-related thrombocytopenia in the absence of overt AIDS have been no more common than in non-HIV-infected persons.

Studies of zidovudine therapy in patients with ITP have shown promising results. The Swiss Group for Clinical Studies on AIDS performed a prospective, controlled, blinded, cross-over study of the effect of zidovudine on 10 HIV-seropositive patients with thrombocytopenia and no AIDS diagnosis. They found that platelet counts increased from a mean of 53,000 to 107,000 per liter while patients received zidovudine and that counts were not affected by placebo.[26] A group of French researchers also found an improvement in HIV-associated thrombocytopenia with the use of zidovudine.[20]

Numerous reports of the success of high-dose intravenous gammaglobulin (400 mg/kg/d for 5 days) have appeared in the literature.[21] These responses have been transient, lasting 2 to 3 weeks. The mechanism is thought to be transient blockade of the reticuloendothelial system. Consequently, platelets coated with immunoglobulin are not prioritized for clearance. Once the immunoglobulin load clears, thrombocytopenia ensues. The high cost and transient nature of the immunoglobulin therapy limit its use to situations in which acute bleeding is occurring or to preoperative intervention for patients undergoing splenectomy when elevation of the platelet count is necessary. Although platelet transfusions are generally contraindicated in patients with thrombocytopenia of immune origin, treatment with intravenous gammaglobulin before transfusion in emergency situations may ensure platelet elevation.

Early reports suggested that the nonandrogenizing testosterone danazol was efficacious in reversing HIV-related thrombocytopenia. No large-scale clinical trial has confirmed these early anecdotal impressions. Six patients treated at San Francisco General Hospital showed no reversal of their thrombocytopenia. Intravenous vincristine and plasmapheresis have anecdotally been reported to be effective in certain situations; however, their success rates do not warrant their use as a first-line approach.

Patients with isolated thrombocytopenia are generally the most healthy among the HIV-infected individuals. Clinical bleeding is minimal, and responses to therapeutic interventions have been suboptimal. Thus a viable alternative is to withhold therapeutic intervention and monitor the patient closely. However, zidovudine therapy may be initiated in patients with evidence of CD4+ lymphocyte depletion.

Thrombotic Thrombocytopenic Purpura

Several reports in the literature describe thrombotic thrombocytopenic purpura (TTP) in HIV-infected patients.[13,19] TTP is a relatively rare disease characterized by fever, neurologic abnormalities, renal abnormalities, purpura, microangiopathic hemolysis, and thrombocytopenia. The exact pathogenesis of this disease is unknown, but it seems to arise from vascular injury caused by immune complexes, endotoxin, or other causes of endothelial injury. The disorder has been associated with increased platelet agglutination and abnormally large, circulating von Willebrand factor complexes.

At present, it is unclear whether the occurrence of TTP in HIV-infected individuals is related to circulating immune complexes or to immunoglobulin dysregulation associated with HIV disease. As in the non-HIV-infected population, this disease has a high mortality rate, and therapy should be directed toward high-dose steroids, plasma transfusion, and plasmapheresis.

Coagulation Abnormalities

Patients with factor VIII and IX deficiencies have been greatly affected by the HIV epidemic. Because of the contamination of pooled factor replacement products, more than 50 percent of this population has undergone seroconversion. Unfortunately, the exorbitant price of many recombinant products leaves many patients at continued risk.

In a variety of disease states and situations, such as systemic lupus erythematosus, AIDS, intravenous drug use, taking of certain drugs (for example, chlorpromazine), and lymphoproliferative malignancies, a circulating inhibitor of coagulation may be noted. The lupus anticoagulant is thought to be an acquired immunoglobulin, either IgG or IgM, that interferes with phospholipid-dependent coagulation assays, prolonging the partial thromboplastin time (PTT). In general, the lupus anticoagulant is an in vitro phenomenon. Further laboratory testing has revealed abnormal results of a mixing study and an abnormal Russell viper venom time.[4]

Paradoxically, lupus anticoagulant is associated with increased thrombosis in non-HIV-infected individuals, but clinical significance has not yet been documented in the HIV-infected population. Its frequency has been noted to be greater during HIV-related infections, and it commonly disappears with treatment of the infection.[23,31] If a patient has a prolonged PTT with no history of bleeding, the lupus anticoagulant should be suspected. Invasive procedures may be performed in the presence of the lupus anticoagulant without increased bleeding diathesis.[4]

HEMATOLOGIC CONSEQUENCES OF ANTI-HIV THERAPY

Many therapeutic interventions contribute to HIV-related hematologic disorders. Zidovudine, a thymidine analog and the most widely used drug in the care of AIDS patients, greatly affects hematopoiesis. The primary action of zidovudine is termination of reverse-transcriptase DNA synthesis. It may also inhibit DNA polymerases to some extent, which then impairs normal hematopoiesis.[22,23] In a large-scale collaborative study, all three cell lines were shown to be affected by zidovudine therapy. Significant anemia developed in 34 percent of patients, and blood transfusions were required in 21 percent; neutropenia developed in 16 percent of patients; and thrombocytopenia developed in 12 percent.[22] Advanced HIV disease, preexisting cytopenias, and low vitamin B_{12} levels were associated with a greater risk of zidovudine-induced hematologic toxic effects. Although zidovudine increases the mean corpuscular volume in most patients, bone marrow examination usually reveals hypoplasia, aplasia, or maturation arrest.[7,22,23,30] Overt megaloblastic changes are not always noted.

In general, the myelosuppression seen with zidovudine therapy is reversed after the drug is discontinued,[22,30] but close observation with monitoring of blood counts is necessary. Ongoing trials are evaluating the efficacy of lower-dose zidovudine therapy, which would result in fewer side effects.

Other drugs used commonly in treating HIV infections also cause myelosuppression. These include ganciclovir (DHPG), foscarnet, sulfa derivatives used to treat toxoplasmosis or *Pneumocystis* infections, and pentamidine.

COLONY-STIMULATING FACTORS IN HIV DISEASE

Experience with colony-stimulating factors is in its infancy; however, their importance in the treatment of HIV-related cytopenias is increasing. In several trials neutropenic patients with AIDS have responded to granulocyte-macrophage colony–stimulating factor (GM-CSF) with a rapid increase in neutrophils and their precursors in conjunction with improved qualitative neutrophil functions.[3,8] Erythropoietin has also been administered to HIV-infected patients with anemia resulting from zidovudine therapy. The best response occurs in patients whose intrinsic erythropoietin levels are less than 500 mU/dl.[23]

Wide-scale clinical trials are being conducted to evaluate the use of GM-CSF and erythropoietin in conjunction with zidovudine therapy. The trials are aimed at limiting the hematologic toxicity of this drug. Ongoing studies are also evaluating the role of GM-CSF therapy in patients receiving chemotherapy for HIV-related malignancies. Certainly, progress in this arena will be forthcoming.

REFERENCES

1. Abrams D, Chinn E, Lewis B, et al: Hematologic manifestations in homosexual men with Kaposi's sarcoma. Am J Clin Pathol 81:13-18, 1984
2. Abrams D, Kiprov D, Goedert J: Antibodies to human T lymphotropic virus type III and development of the acquired immunodeficiency syndrome in homosexual men presenting with immune thrombocytopenia. Ann Intern Med 104:47-50, 1986
3. Baldwin C, Gasson J, Quan S, et al: Granulocyte-macrophage colony–stimulating factor enhances neutrophil function in acquired immunodeficiency syndrome patients. Proc Natl Acad Sci USA 85:2763-2766, 1988
4. Bloom E, Abrams D, Rodgers G: Lupus anticoagulant in the acquired immunodeficiency syndrome. JAMA 256:491-493, 1986
5. Castella A, Croxson T, Mildvan D, et al: The bone marrow in AIDS: A histologic, hematologic, and microbiologic study. Am J Clin Pathol 84:425-432, 1985
6. Donahue R, Johnson M, Zon L, et al: Suppression of in vitro haematopoiesis following human immunodeficiency virus infection. Nature 326:200-203, 1987
7. Gill P, Rarick M, Brynes R, et al: Azidothymidine associated with bone marrow failure in the acquired immunodeficiency syndrome. Ann Intern Med 107:502-505, 1987
8. Groopman J, Mitsuyasu R, DeLeo M, et al: Effect of recombinant human granulocyte-macrophage colony–stimulating factor on myelopoiesis in the acquired immunodeficiency syndrome. N Engl J Med 317:593-598, 1987
9. Harriman G, Smith P, Horne M, et al: Vitamin B_{12} malabsorption in patients with acquired immunodeficiency syndrome. Arch Intern Med 149:2039-2041, 1989
10. Hirsch M: Azidothymidine. J Infect Dis 157:427-431, 1988
11. Karpatkin S: Immunologic thrombocytopenic purpura in HIV: Seropositive homosexuals, narcotic addicts and hemophiliacs. Semin Hematol 25:219-229, 1988
12. Krumholz H, Sande M, and Lo B: Community-acquired bacteremia in patients with acquired immunodeficiency syndrome: Clinical presentation, bacteriology, and outcome. Am J Med 86:776-779, 1989
13. Leaf A, Laubenstein L, Raphael B, et al: Thrombotic thrombocytopenic purpura associated with human immunodeficiency virus type 1 infection. Ann Intern Med 109:194-197, 1988
14. Leiderman I, Greenberg M, Adelsberg B, et al: A glycoprotein inhibitor of in vitro granulopoiesis associated with AIDS. Blood 70:1267-1272, 1987
15. McCance-Katz E, Hoecker J, Vitale N: Severe neutropenia associated with anti-neutrophil antibody in a patient with acquired immunodeficiency syndrome–related complex. Pediatr Infect Dis J 6:417-418, 1987
16. McGinniss M, Macher A, Rook A, et al: Red cell autoantibodies in patients with acquired immune deficiency syndrome. Transfusion 26:405-409, 1986
17. Murphy M, Metcalfe P, Waters A, et al: Incidence and mechanism of neutropenia and thrombocytopenia in patients with human immunodeficiency virus infection. Br J Haematol 66:337-340, 1987
18. Murphy P, Lane C, Fauci A, et al: Impairment of neutrophil bactericidal capacity in patients with AIDS. J Infect Dis 158:627-630, 1988
19. Nair J, Bellevue R, Bertoni M, et al: Thrombotic thrombocytopenic purpura in patients with the acquired immunodeficiency syndrome-related complex. Ann Intern Med 109:209-212, 1988
20. Oksenhendler E, Bierling P, Ferchal F, et al: Zidovudine for thrombocytopenic purpura related to human immunodeficiency virus infection. Ann Intern Med 110:365-368, 1989
21. Perret B, Baumgartner C: Workshop on immunoglobulin therapy of lymphoproliferative syndromes, mainly AIDS-related complex, and AIDS. Vox Sang 52:1-14, 1986
22. Richman D, AZT Collaborative Working Group: The toxicity of azidothymidine in the treatment of patients with AIDS and AIDS-related complex. N Engl J Med 317:192-197, 1987
23. Scadden DT, Zon LI, Groopman JE: Pathophysiology and management of HIV-associated hematologic disorders. Blood 74:1455-1463, 1989

24. Schneider P, Abrams D, Rayner A, et al: Immunodeficiency-associated thrombocytopenic purpura: Response to splenectomy. Arch Surg 122:1175-1178, 1987
25. Stricker R, Abrams D, Corash L, et al: Target platelet antigen in homosexual men with immune thrombocytopenia. N Engl J Med 313:1375-1380, 1985
26. Swiss Group for Clinical Studies on AIDS: Zidovudine for the treatment of thrombocytopenia associated with human immunodeficiency virus. Ann Intern Med 109:718-721, 1988
27. Toy P, Reid M, Burns M: Positive direct antiglobulin test associated with hyperglobulinemia in acquired immunodeficiency syndrome. Am J Hematol 19:145, 1985
28. Treacy M, Lai L, Costello C, et al: Peripheral blood and bone marrow abnormalities in patients with HIV related disease. Br J Haematol 65:289-294, 1987
29. Valone F, Payan D, Abrams D, et al: Defective polymorphonuclear leukocyte chemotaxis in homosexual men with persistent lymph node syndrome. J Infect Dis 150:267-271, 1984
30. Walker R, Parker R, Kovacs J, et al: Anemia and erythropoiesis in patients with the acquired immunodeficiency syndrome and Kaposi sarcoma treated with zidovudine. Ann Intern Med 108:372-376, 1988
31. Zon L, Groopman J: Hematologic manifestations of the human immune deficiency virus. Semin Hematol 25:208-218, 1988

14

CARDIAC, ENDOCRINE, AND RENAL COMPLICATIONS OF HIV INFECTION

JOHN D. STANSELL, MD

During the early years of the AIDS epidemic, clinicians viewed pulmonary, gastrointestinal, hematologic, and neurologic dysfunction as the principal, if not exclusive, manifestations of HIV infection. As experience with HIV infection broadened, the pace of the epidemic increased, and longevity improved because of more effective treatment and prophylaxis of opportunistic infections, it became clear that no organ system eludes the ravages of HIV. This chapter focuses on the cardiac, endocrine, and renal manifestations of HIV disease. Although these manifestations still play a minor role in the clinical course of most HIV-infected patients, clinicians will probably encounter abnormalities of these organ systems as the AIDS epidemic evolves.

CARDIAC DISEASE

Many autopsy studies have documented cardiac involvement in AIDS and ARC.[2,9,21,30,52] These studies, however, differ widely on the prevalence of cardiac disease and the type of cardiac lesion. Early in the epidemic, Welsh et al described 11 of 36 patients (31 percent) with cardiac lesions at necropsy.[52] Similarly, Cammarosano and Lewis found cardiac disease in 10 of 41 patients (25 percent) dying of AIDS.[9] Fink et al described a 73 percent prevalence of cardiac disease in a small series of AIDS patients. Moreover, Fink et al were among the first to note the asymptomatic nature of these

195

cardiac abnormalities.[21] More recently, Anderson et al retrospectively evaluated 71 consecutive necropsy patients who died of AIDS between 1982 and 1986; 52 percent demonstrated evidence of cardiac disease.[2]

Findings in the preceding studies included myocarditis, pericarditis, pericardial effusion, ventricular dilatation, nonbacterial thrombotic endocarditis, metastatic Kaposi's sarcoma, and lymphoma.

Myocarditis

Several observers have noted a high incidence of myocarditis in autopsy findings of AIDS patients.[2,35] In general, histologic findings include nonspecific interstitial inflammatory infiltrates or interstitial edema. Myocyte necrosis is uncommon. Lafort et al reviewed 137 consecutive autopsies of AIDS patients and found 56 (41 percent) with myocarditis.[35] Anderson et al described similar changes in 52 percent of 71 patients.[2] However, only a small percentage of patients with histologic evidence of myocarditis demonstrated signs of ventricular dysfunction before death.

Significantly, myocarditis was not associated with any one or combination of possible etiologic organisms. Opportunistic organisms most frequently encountered include *Cryptococcus*,[9,35,36] *Toxoplasma*,[35,39] and *Mycobacterium*.[2] More important, the large majority of cases show no specific organism. Thus the etiology of myocarditis in most cases remains unclear.

In the absence of demonstrable organisms, known toxic exposures, or hypersensitivity, Anderson et al suggest that most patients with AIDS and myocarditis have disease with the histologic characteristics of viral infection.[2]

The list of *viral* causes of myocarditis in AIDS patients is long. Cytomegalovirus, (CMV), coxsackie B virus, and HIV itself have received close attention. Most AIDS patients are infected with CMV. Myocardial tissue, however, rarely shows evidence of CMV inclusions.[9] In short, there is no demonstrated cause-and-effect relationship between CMV and myocardial inflammation. Coxsackie A and B viruses most commonly cause myocarditis in the United States,[10] and Dittrick et al found rising coxsackie B virus titers in an AIDS patient dying of refractory congestive heart failure.[19] Finally, HIV itself may damage myocardium either by direct cytolytic infection or by "innocent bystander destruction." Although several investigators have grown HIV in cultures of myocardial biopsy specimens, direct evidence of myocyte infection using DNA hybridization or immunocytochemical techniques is lacking. The "innocent bystander" theory, as proposed by Ho et al,[29] suggests that HIV replication in lymphocytes or macrophages releases enzymes or lymphokines toxic to surrounding myocytes.

No series as yet have defined optimal workup and treatment of AIDS-related myocarditis. The roles of myocardial biopsy, immunosuppressive therapy, and antiviral therapy remain undefined.

Dilated Cardiomyopathy

Investigators have not described isolated right ventricular hypertrophy outside a setting of significant pulmonary disease. Predictably pulmonary vascular compromise from severe or recurrent infection gives rise to pulmonary hypertension and resulting right ventricular failure.

Many case reports document congestive cardiomyopathy in AIDS.[8,12,15,33] The pathologic hallmark of these cases is biventricular dilatation. Anderson et al found pathologic features of myocarditis present in all such cases.[2] Thus they postulate that a congestive cardiomyopathy is the end result of viral infection. Evidence from non-AIDS-associated cardiomyopathy supports this hypothesis. Biopsy specimens from patients with non-AIDS myocarditis and dilated cardiomyopathy have exhibited high antiviral titers against coxsackie B virus and virus-specific RNA sequences. As previously discussed, culture studies have found HIV in endomyocardial biopsy specimens from patients with congestive cardiomyopathy.[8,19] Speculation arises, however, about the inevitable contamination of myocardial tissue with mononuclear cells. At this writing, neither electron microscopy nor sensitive DNA probes have demonstrated virus or viral DNA in myocytes themselves.

Nutritional deficiency, cardiotoxins, and immunologic mechanisms, in addition to infection, can cause dilated cardiomyopathy. Although marked cellular and humoral immune dysfunction define AIDS, no convincing evidence has emerged implicating autoimmune mechanisms in AIDS-associated heart disease. Similarly, wasting syndrome and cachexia are common manifestations of advanced HIV disease, but investigators have failed to show a clear cause-and-effect association between protein-calorie malnutrition, vitamin or trace element deficiency, and AIDS-associated cardiomyopathy. A recent report by Kavanaugh-McHugh presented evidence of decreased ejection fraction or ventricular dilatation in four of five pediatric AIDS patients with selenium deficiency.[34] Clarification of the role of nutritional deficiency in AIDS cardiomyopathy awaits further study.

Drug toxicity is a well-documented source of myocardial damage. Physicians frequently prescribe drugs from several categories in the treatment of patients with HIV disease: anti-infectives, including antifungal and antiviral agents; immune modulators; and chemotherapeutic agents. Although AIDS patients have a high incidence of drug-related adverse reactions, drugs commonly used in treating opportunistic infections have not shown significant cardiotoxicity. Similarly, the known cardiotoxins cyclophosphamide, adriamycin, bleomycin, and vinca alkaloids are prominently used in treatment of AIDS-related non-Hodgkin's lymphoma and Kaposi's sarcoma. Investigators, however, describe no increased incidence of toxic effects on the heart (L. Kaplan, personal communication). While experience with antiviral agents (such as acyclovir and ganciclovir) is rapidly accumulating, research has not revealed significant cardiotoxicity. Despite widespread use of zidovudine since 1987, investigators have not reported major cardiac complications (P. Volberding, personal communication). Similarly, in stages 1 and 2 of clinical testing, dideoxycytidine (DDC) and dideoxyinosine (DDI) have not shown significant cardiac side effects (T. Merigan, personal communication).

In contrast, Deyton et al recently described three patients with AIDS and Kaposi's sarcoma who had reversible cardiac dysfunction in association with interferon alfa therapy.[18] Endomyocardial biopsy studies of one patient did not show any inflammatory infiltrate. In all three patients cardiac motion and contractility improved after interferon was withdrawn.

Clinical presentation of AIDS-associated dilated cardiomyopathy is similar to that of dilated cardiomyopathy of any cause. Providers should evaluate by echocardiogram or multiple gated acquisition (MUGA) scan any AIDS patient with progressive breathlessness, edema, auscultatory findings of congestive heart failure, or increased cardiac silhouette on chest roentgenogram. The mainstays of therapy continue to be afterload reduction, diuretics, and perhaps digoxin.

Endocarditis

Autopsies of AIDS patients frequently reveal nonbacterial, thrombotic (marantic) endocarditis. Lesions, found frequently in chronically ill patients and particularly in patients with malignancy, consist of sterile thrombi. These lesions may be located on any valve and may embolize systemically.[9]

Early evidence suggests that HIV-seropositive persons may have increased skin and nasopharyngeal carriage of *Staphylococcus aureus*. Furthermore, preliminary evidence suggests an increased incidence of staphylococcal endocarditis among HIV-seropositive intravenous drug users. However, HIV-seropositive patients with endocarditis display no altered therapeutic response to antibiotics (H. Chambers, personal communication). Opportunistic organisms have not proved to be a major cause of endocarditis in AIDS patients, although a few case reports exist.[27,39]

Pericardial Disease

Early reports confirmed pericardial effusion, including tamponade, a major cardiac manifestation of AIDS.[9,21] Although most of these effusions are sterile,[9,39] specific organisms associated with pericarditis and effusion include *Mycobacterium tuberculosis*,[39] *Mycobacterium avium* complex,[39] and *Cryptococcus*.[9] Since most patients with pericarditis have myocardial inflammation,[1] clinicians should become familiar with this AIDS complication and early pericardiocentesis.

Malignancy

Early in the AIDS epidemic 15 percent of patients were found to have Kaposi's sarcoma. Although Kaposi's sarcoma remains the most common malignancy in AIDS, its incidence has decreased over the ensuing years.

Kaposi's sarcoma shows a tendency to metastasize widely to the skin, mucosa, lung, lymph nodes, and gastrointestinal tract. Several investigators have described myocardial or pericardial infiltration with the malignancy.[8,49] Silver et al found cardiac involvement in 5 of 18 patients (28 percent) with widely disseminated disease.[49] All were clinically silent before the patients' deaths.

As the incidence of Kaposi's sarcoma declines, the incidence of lymphoma rises. Most of the lymphomas are high-grade B-cell lymphomas presenting as stage IV disease. Although cardiac involvement usually indicates widely metastatic disease, investigators have described primary cardiac lymphoma.[14]

Conclusion

Autopsy studies clearly document a high incidence of cardiac disease among patients dying of AIDS. Yet, despite more than 100,000 AIDS cases in the United States alone, cardiac complications have only rarely played a major role in AIDS patient management. The clinically silent nature of cardiac involvement in AIDS must give way to a heightened awareness of possible cardiac sources of morbidity and mortality. As the prognosis improves, we are likely to encounter cardiac manifestations of HIV disease more frequently.

ENDOCRINE DISEASE

Autopsy studies of AIDS patients have documented diffuse endocrine disease, usually involving opportunistic organisms or neoplasia.[30,52] Mounting evidence suggests significant morbidity with HIV-associated endocrine dysfunction, initially thought to be clinically slient.

Pituitary Gland

Sano et al recently reviewed pituitary morphology in autopsies of 49 AIDS patients.[47] Six patients (12 percent) demonstrated direct infectious involvement of the anterior pituitary gland: five with CMV and one with *Pneumocystis carinii* pneumonia. In addition the authors noted two cases (4 percent) of posterior pituitary infection. Significantly, infection was not associated with an inflammatory response. Moreover, adenomas and nodular hyperplasia were similar to those in age-matched control subjects. Functional pituitary insufficiency was uncommon. Membreno et al describe four AIDS patients with adrenal insufficiency and low levels of adrenocorticotropic hormone (ACTH).[38] The authors (see following discussion) postulated possible pituitary lesions in AIDS based on their findings and blunted 17-deoxysteroid response to sustained ACTH. Similarly, inappropriately low gonadotropin levels in conjunction with a low testosterone level led Dobs et al to suggest a hypothalamic-pituitary abnormality in AIDS.[20]

Thyroid Gland

Thyroid function abnormalities in chronic illness are common and well documented. This pattern usually presents as a fall in triiodothyronine (T_3) and a reciprocal rise in reverse T_3 (rT_3). Circulating thyroxine (T_4) and thyroid-stimulating hormone levels usually remain normal. Two recent reports suggest a uniquely different pattern in HIV-related illness. Dobs et al reported surprisingly normal thyroid function in 70 men with HIV seropositivity, ARC, or AIDS.[20] More recently Lo Presti et al presented intriguing evidence suggesting AIDS and ARC patients have high levels of T_3, T_4, and thyroid-binding globulin and low levels of rT_3.[37] The rise in thyroid-binding globulin appeared to parallel the advance in HIV infection. The authors speculated that immune dysfunction removed a physiologic check on thyroid hormone metabolism. Sato et al further speculated that failure to down-regulate enzymes responsible for conversion of T_4 to T_3 might contribute to the wasting seen in end-stage HIV illness. They suggested that this failure to down-regulate might be secondary to HIV-related cytokine dysregulation. Corroboration awaits further study.

Adrenal Gland

Autopsy studies have consistently found the adrenal gland the most commonly affected endocrine gland in AIDS. Glasgow et al surveyed 41 autopsies for evidence of adrenal disease.[23] Findings included lipid depletion typical of chronic illness, infection with *Cryptococcus* and *Mycobacterium*, and infiltration with Kaposi's sarcoma. Most important, CMV adrenalitis, characterized by intranuclear and cytoplasmic inclusions, was the most common infection of the adrenal gland, occurring in 51 percent of cases. No patient had necrosis involving more than 70 percent of the adrenal gland, and most had less than 50 percent necrosis. Although 32 of the 41 patients showed nonspecific antemortem findings consistent with hypocortisolism, only one patient had documented partial adrenal insufficiency. None had hyperpigmentation. Adrenal function is usually not impaired until 80 to 90 percent of glandular tissue is compromised. Although pathologic involvement of the adrenal gland in AIDS is common, clinical adrenal insufficiency is not.

Multiple reports chronicle isolated clinical adrenal insufficiency since the beginning of the HIV epidemic.[24–26,51] In a small series Hilton et al found normal cortisol response to rapid ACTH stimulation in AIDS and ARC patients.[28] Dobs et al similarly found a normal cortisol rise to rapid cosyntropin testing in 92 percent of HIV-infected men.[20] The 8 percent with blunted responses had no clinical symptoms of hypocortisolism. In the largest study of its kind, Membreno et al examined adrenal response and reserve in 93 HIV-infected men (74 AIDS patients and 19 ARC patients) compared with 25 normal control subjects.[38] AIDS patients showed elevated basal cortisol levels compared with unstressed control subjects. Cosyntropin testing revealed that 86 percent of AIDS patients have cortisol levels within 2 standard deviations of mean normal value, but only 48 percent within 1 standard deviation. Although basal 17-deoxysteroid (corticosterone, deoxycorticosterone, 18-hydroxydeoxycorticosterone) levels were normal, they failed to rise normally in response to rapid ACTH administration. ACTH infusion for 3 days confirmed the depressed 17-deoxysteroid response but demonstrated a rise in cortisol to normal levels. The plasma ACTH level at 8 AM was normal in 19 AIDS patients. ARC patients showed basal plasma cortisol levels similar to those of control subjects. The 19 patients with ARC, however, responded to consyntropin testing with subnormal rises in cortisol, similar to AIDS patients. In contrast, ARC patients responded to prolonged ACTH stimulation with normal rises in cortisol and 17-deoxysteroid levels. Zona glomerulosa function was normal in AIDS and ARC patients. These data suggest that AIDS patients have limited adrenal capacity to respond to stress. Membreno et al[38] and Biglieri[5] recommended 3-day ACTH stimulation for patients who fail to achieve a plasma cortisol level of 685 nmol/L after consyntropin administration. Patients who fail to achieve 994 nmol/L after 3-day ACTH infusion should be considered to have partial adrenal insufficiency and should be treated with steroids at times of stress. Biglieri suggests that measurement of 17-deoxysteroid levels after acute ACTH stimulation might be of value in identifying patients with incipient adrenal abnormality.[5] Again, confirmation awaits further study.

Clouding the issue of adrenal function in AIDS and ARC is the frequent use of drugs that affect steroidogenesis and steroid metabolism. Ketoconazole, a frequently used antifungal agent, interferes with glucocorticoid, mineralocorticoid, and sex hormone production (see Chapter 17). Rifampin, widely used in treating mycobacterial disease, is a powerful inducer of hepatic enzymes that metabolize steroids. In the face of a limited ability to increase steroid production, either drug may precipitate clinical adrenal insufficiency.

Pancreas

Pathologic changes in the pancreas mirror those found in other endocrine tissue. Abnormalities in carbohydrate metabolism most frequently result from administration of pentamidine for *P. carinii* pneumonia (see Chapter 15). Pentamidine is directly toxic to pancreatic islet cells, producing hypoglycemia by the aberrant release of insulin from injured cells. If injury is sufficiently severe or sustained, type I diabetes mellitus and hyperglycemia may develop.

Testes

Histologic testicular abnormalities are common in AIDS patients, usually in combination with markedly decreased or absent spermatogenesis. Several studies have documented low testosterone levels in AIDS and ARC patients in association with high levels of luteinizing hormone or follicle-stimulating hormone and normal gonadotropin response to releasing factors.[16,20] These data suggest a pattern of primary testicular failure in AIDS and probably account for the decreased libido and impotence. As discussed previously, ketoconazole is a powerful inhibitor of androgen production in the testes. In addition, ketoconazole displaces testosterone from sex hormone–binding globulin. Gynecomastia may result.

RENAL DISEASE

Throughout the course of their illness, AIDS patients are at high risk for renal complications. Systemic infection, sepsis, dehydration, hypoxia and nephrotoxic drugs (Table 14–1) combine to disturb renal function. Emerging from this background of renal injury, however, is evidence of an HIV disease-specific nephropathy.[6,22,31,44] In 1984 Rao et al reported a series of 11 AIDS patients with proteinuria or azotemia at initial examination.[44] Nine of 11 AIDS patients rapidly progressed to end-stage renal disease. Renal histologic examination revealed focal and segmental glo-

**TABLE 14–1.   NEPHROTOXIC DRUGS COMMONLY USED
IN AIDS PATIENTS**

Commonly Nephrotoxic
Amphotericin B
Pentamidine
Foscarnet
Aminoglycosides
Radiocontrast dyes
Potentially Nephrotoxic
Trimethoprim-sulfamethoxazole
Pyrimethamine-sulfadiazine
Rifampin
Acyclovir
Nonsteroidal anti-inflammatory drugs
Dapsone

merulosclerosis with intraglomerular deposition of immunoglobulin M and C3 in 10 of 11 cases.

Subsequent studies identified focal segmental glomerulosclerosis (FSGS) and mesangial hyperplasia as the glomerular lesions commonly associated with AIDS. FSGS, however, is not specific to AIDS, since 20 percent of patients with adult idiopathic nephrotic syndrome and patients with heroin nephropathy also show evidence of FSGS. The association of heroin nephropathy with FSGS raises the question of whether intravenous drug use predisposes patients to renal dysfunction in AIDS. This conclusion is supported by epidemiologic studies that show a disproportionate prevalence of nephropathy among intravenous drug users and by autopsy studies that fail to find renal disease in homosexual AIDS patients.[52] Pardo et al also found a strong association between a history of drug use, AIDS, and renal disease.[41] This association cannot account for FSGS seen in Haitian AIDS patients with no history of intravenous drug use. Moreover, the clinical courses of heroin nephropathy and HIV nephropathy are markedly discordant. Non-HIV-infected patients with heroin nephropathy show slow progression of their disease over months to years and have prolonged survival with hemodialysis. In contrast, patients with AIDS nephropathy have rapid progression to end-stage disease over weeks to months and poor prognosis for survival.

Rao et al reexamined their accumulated data in 1987.[45] Drawing on 750 AIDS cases, they identified 78 patients with renal disease. Of 55 patients with massive proteinuria, azotemia, or both, 43 had progression to irreversible uremia. All were black, and 55 percent had a history of intravenous drug use. Thirty-one received maintenance hemodialysis. Despite dialysis, 26 died in less than 3 months, three lived for 3 to 6 months, and two lived for less than 1 year. Death resulted from progressive inanition despite vigorous nutritional support and opportunistic infections. AIDS was diagnosed in 18 patients after initiation of maintenance dialysis; their course was similar to the preceding with a median survival of less than 1 month. The authors inferred that hemodialysis is of no value in prolonging life in AIDS and irreversible uremia. Lending support to this is a recent report by Ortiz et al, which found a median survival of 30 days in AIDS patients receiving dialysis.[30] In contrast to their experience with AIDS patients, however, the authors reported prolonged survival in HIV-seropositive and ARC patients undergoing maintenance dialysis.

A recent letter reported that zidovudine produced sustained improvement in proteinuria in a patient with HIV-associated focal and segmental glomerulosclerosis.[4] The same letter reported another patient in whom AZT therapy permitted temporary discontinuation of hemodialysis therapy. These intriguing first reports await further study and experience with antiviral therapy.

Acknowledgement

I thank Clint C. Hockenberry for his editorial assistance and technical support.

REFERENCES

1. Acierno L: Cardiac complications in acquired immunodeficiency syndrome (AIDS): A review. J Am Coll Cardiol 13:1144–1154, 1989
2. Anderson D, Virmani R, Reilly J, et al: Prevalent myocarditis at necropsy in the acquired immunodeficiency syndrome. J Am Coll Cardiol 11:792–799, 1988
3. Aron D: Endocrine complications of the acquired immunodeficiency syndrome. Arch Intern Med 149:330–333, 1989
4. Babut-Gay M, Echard M: Zidovudine and nephropathy with human immunodeficiency virus (HIV) infection. (Letter.) Ann Intern Med 111:856–857, 1989
5. Biglieri E: Adrenocortical function in the acquired immunodeficiency syndrome (AIDS) (medical staff conference). West J Med 148:70–73, 1988
6. Bourgoigine J, Meneses R, Pardo V: The nephropathy related to the acquired immune deficiency syndrome. Adv Nephrol 17:113–126, 1988
7. Cacoub P, Deray G, Baumelou A, et al: Acute renal failure induced by Foscarnet: 4 cases. Clin Nephrol 29:315–318, 1988
8. Calabrese L, Proffitt M, Yen-Lieberman B, et al: Congestive cardiomyopathy and illness related to the acquired immunodeficiency syndrome (AIDS) associated with isolation of retrovirus from myocardium. Ann Intern Med 107:691–692, 1987
9. Cammarosano C, Lewis W: Cardiac lesions in acquired immune deficiency syndrome (AIDS). J Am Coll Cardiol 5:703–706, 1985
10. Chabon A, Stnger R, Grabstald H: Histopathology of testis in acquired immune deficiency syndrome. Urology 29:658–663, 1987
11. Chander P, Soni A, Suri A, et al: Renal ultrastructural markers in AIDS-associated nephropathy. Am J Pathol 126:513–526, 1987
12. Cohen I, Anderson D, Virmani R, et al: Congestive cardiomyopathy in association with the acquired immunodeficiency syndrome. N Engl J Med 315:628–630, 1986
13. Coplan N, Bruno M: Acquired immunodeficiency syndrome and heart disease: The present and the future. (Editorial.) Am Heart J 117:1175–1177, 1989

14. Constantino A, West T, Gupta M, et al: Primary cardiac lymphoma in a patient with acquired immune deficiency syndrome. Cancer 60:2801–2805, 1987
15. Corboy J, Fink L, Miller W: Congestive cardiomyopathy in association with AIDS. Radiology 165:139–141, 1987
16. Croxson T, Chapman W, Miller L, et al: Changes in the hypothalamic-pituitary-gonadal axis in human immunodeficiency virus–infected homosexual men. J Clin Endocrinol Metab 68:317–321, 1989
17. D'Agati V, Suh J, Carbone L, et al: Pathology of HIV-associated nephropathy: A detailed morphologic and comparative study. Kidney Int 35:1358–1370, 1989
18. Deyton L, Walker R, Kovacs J, et al: Reversible cardiac dysfunction associated with interferon alfa therapy in AIDS patients with Kaposi's sarcoma. N Engl J Med 321:1246–1249, 1989
19. Dittrich H, Chow L, Denaro F, et al: Human immunodeficiency virus, coxsackievirus, and cardiomyopathy. (Letter.) Ann Intern Med 108:308–309, 1988
20. Dobs A, Dempsey M, Ladenson P, et al: Endocrine disorders in men infected with human immunodeficiency virus. Am J Med 84:611–616, 1988
21. Fink L, Reichek N, St John Sutton M: Cardiac abnormalities in acquired immune deficiency syndrome. Am J Cardiol 54:1161–1163, 1984
22. Gardenswartz M, Lerner C, Seligson G, et al: Renal disease in patients with AIDS: A clinicopathologic study. Clin Nephrol 21:197–204, 1984
23. Glasgow B, Steinsapir K, Anders K, et al: Adrenal pathology in the acquired immune deficiency syndrome. Am J Clin Pathol 84:594–597, 1985
24. Greene L, Cole W, Greene J, et al: Adrenal insufficiency as a complication of the acquired immunodeficiency syndrome. Ann Intern Med 101:497–498, 1984
25. Guenthner E, Rabinowe S, Van Niel A, et al: Primary Addison's disease in a patient with the acquired immunodeficiency syndrome. Ann Intern Med 100:847–848, 1984
26. Guy R, Turberg Y, Davidson R, et al: Mineralocorticoid deficiency in the HIV infection. Br Med J 298:496–497, 1989
27. Henochowicz S, Mustafa M, Lawrinson W, et al: Cardiac aspergillosis in acquired immune deficiency syndrome. Am J Cardiol 55:1239–1240, 1985
28. Hilton D, Harrington P, Prasad C, et al: Adrenal insufficiency in the acquired immunodeficiency syndrome. South Med J 81:1493–1495, 1988
29. Ho D, Pomerantz R, Kaplan J: Pathogenesis of infection with human immunodeficiency virus. N Engl J Med 317:278–286, 1987
30. Hui A, Koss M, Meyer P: Necropsy findings in acquired immunodeficiency syndrome: A comparison of premorten diagnoses with postmortem findings. Hum Pathol 15:670–676, 1984
31. Humphreys M, Schoenfeld P: Renal complications in patients with the acquired immune deficiency syndrome (AIDS). (Editorial.) Am J Nephrol 7:1–7, 1987
32. Kaplan M, Wechsler M, Benson M: Urologic manifestations of AIDS. Urology 30:441–443, 1987
33. Kaminski H, Katzman M, Wiest P, et al: Cardiomyopathy associated with the acquired immune deficiency syndrome. J AIDS 1:105–110, 1988
34. Kavanaugh-McHugh A, Rowe S, Benjamin Y, et al: Selenium deficiency and cardiomyopathy in malnourished pediatric AIDS patients (Abstract No.TBP-256). Presented at the Fifth International Conference on AIDS, Montreal, Canada, June 4–9, 1989
35. Lafont A, Marche C, Wolff M, et al: Myocarditis in acquired immunodeficiency syndrome (AIDS): Etiology and prognosis (Abstract). J Am Coll Cardiol 11:196A, 1988
36. Lewis W, Lipsick J, and Cammarosano C: Cryptococcal myocarditis in acquired immune deficiency syndrome. Am J Cardiol 55:1240, 1985
37. LoPresti J, Fried J, Spencer C, et al: Unique alterations of thyroid hormone indices in the acquired immunodeficiency syndrome (AIDS). Ann Intern Med 110:970–975, 1989
38. Membreno L, Irony I, Dere W, et al: Adrenocortical function in the acquired immunodeficiency syndrome, J Clin Endocrinol Metab 65:482–487, 1987
39. Monsuez J, Dinney E, Vittecoq D, et al: AIDS heart disease: Results in 85 patients (Abstract). J Am Coll Cardiol 11:195A, 1988
40. Ortiz C, Meneses R, Jaffe D, et al: Outcome of patients with human immunodeficiency virus on maintenance hemodialysis. Kidney Int 34:248–253, 1988

41. Pardo V, Aldana M, Colton R, et al: Glomerular lesions in the acquired immunodeficiency syndrome. Ann Intern Med 101:429–434, 1984
42. Paepe M, Waxman M: Testicular atrophy in AIDS: A study of 57 autopsy cases. Hum Pathol 20:210–214, 1989
43. Pardo V, Meneses R, Ossa L, et al: AIDS-related glomerulopathy: Occurrence in specific risk groups. Kidney Int 31:1167–1173, 1987
44. Rao TKS, Fillippone E, Nicastri A, et al: Associated focal and segmental glomerulosclerosis in the acquired immunodeficiency syndrome. N Engl J Med 310:669–673, 1984
45. Rao TKS, Friedman E, Nicastri A: The types of renal disease in the acquired immunodeficiency syndrome. N Engl J Med 316:1062–1067, 1987
46. Reitano J, King M, Cohen H, et al: Cardiac function in patients with acquired immune deficiency syndrome (AIDS) or AIDS prodrome (Abstract). J Am Coll Cardiol 3:525A, 1984
47. Sano T, Kovacs K, Scheithauer B, et al: Pituitary pathology in the acquired immunodeficiency syndrome. Arch Pathol Lab Med 113:1066–1070, 1989
48. Sato K, Ozawa M, Demura H, et al: Thyroid function in the acquired immunodeficiency syndrome (AIDS). (Letter.) Ann Intern Med 111:857–858, 1989
49. Silver M, Macher A, Reichert C, et al: Cardiac involvement by Kaposi's sarcoma in acquired immune deficiency syndrome (AIDS). Am J Cardiol 53:983–985, 1984
50. Soni A, Agarwal A, Chander P, et al: Evidence for an HIV-related nephropathy: A clinicopathological study. Clin Nephrol 31:12–17, 1989
51. Tapper M, Rotterdam H, Lerner C, et al: Adrenal necrosis in the acquired immunodeficiency syndrome. Ann Intern Med 100:239–240, 1984
52. Welch K, Finkbeiner W, Alpers C, et al: Autopsy findings in the acquired immune deficiency syndrome. JAMA 252:1152–1159, 1984

III

SPECIFIC INFECTIONS AND MALIGNANT CONDITIONS

15

PNEUMOCYSTIS CARINII PNEUMONIA

PHILIP C. HOPEWELL, MD

Pneumocystis carinii was first identified in guinea pig lungs by Chagas in 1909 and in human lung tissue in 1911. Although originally the organism was thought to cause disease in humans, it was not until the early 1950s that the clinical illness produced by *P. carinii* was described.[34] The first reports of *P. carinii* pneumonia causing what was then known as interstitial plasma cell pneumonia originated in central Europe and involved premature or debilitated infants 6 weeks to 4 months of age. However, North American physicians did not initially accept *P. carinii* as the etiologic agent of the disease.[21,34] Nearly all the early patients reported were infants, but *P. carinii* pneumonia was diagnosed subsequently in older children and adults.[40] Each patient with the disease had a recognized condition that impaired host responsiveness, leading to the classification of the organism as an opportunist.[25,34]

Presumably because the wartime conditions and postwar food shortages that led to malnutrition among infants in Europe abated by the late 1950s, the near epidemics in orphanages that characterized the epidemiology of *P. carinii* pneumonia disappeared. The pattern seen later was one of sporadic cases occurring in patients with congenital or acquired immunodeficiency states.[64] Between 1955 and 1967, 130 cases were reported in the American literature.[112] With few exceptions, until 1981 *P. carinii* pneumonia continued to be a sporadic opportunistic infection mainly involving patients who had hematologic or lymphoreticular malignancies or who were receiving immunosuppressive therapy.[99,116] In fact, although supporting data are lacking, the incidence of *P. carinii* pneumonia was probably decreasing because of the routine use of trimethoprim-sulfamethoxazole to prevent the disease.[49]

Beginning in 1981 the epidemiology of *P. carinii* pneumonia changed drastically with the recognition of its frequent occurrence in patients with what subsequently came to be known as AIDS.[38,71] Consistently, since data describing the incidence of AIDS began to be collected and reported, *P. carinii* pneumonia has been the most common index diagnosis.[19] More than 60 percent of the reported cases of AIDS have *P. carinii* pneumonia either alone or in combination with Kaposi's sarcoma as the index diagnosis.[1] Another 20 percent of AIDS patients are estimated to have development of the disease later in their course. Moreover, many patients have more than one episode of the illness. In the face of these data it is obviously of considerable importance for physicians to be aware of the clinical features of *P. carinii* pneumonia, to understand the most expeditious and efficient diagnostic approaches, and to be able to use the available treatment and prevention measures effectively.

TAXONOMY AND CHARACTERISTICS OF THE ORGANISM

The confusion regarding the taxonomy of *P. carinii* that began with its initial identification as a trypanosome by Chagas has persisted. Although most taxonomists agree that the organism is either a protozoan or a fungus, the category to which *P. carinii* belongs is not yet clear. Granted the determination of a correct taxonomic position is of little clinical relevance, establishing the correct assignment might provide important insights into some of the vexing problems the organism presents, such as its inability to be grown on cultures of artificial media.

Perhaps the most convincing data concerning the classification of *P. carinii* have been presented by Edman and associates, who characterized the DNA sequence that encodes the organism's unique ribosomal RNA subunit.[26] Analysis of these data suggests that *P. carinii* fits within the fungi and is most closely related to the yeasts.

Although a great deal is known about the features of *P. carinii*, investigators have been hampered by the inability to culture the organism on cell-free media and to maintain cultures in cell lines. Details of the various approaches to cultivation of the organism in cell culture have been summarized by Hughes[46] and are beyond the scope of this chapter. The lack of reliable means for culture of the organism has at least two important clinical implications. First, the clinical material must contain enough organisms for their detection by microscopic examination. If the sensitivity of microscopic examination for *Mycobacterium tuberculosis* applies to *P. carinii*, the threshold for visualization would be in the range of 10^4 organisms per milliliter of respiratory secretions. Thus it is certainly possible that earlier stages of infection are not detected. Second, *P. carinii* cannot be tested for susceptibility to anti-*Pneumocystis* agents and the evaluation of new drugs must be performed largely in animal models.

Morphologic studies suggest that *P. carinii* has a life cycle comprising three developmental forms: cysts, which are spherical or crescent-shaped forms 5 to 8 μm in diameter; sporozoites or intracystic bodies found only within the cyst; and trophozoites, found outside the cyst and thought to be intermediate between the sporozoite and the cyst.[46] Trophozoites are 2 to 5 μm in diameter and have eccentric nuclei and reticular cytoplasm. The clinical relevance of the developmental stages is related to their different staining properties. Some stains, such as methenamine silver and toluidine blue O, stain only the cyst wall, and thus only cysts can be identified in preparations stained by these methods. The Giemsa stain is taken up by both the intracystic sporozoites and extracystic trophozoites. Cysts can be seen only as negative images or "ghosts" within the matrix of a clump of trophozoites. The Gram-Weigert stain also stains sporozoites and trophozoites but not the cyst wall.

PATHOGENESIS OF *P. CARINII* PNEUMONIA

Substantial albeit inferential evidence suggests that *P. carinii* pneumonia results from recrudescence of infection that occurred early in life and was easily suppressed by normal host defense mechanisms. In animals, especially rats and mice, *P. carinii* pneumonia develops as a consequence of corticosteroid administration without obvious exposure to exogenous sources of infection.[33,50,109,110]

In humans evidence for early infection comes from serologic testing. Studies using several different antigen and antibody detection systems have suggested that most children have acquired *P. carinii* infection by 4 years of age. Meuwissen and associates, using an indirect fluorescent antibody (IFA) test with antigen prepared from *P. carinii* cyst walls, found immunoglobulin M and immunoglobulin G (IgM and IgG) antibody titers of greater than 1:40 in nearly all tested children 2 to 4 years of age.[77] Pifer and coworkers used IFA tests to identify antibody and counterimmunoelectrophoresis to detect circulating antigen in normal children.[91] Although antigenemia was not found in any of the normal children, 83 percent of those 3 to 4 years old had antibody titers of 1:16 or greater. In a separate group of 23 children studied longitudinally, discounting maternal antibody, antibody development began at 7 months of age and increased to a peak of 63 percent of the subjects by 4 years of age. Sheppard and colleagues, using similar techniques, found antibody to *P. carinii* in 53 percent of a group of normal subjects.[97] Hofmann and coworkers found IgM antibodies to *P. carinii* in 72 percent, IgG in 38 percent, and IgA in 31 percent of healthy subjects.[42]

More recently Kovacs and associates using Western blot analysis to detect antibodies against human *P. carinii* antigens, reported findings similar to those summarized previously.[58] Seven of eight healthy adults had anti-*Pneumocystis* antibodies detected in their sera, as did all 10 immunosuppressed patients without a history of *P. carinii* pneumonia and all 19 patients who had had *P. carinii* pneumonia. Conversely, none of seven healthy infants had circulating antibodies detected. These data from studies using more specific antigens and more precise detection methods tend both to confirm the postulated pathogenetic sequence and to demonstrate that antibody measurement will not be useful in diagnostic evaluations.

Countering the hypothesis that *P. carinii* pneumonia is recrudescence of a latent infection is the infrequency with which the organisms have been found at autopsy in the lungs of persons dying of nonimmunosuppressive conditions.[16,27,39,77] These findings however, may result from the small number of organisms present and the use of relatively insensitive techniques.

Despite evidence suggesting that latent infection is responsible for most clinical pneumonia caused by *P. carinii*, some reports of case clusters imply that horizontal transmission may also play a role.[25,99,111,116] Although transmission from person to person could be important in some instances, the lack of a consistent epidemiologic pattern seems to argue against a significant role for recent infection in causing the clinical illness.

P. carinii seems to be acquired via the airborne route. Hughes demonstrated that, when germ-free rats without *P. carinii* were isolated and given sterile food and water but exposed to nonsterile air, they acquired the organism.[45] When the air the animals breathed was filtered, they remained uninfected with *P. carinii*. This observation again suggests that horizontal transmission may occur via the air from potential sources of infection to susceptible persons in the vicinity.

The specific abnormalities of host defenses that predispose to *P. carinii* pneumonia are not well understood. Apparently, however, defects in cellular immunity are the major factors involved. Corticosteroid-treated rats are the experimental model in which *P. carinii* pneumonia has been studied most commonly. However, because corticosteroids have multiple effects on host defenses in addition to depressing cell-mediated immunity, a precise determination of the most important affected components has not been possible. Recently, using monoclonal antibodies against the murine L3 and L4 (CD4) receptors, Shellito and associates produced a mouse model of *P. carinii* pneumonia in which the only defect is in T-helper lymphocytes.[96] This suggests that T-helper cell depletion is by far the most important factor predisposing to *P. carinii* in HIV infection. Studies using rat macrophages have suggested, however, that both specific anti-*Pneumocystis* antibody and intact macrophage function are necessary for ingestion and killing of *P. carinii*.[70,103] The clinical conditions with which *P. carinii* pneumonia has most commonly been associated are those that predominantly affect T lymphocytes and the expression of cell-mediated immunity.[9,25] However, the role of humoral antibodies is suggested by reports of *P. carinii* pneumonia in children with congenital agammaglobulinemia or hypogammaglobulinemia.[9]

A major aspect of the natural history of HIV infection is progressive depletion of CD4+ lymphocytes.[86] Because *P. carinii* is not a particularly pathogenic organism, severe immunocompromise, indicated by a marked reduction in CD4+ lymphocytes, must be present for the organism to proliferate and cause disease. Masur and associates have examined the circulating CD4+ lymphocyte counts of patients infected with HIV and related diseases diagnosed at the time the counts were performed.[72] Patients found to have *P. carinii* pneumonia had a median CD4+ cell count of 26/mm³ with an interquartile cell count range of 12 to 62.5/mm³. In only two of 46 episodes of *P. carinii* pneumonia were the CD4+ cell counts greater than 200/mm³.

In addition to depleting CD4+ lymphocytes, HIV infection produces B cell defects causing abnormalities in circulating antibody production and impairs alveolar macrophage function. Macrophage function is altered both by direct viral infection of the cells and by a reduction in macrophage-activating cytokines caused by the CD4+ lymphocyte depletion.[4] Thus patients with advanced HIV infection have substantial reductions of all aspects of host defenses thought to be necessary for continued suppression of *P. carinii,* thereby setting the stage for the organism's emergence as a cause of lung disease. In addition to lung involvement, extrapulmonary pneumocystosis may occur, presumably because of failure to control *P. carinii* growth in the lungs and subsequent hematogenous dissemination of the organism from a primary pulmonary site to other organs.

DIAGNOSIS

Clinical Presentation

Although *P. carinii* pneumonia is the most common index diagnosis in patients with AIDS, these patients usually have had nonspecific symptoms such as fever, fatigue, and weight loss for weeks to months before respiratory symptoms develop. In addition, HIV-related disorders such as oral candidiasis, indicative of severe immunocompromise, are commonly present. The most frequent symptoms of *P. carinii* pneumonia are fever, cough, and shortness of breath. The shortness of breath usually progresses from being present only with exertion to being present at rest. Cough is generally nonproductive but may produce sputum in patients who smoke cigarettes or who have bacterial bronchitis or pneumonia as well as *P. carinii* pneumonia. The respiratory symptoms may be prominent or relatively minor when the patient is evaluated for *P. carinii.* Since both zidovudine and aerosol pentamidine prophylaxis decrease the severity of *P. carinii* pneumonia if it does develop, the presenting symptoms may be subtle. Conversely, patients who have not been under medical care and do not readily seek medical attention may have advanced pneumonia and marked symptoms when first examined.

The physical examination in patients with *P. carinii* pneumonia is not particularly helpful in diagnosing the disease and may be dominated by other HIV-associated diseases. Patients with advanced HIV infection may be somewhat wasted and are generally febrile. Those with more severe pulmonary involvement may be tachypneic. Diffuse lymphadenopathy may be noted, and a substantial percentage have oral candidiasis or hairy leukoplakia. Cutaneous lesions of Kaposi's sarcoma may be present. Pulmonary findings generally are not striking. Dry rales may be heard, but evidence of consolidation is unusual.

Initial laboratory evaluation is also not especially helpful. Lyphopenia is common but not invariable. As noted earlier, CD4 + cell counts may be useful in identifying patients who have severe immunocompromise and therefore are at risk of opportunistic infection. A variety of other hematologic abnormalities, including anemia, leukopenia, and thrombocytopenia, may also occur.

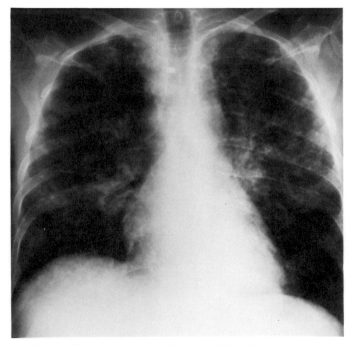

FIGURE 15–1.   Chest radiograph showing diffuse interstitial infiltration typical of *Pneumocystis carinii* pneumonia.

Radiographic Findings

In patients with respiratory symptoms the initial diagnostic study generally is a chest radiograph. This provides information useful in directing subsequent evaluations. The radiograph may show abnormalities unlikely to be caused by an opportunistic process, such as hyperinflation from asthma or focal consolidation consistent with a pyogenic bacterial pneumonia (although this may be opportunistic). The radiographic patterns of the opportunistic processes are nonspecific, although some diagnoses are made more likely by the radiographic findings.[13]

P. carinii pneumonia most often causes diffuse interstitial infiltration involving all portions of the lungs rather evenly (Fig. 15–1).[13,100] Several variations of the basic pattern may be seen: the infiltration may be heterogeneously distributed throughout the lung or may be more miliary in appearance. *P. carinii* pneumonia may cause diffuse and focal airspace consolidation, especially as the disorder becomes more severe (Fig. 15–2).

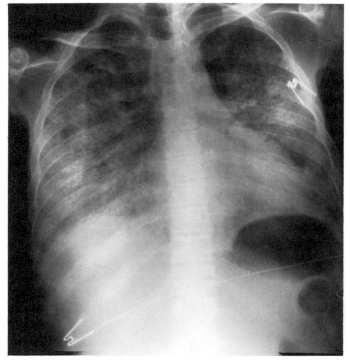

FIGURE 15–2. Chest radiograph demonstrating diffuse airspace consolidation in patient with severe *Pneumocystis carinii* pneumonia.

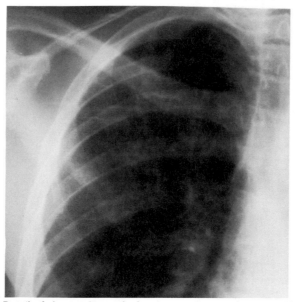

FIGURE 15—3.   Detail of chest radiograph showing pneumatoceles caused by *Pneumocystis carinii.*

Cystic changes or pneumatoceles (Fig. 15–3) have been noted, particularly during the healing process, and cavitation may take place within preexisting nodular lesions. Spontaneous pneumothorax may occur, probably as an extension of the cystic or cavitary processes. Pleural effusions and intrathoracic adenopathy are uncommon with *P. carinii* pneumonia. Adenopathy in a patient with *P. carinii* pneumonia is probably due to another process. Likewise, when significant amounts of pleural fluid are present, other diagnoses should be considered. There seems to be a general perception among clinicians caring for patients with *P. carinii* pneumonia that the frequency of unusual or atypical radiographic findings is increasing. If true this perception could simply be related to increasing experience with the disease, to the effects of antiviral therapy, or to the use of aerosol pentamidine prophylaxis.

If no radiographic abnormalities are found, the patient's respiratory symptoms are not being caused by lung disease or the disease is not sufficiently advanced to cause radiographic findings. Approximately 5 to 10 percent of AIDS patients with proven *P. carinii* pneumonia have normal chest radiographs. Other pathogens such as cytomegalovirus and *Mycobacterium avium* complex may also be present without causing abnormal chest radiographs. For this reason, if the symptoms are judged to be significant, further evaluation is warranted.

Pulmonary Function Tests

Abnormalities in lung function are found commonly in patients with *P. carinii* pneumonia, although, as with radiographic abnormalities, the changes cannot be viewed as specific. Typical findings include reductions in vital capacity, total lung capacity, and single breath diffusing capacity for carbon monoxide (DLco). It should be noted that intravenous drug abuse, an AIDS risk factor, may cause abnormalities on the chest radiograph as well as a reduction in DLco and thus confound the evaluation of patients in this risk group.

Arterial blood gas measurements are helpful in determining the severity of pulmonary involvement. Hypoxemia is common but not invariable, and hypocarbia may also be found. An increase in the alveolar-to-arterial oxygen tension difference, especially with exercise, has been reported to be common in patients with *P. carinii* pneumonia.[100]

Gallium Lung Scans

Gallium lung scanning has proved to be a sensitive, although nonspecific, test for the presence of *P. carinii* pneumonia.[15] At San Francisco General Hospital, only 4 of 65 patients shown to have *P. carinii* on lung biopsy had a normal gallium lung scan.[20]

Table 15–1 shows the overall diagnostic value of screening tests for *P. carinii* pneumonia used at San Francisco General Hospital.[20] As can be seen, both the DLco and the gallium lung scan are very sensitive to the presence of *P. carinii* but have a low specificity. None of the studies alone has a high enough positive or negative predictive value to be definitive. However, when grouped together, the noninvasive tests enable identification of persons who should have further diagnostic studies.

TABLE 15–1.   DIAGNOSTIC VALUE OF NONINVASIVE TESTS FOR *P. CARINII* PNEUMONIA

	VC	TLC	DLco	CXR	GAL
Sensitivity (%)	85.2	71.4	89.3	82.8	90.7
Specificity (%)	52.2	64.4	23.8	45.4	40.9
Positive predictive value (%)	75.8	77.5	67.7	68.8	75.0
Negative predictive value (%)	66.7	56.9	55.6	64.5	69.2

VC, Vital capacity; *TLC*, total lung capacity; *DLco*, single breath diffusing capacity for carbon monoxide; *CXR*, chest radiograph; *GAL*, gallium-67 citrate lung scan.
From Curtis J, Goodman P, Hopewell PC: Noninvasive tests in the diagnostic evaluation for *P. carinii* pneumonia in patients with or suspected of having AIDS. Am Rev Respir Dis 133:A182, 1986.

Means to Identify *P. carinii*

Sputum Examination

Although patients with *P. carinii* pneumonia often complain of cough, they rarely produce sputum that is suitable for examination. However, adequate specimens can be obtained by having patients inhale a mist of 3 percent saline solution produced by an ultrasonic nebulizer. Both Pitchenik and coworkers[92] and Bigby and colleagues[5] showed that sputum examination provides diagnoses in a substantial number of patients with AIDS. In both studies *P. carinii* was found in 40 to 50 percent of the specimens examined and the sensitivity was between 50 and 60 percent. In the group studied by Bigby et al no features predicted which patients would have *P. carinii* found in sputum, although those whose sputum tests were positive tended to have a lower arterial oxygen tension (PaO_2) and DL_{CO}.[5]

Since early 1986 at San Francisco General Hospital, examination of induced sputum has been used routinely as the first test in patients suspected to have *P. carinii* pneumonia because of clinical findings. For the 10-month period September 1986 through June 1987, 404 episodes of HIV-associated lung disease were evaluated with sputum examination as the first potentially definitive study.[88] *P. carinii* was identified in 222 specimens (55 percent). The sensitivity of sputum examination for detecting *P. carinii* was 77 percent, and the negative predictive value was 64 percent. These results reflect the operational utility of sputum examination in routine practice and demonstrate the considerable savings in resources and patient discomfort provided by this examination.

Nevertheless, because of the sensitivity and negative predictive values of sputum examination, a negative result cannot be regarded as definitively excluding *P. carinii*. Recently immunofluorescent stains for *P. carinii* using monoclonal antibodies were developed and evaluated. Preliminary reports suggested that using these staining procedures for induced sputum will increase the sensitivity of the test, although in routine practice the sensitivity may not be greater than use of the modified Wright-Giemsa stain (Color Plate IC) by an experienced practitioner.[59,89]

Bronchoalveolar Lavage and Transbronchial Lung Biopsy

Bronchoalveolar lavage and transbronchial lung biopsy have proved highly sensitive in identifying pulmonary infections in patients with AIDS.[8,14] Stover et al reported the results of bronchoscopic procedures in 72 patients with AIDS.[101] Both transbronchial biopsy and bronchoalveolar lavage had high yields (88 and 85 percent, respectively), and when they were used together, the yield was 94 percent. The yield was especially high for *P. carinii* (94 percent). Similar results were reported by Broaddus and coworkers, who described the efficacy of bronchoalveolar lavage and transbronchial biopsy in detecting pulmonary pathogens in 276 fiberoptic bronchoscopic examinations performed on 171 patients with known or suspected AIDS.[8] Of 173 pathogens identified during the initial evaluation or in the subsequent month, 166 (96 percent) were detected in the initial bronchoscopy. Bronchoalveolar lavage and transbronchial biopsy had similar sensitivities of 86 percent (124 of 145) and 87 percent (133 of 153), respectively. For *P. carinii*, lavage had an 89 percent sensitivity and transbronchial biopsy a 97 percent sensitivity. In patients who had both procedures performed the sensitivity was 100 percent. Possibly the use of aerosol pentamidine makes the procedures less sensitive in patients who have mild forms of the disease.

More recently Golden and coworkers reported bronchoalveolar lavage alone to have a 97 percent sensitivity for *P. carinii*.[35] At the San Francisco General Hospital we have reviewed our experience subsequent to the report by Broaddus et al[8] and found that only rarely was *P. carinii* identified in transbronchial biopsy specimens when it was not seen in bronchoalveolar lavage fluid. Thus, as a matter of routine in patients known or suspected to have AIDS but in whose sputum *P. carinii* is not found, we perform only bronchoalveolar lavage. If that procedure does not establish the diagnosis, the lavage is repeated and a transbronchial biopsy is performed to look for other diagnoses.

Fiberoptic bronchoscopy with bronchoalveolar lavage and transbronchial biopsy can be safely performed via a transnasal or transoral approach without an endotracheal tube, using local anesthesia. Unless a focal abnormality is present on the chest film, the procedure can be done without fluroscopic guidance, saving time, cost, and discomfort to the patient.[80] The bronchoscopic procedure should involve inspection of the hypopharynx, vocal cords, and airways from the trachea to subsegmental bronchi.

Bronchoalveolar Lavage.   After inspection of the airways the bronchoscope is positioned in a peripheral airway, usually in the right middle lobe, and 80 to 100 ml of sterile, nonbacteriostatic saline solution in 20 ml aliquots is instilled. Suction is applied after each bolus. The aspirated return is usually 40 to 50 ml. Bronchoalveolar lavage can also be performed with a fiberoptic catheter or a double-lumen balloon-tipped catheter, neither of which requires bronchoscopy.[115]

Transbronchial Biopsy.   If a transbronchial biopsy is to be performed, it should be done after the lavage. The bronchoscope is repositioned, generally in the right lower lobe. If the radiographic abnormality is localized, the biopsy specimens should be taken from the area of greatest abnormality. Multiple specimens are generally obtained. At our institution the specimens for microbiologic evaluation are placed on a moistened gauze sponge and transported in a tightly capped specimen jar. Specimens for histologic study are placed in formalin. Staining of touch imprints made from unfixed tissue specimens and smears of lavage sediment for *P. carinii* has the advantage of being rapid, in contrast to the slower methenamine silver staining of fixed tissue sections.[6] Routine tissue histopathologic studies with hematoxylin and eosin staining provide only inferential information concerning *P. carinii*. Typically, eosinophilic material fills the alveoli. The amount of cellular infiltration is variable, and *P. carinii* cannot be seen.

The most common complications of transbronchial biopsy are hemorrhage and pneumothorax. In the series of transbronchial biopsies in patients with AIDS or suspected AIDS reported by Broaddus et al, pneumothorax occurred in 9 percent (23 of 253) and 5.9 percent (15) required placement of a chest tube for reexpansion.[8] Hemoptysis sufficient to cause respiratory compromise or to necessitate blood transfusion did not occur and there were no deaths. The presence of an uncorrectable coagulopathy is an absolute contraindication to transbronchial biopsy, and respiratory failure sufficiently severe to require mechanical ventilation is usually viewed as a relative contraindication. However, bronchoalveolar lavage can be performed safely in these situations.

Open Lung Biopsy

Open lung biopsy in patients with AIDS should be reserved for several infrequently encountered situations: (1) a patient with progressive pulmonary disease in whom sputum induction and a carefully performed fiberoptic bronchoscopy with bronchoalveolar lavage and transbronchial biopsy were nondiagnostic; (2) a patient with an uncorrectable coagulopathy in whom lavage has been nondiagnostic; and (3) a patient who is requiring mechanical ventilation in whom biopsy and or lavage has been nondiagnostic. Even in these situations a second bronchoscopic procedure may be indicated before open lung biopsy. If possible the physician should wait until the results of all microbiologic evaluations of the initial specimens have been returned before performing an open biopsy.

Presumptive Diagnosis

In some cases an empiric treatment trial may be used to infer a diagnosis. Generally, however, this is unsatisfactory, first because another treatable process may be missed, and second because such an approach exposes the patient to the risks of therapy, perhaps without benefit. However, if a patient has classic clinical features, an experienced clinician can establish a presumptive diagnosis with a high degree of accuracy.[79] This approach may be useful in institutions not capable of making diagnoses from induced sputum but does not seem justified when the majority of diagnoses can be established by this noninvasive and relatively inexpensive test.

Diagnostic Strategy

The results of the studies described previously enable formulation of a logical sequence for evaluating patients suspected of having *P. carinii* pneumonia. This scheme is shown in Figure 15–4. Although several modifications are possible, a logical, orderly approach of this sort should result in a more expeditiously reached diagnosis and more efficient use of resources. Using more invasive studies only after less invasive approaches have failed minimizes patient discomfort. Obviously, clinical circumstances and institutional experience and resources influence the determination of a diagnostic approach. Institutions should periodically evaluate their results to determine the most effective diagnostic strategy based on prevailing local conditions.

TREATMENT

Evolution of Treatment

Although many agents were used in attempts to treat *P. carinii* pneumonia, none was successful until 1958 when Ivady and Paldy began trials

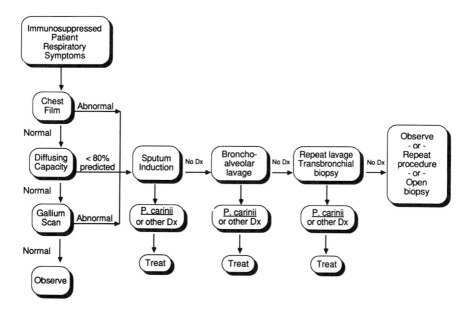

FIGURE 15–4. Flow diagram of sequence of diagnostic studies for evaluation of patients suspected of having *Pneumocystis carinii* pneumonia or other opportunistic pulmonary infection.

of pentamidine.[52] In 1967 pentamidine became available in the United States through the Parasitic Disease Drug Service of the National Communicable Disease Center and was used routinely in treating *P. carinii* pneumonia. In 1971 Kirby and associates reported successful treatment with pyramethamine and sulfadiazine in two of three patients with *P. carinii* pneumonia.[55] None of four previous patients treated with these agents had survived. Further experience with this combination has been limited. Hughes et al in 1974 first showed the combination of trimethoprim (TMP) and sulfamethoxazole (SMX) to be effective in treating and preventing *P. carinii* pneumonia in cortisone-treated rats.[44] Subsequent clinical studies documented the usefulness of this combination in humans.[47,48,62,63] Currently both TMP-SMX and pentamidine isethionate are approved for treating *P. carinii* pneumonia.

Specific Anti-*Pneumocystis* Agents

Pentamidine

Pharmacology.   Pentamidine is an aromatic diamidine that was first used in the 1940s to treat African trypanosomiasis and leishmaniasis. Its spectrum of activity includes only *Trypanosoma rhodesiense, Trypanosoma gambiense, Leishmania donovani,* and *P. carinii.*[24]

Pentamidine's mechanism of action against *P. carinii* has not been firmly established. It inhibits dihydrofolate reductase in vitro, although it is not so potent in this regard as other folate antagonists.[105] In addition, it interferes with anerobic glycolysis, inhibits oxidative phosphorylation, and limits nucleic acid and protein synthesis.[7] Data described more recently indicate that pentamidine also inhibits the metabolism of para-aminobenzoic acid and the eventual synthesis of dihydrofolate.[57]

Until recently the pharmacokinetics of pentamidine had not been well studied; however, the development of a specific and sensitive assay has enabled more accurate studies.[67] Conte and colleagues measured plasma and urine pentamidine concentrations in six patients who received 4 mg/kg body weight intravenously and in six with the same dose given intramuscularly.[18] Mean peak concentrations occurred at 0.67 hour after intramuscular administration and at 2 hours after initiation of a 2-hour intravenous infusion. A wide range of concentrations occurred in each group, but the mean peak values were 209 ng/ml and 612 ng/ml with intramuscular and intravenous administration, respectively. The elimination halftime was 9.36 hours in the intramuscular group and 6.40 hours in patients given the drug intravenously. The apparent volume of distribution was very large in both groups, indicating tissue sequestration. All patients had measurable concentrations 24 hours after administration. Urinary excretion in 24 hours was 2.5 to 4.1 percent of the total dose.

Previous studies in animals have shown high concentrations in the kidneys and liver with lower concentrations in the lungs after systemic administration of pentamidine.[104,106] Waldman and coworkers also demonstrated selective sequestration of pentamidine in the lungs of rats given the drug by aerosol.[106] More recently, Debs and associates showed lung uptake with little or no systemic absorption when the drug was given as an aerosol.[23] In addition, these investigators reported that rats with *P. carinii* pneumonia could be treated successfully with aerosolized pentamidine.[22] Extending the observations on aerosol delivery of pentamidine to humans, Montgomery and colleagues measured very high concentrations of the drug in bronchoalveolar lavage fluid with little or no drug in the plasma after aerosol administration in patients with *P. carinii* pneumonia.[83] Both Conte and coworkers[17] and Montgomery and associates[84,85] reported high rates of successful initial and second-line treatment with no systemic toxic effects in pilot studies of aerosol pentamidine given to AIDS patients with *P. carinii* pneumonia.

Dosage and Administration.   The standard dosage of pentamidine isethionate is 4 mg/kg body weight per day, although in a pilot study Conte and coworkers reported successful treatment with 3 mg/kg/d.[17] The dosage is based loosely on animal studies and empiric observations. Because *P. carinii* cannot be maintained in culture, a minimum inhibitory concentration of pentamidine cannot be determined. Using a determination of dye uptake by *P. carinii* as an index of viability, Pesanti showed that pentamidine concentrations of 5μg/ml and 10 μg/ml sharply decreased uptake of neutral red dye after a lag of 6 hours.[90] The 5 μg/ml concentration corresponds roughly to the plasma concentrations produced by intramuscular or intravenous administration of pentamidine isethionate 4 mg/kg.[18,104] Because of the tissue tropism of the drug, concentrations probably are substantially greater in the lung than in serum and perhaps lower doses could be used effectively.[106]

Because pentamidine is not absorbed from the gastrointestinal tract, parenteral administration is necessary. The preferred route of administration is intravenous, but the drug may be given intramuscularly. It should be administered intravenously only if the patient can be observed and the blood pressure measured. The drug should be dissolved in 250 ml of 5 percent dextrose in water and administered at a constant infusion rate for 1 hour. The dosage interval of 24 hours should be increased for patients with impaired renal function if no alternative agent is suitable.

The minimum duration of treatment with pentamidine has not been established, but in most trials the drug was given for 14 to 21 days. In addition, for patients with AIDS retrospective analysis has suggested that 21 days of administration is superior to 14 days.[41]

Adverse Reactions.   Western and coworkers reported the first systematic compilation of the adverse reactions to pentamidine.[112] Of 164 patients given the drug, 69 (42 percent) had untoward effects. Walzer and associates extended these observations to include 404 patients of whom 190 (47 percent) had adverse reactions.[108] The most common reactions were azotemia, pain at the injection site, hypoglycemia, and sterile abscesses. A variety of other reactions, including hypotension, nausea, vomiting, skin rashes, and hypocalcemia, also were reported.

In most studies adverse reactions to pentamidine occurred with approximately the same frequency in AIDS patients as described in non-AIDS patients, but the array has broadened. In the study by Wharton and colleagues 14 (44 percent) of 32 patients given pentamidine for any period of time had a major adverse reaction that necessitated changing to a different drug.[113] All patients given pentamidine had minor adverse reactions. In this group the most common major adverse reaction was neutropenia (polymorphonuclear leukocyte count $<1000/\mu l$), whereas hyponatremia, abnormal liver function, and azotemia were the most common minor reactions. Most reactions in these patients occurred between days 7 and 14 of treatment. Sattler and associates also reported a high frequency of adverse reactions in pentamidine-treated AIDS patients, but in only one patient was the reaction severe (fatal hypoglycemia).[94] Discontinuation of the drug was not necessary in any patients, at least in part because the threshold for changing therapy was higher than in the study by Wharton et al.[113]

Reported Effectiveness.   The use of pentamidine clearly decreased the mortality rate in the epidemic form of *P. carinii* pneumonia reported from Europe. Without treatment the estimated case fatality rate was 50 percent, whereas with pentamidine therapy deaths were reduced to 3.5 percent.[52]

In the United States, Western and associates demonstrated a 76.7 percent rate of successful treatment for patients who received 9 or more days of pentamidine treatment.[112] Overall 36 (48 percent) of 75 patients recovered. Subsequently, Hughes and coworkers prospectively evaluated 24 immunosuppressed children treated with pentamidine, 18 (75 percent) of whom recovered.[47] In a similar study Siegal and colleagues reported recovery in 9 of 10 children treated with pentamidine.[98] In a prospective study of *P. carinii* pneumonia in patients with AIDS, Wharton et al reported success in all but 1 of 20 patients selected at random to receive pentamidine.[113] Similar results in AIDS patients were reported by Klein and coworkers.[56] In the prospective randomized study by Sattler and coworkers, however, only 61 percent of patients who received pentamidine survived.[94]

Trimethoprim-Sulfamethoxazole

Pharmacology.   Sulfonamides were first synthesized in 1932 and used as anti-infective agents in 1935. TMP was synthesized in 1956 as a result of a systematic search for potential antimicrobial agents. The combination of TMP and SMX has activity against a broad range of organisms, including many gram-positive and aerobic gram-negative bacteria. These two agents act on separate sites to inhibit purine synthesis.[60] Sulfonamides inhibit dihydrofolic synthetase, preventing the conversion of microbial para-aminobenzoic acid to dihydrofolic acid. TMP acts on dihydrofolic acid reductase (DHFR), thereby decreasing synthesis of tetrahydrofolic acid.

Both drugs are well absorbed from the gastrointestinal tract. After an oral TMP dose of 240 mg, peak serum levels of 2 to 3 μg/ml are reached in 1 to 2 hours. The serum half-life of TMP is approximately 13 hours with measurable concentrations present 24 hours after administration. SMX reaches a peak concentration of approximately 60 μg/ml 2 hours after an oral dose of 1200 mg. Its serum half-life is 9 to 12 hours, and measurable concentrations of the drug are present 24 hours after administration. Because the absorption rates and half-lives of the drugs are similar, they can be administered simultaneously.

Concentrations of TMP and SMX are generally higher in tissues than in serum. In sputum the TMP concentration is approximately twice the serum concentration but the SMX concentration is only half that in serum.[43]

Dosage and Administration.   As with pentamidine, minimal inhibitory concentrations of TMP and SMX for *P. carinii* have not been determined. In the studies of *P. carinii* pneumonia in the rat model that first documented the effectiveness of TMP-SMX, Hughes and coworkers used a dose of 50 mg/kg/d for TMP and 250 mg/kg/d for SMX.[50] Serum concentrations of the drugs were not measured. In the first report of treatment of patients with TMP-SMX, two doses were used, 4 to 7 mg/kg/d of TMP with 20 to 35 mg/kg/d of SMX and 20 and 100 mg/kg/d of the respective agents.[48] Peak serum concentrations of TMP were approximately 2 μg/ml at the lower dose and 7 to 10 μg/ml at the higher dose. The peak SMX concentrations were 50 to 60 μg/ml and 80 to 120 μg/ml for the low and high doses, respectively. Two of six patients treated with low doses died, as did two of 14 who received high doses.

Based on this experience, Hughes and coworkers conducted a prospective randomized study comparing TMP-SMX (TMP 20 mg/kg/d; SMX 100 mg/kg/d) with pentamidine in immunosuppressed children who had *P. carinii* pneumonia.[47] Serum levels of both TMP and SMX were measured 2 hours and 6 hours after oral ingestion of one fourth of the daily dose (5 mg/kg and 25 mg/kg) on days 1, 3, 6, 9, and 12. The concentrations of both drugs tended to remain constant from the third day, although moderate variability occurred from day to day. The 2-hour and 6-hour mean concentrations were not substantially different for either drug: for TMP the mean concentrations ranged from approximately 4 to 6.5 μg/ml, and for SMX the range was approximately 115 to 175 μg/ml. Nearly all studies reported since the 1975 paper by Hughes and associates[48] have used these doses. However, Sattler et al reported no loss of efficacy with a lower dose of trimethoprim if serum levels were maintained at 5 to 8 μg/ml.[94]

Although in the earlier reports oral administration was used, concern about absorption prompted investigators to administer the drug intravenously.[56,95,113,114] The current daily dosage recommendation is four doses at 6-hour intervals. If there is no suggestion that the drug will not be completely absorbed, it can be given orally, usually in the form of tablets containing TMP 160 mg and SMX 800 mg. For parenteral administration the drug should be diluted in 250 ml of 5 percent dextrose in water and given over 30 to 60 minutes at 6-hour intervals. Whether the high dose of TMP-SMX should be continued for the full course of therapy or can be reduced once a response is evident is not clear. The minimum duration of treatment necessary has not been established. Nearly all published experience, however, has been with 14 to 21 days of therapy or occasionally longer depending on the clinical course.

Adverse Reactions.   The major benefit offered by TMP-SMX over pentamidine in the early reports was a much lower incidence of adverse reactions.[47,48,62,63] In the prospective trial conducted by Hughes and colleagues only one patient had therapy changed because of an adverse reaction, an urticarial rash.[47] Three patients had nausea and vomiting but were able to continue with the drug. Winston and coworkers treated 11 patients and reported one with a skin rash and one with nausea and vomiting.[114] Sattler and Remington reported mild rash, phlebitis, and vomiting in 3 of 15 patients.[95] Siegal and associates noted skin rashes in 3 of 15 patients, but in only one was a change in therapy necessary.[98] Also noted were mild transaminasemia and a 50 percent decrease in white blood cell count, each of which occurred in two patients.

In treating AIDS patients the frequency of significant adverse reactions has proved to be much higher than noted in non-AIDS patients. Gordin and colleagues retrospectively reviewed adverse reactions among AIDS patients treated with TMP-SMX.[37] They found that 19 of 35 patients treated for more than 2 days were unable to complete a course of the agent because of adverse reactions. Severe skin rashes often associated with fever were the most common reactions. Leukopenia and thrombocytopenia were the most common reactions. Leukopenia and thrombocytopenia were the next most frequent reasons for discontinuing the drug. Hepatitis occurred in a smaller number. The adverse reactions nearly always occurred between days 6 and 14 of a planned 21-day course of treatment.

In the prospective study conducted by Wharton and associates, adverse reactions to TMP-SMX were encountered frequently.[113] Of 20 patients receiving the drug, 10 had major adverse reactions that necessitated its discontinuation after a median of 11 days. As Gordin et al[37] noted, nearly all adverse reactions occurred between days 6 and 14. Again, the most common major reactions were severe skin rash (20 percent), hepatitis (20 percent), neutropenia (15 percent), and thrombocytopenia (15 percent). All patients had minor adverse reactions that did not necessitate discontinuation of the drug. In addition to lesser degrees of the severe reactions, these minor effects included nausea, vomiting, and hyponatremia. Sattler and colleagues also reported a high frequency of adverse effects from TMP-SMX in their prospective study, but these reactions did not necessitate discontinuation of the agent.[94] In part they attributed the lack of severe reactions to dosage reductions based on serum TMP concentrations (as noted previously).

Reported Effectiveness. Despite the differences in adverse reactions to TMP-SMX between patients without and with AIDS and *P. carinii* pneumonia, rates of success in those who complete therapy are similar. In the two early papers by Hughes et al, survival rates in children were 75 and 77 percent.[47,48] Early experience in adult patients was not so good as in children. Five (62 percent) of eight patients reported by Lau and Young[63] survived, as did 7 (64 percent) of 11 patients reported by Winston et al[114] and 8 (53 percent) of 15 patients reported by Sattler and Remington.[95] In each of these groups of patients the underlying disease processes and their treatment contributed to the mortality rates, reducing the apparent rates of cure. For example, at autopsy lung tissue from five of the seven patients who died in Sattler and Remington's series showed no *P. carinii*, indicating a "microbiologic cure."

Evaluating the success rates of TMP-SMX in AIDS patients is difficult because of the frequency with which adverse reactions lead to discontinuation of the drug. In a retrospective review Haverkos reported 91 percent (40 of 44 patients) survival in patients who were treated with a full course of the agent.[41] In contrast, survival was only 31 percent (11 of 35) in patients whose therapy was changed to pentamidine because of a lack of effect of TMP-SMX and 69 percent in patients whose therapy was changed because of adverse reactions. Overall, 74 (76 percent) of 97 patients who were initially given TMP-SMX survived. This rate was not significantly different from survival rates in adults (65 percent) and children (70 percent) with other forms of immunosuppression reviewed by Haverkos.

Of 107 patients reported in the National Heart, Lung, and Blood Institute workshop on the pulmonary complications of AIDS, 88 (82 percent) treated with TMP-SMX alone survived.[100] Of 37 patients who failed to complete a course of TMP-SMX, only 4 (11 percent) survived, whereas all 41 patients whose treatment was changed to pentamidine because of adverse reactions survived.

In the prospective studies by Wharton and coworkers,[113] Klein and associates,[56] and Sattler and colleagues,[94] survival rates for patients assigned to receive TMP-SMX were 75 percent (15 of 20), 63 percent (22 of 35), and 86 percent (31 of 36), respectively.

Dapsone (Diaminodiphenylsulfone)

Dapsone is a sulfone used nearly exclusively in the treatment of leprosy. In screening a number of agents for anti-*Pneumocystis* effects, Hughes and Smith found that dapsone was effective in both preventing and treating *P. carinii* pneumonia in cortisone-treated rats.[51] A dose of 25 mg/kg/d had an effect similar to TMP-SMX (50 and 250 mg/kg/d, respectively), whereas 5 mg/kg/d had a lesser but still apparent effect.

Based on these experimental results, Leoung and colleagues conducted an open trial of the combination of dapsone 100 mg/d and TMP 20 mg/kg/d in treating mild to moderate *P. carinii* pneumonia in patients with AIDS.[65] All 15 patients recovered. Although 14 of the 15 had minor adverse reactions, only two patients had to discontinue the drug, both because of rash. The most common minor reactions were nausea and vomiting. Subsequently these investigators completed an open trial of dapsone 100 mg without TMP and a prospective comparative trial of dapsone-TMP versus TMP-SMX.[75,81] Treatment with dapsone alone in a dose of 100 mg was associated with treatment failure or lack of improvement in 7 (39 percent) of 18 patients. No adverse effects required stopping the drug. Based on the results of this study, the investigators believed that dapsone was probably less effective than standard therapy and that it should not be used alone to treat *P. carinii* pneumonia.

In the trial comparing TMP-dapsone with TMP-SMX, treatment failure occurred in 2 (7 percent) of 29 patients in each group.[75] Major toxic effects occurred in 16 (55 percent) of 29 patients who received TMP-SMX and 9 (31 percent) of 29 given TMP-dapsone. The adverse effects of TMP-dapsone included skin rash (three patients), nausea and vomiting (two patients), and leukopenia, thrombocytopenia, hepatitis, and methemoglobinemia (all in one patient each). The authors concluded that TMP-dapsone was as effective as TMP-SMX and produced fewer adverse reactions in patients with mild to moderately severe *P. carinii* pneumonia.

α-*Difluoromethylornithine*

α-Difluoromethylornithine (DFMO) inhibits ornithine decarboxylase, thereby decreasing polyamine synthesis. It has been effective in treating African trypanosomiasis and affects other protozoa as well.[73] Although the drug was tested in the rat model of *P. carinii* pneumonia and had no effect, clinical studies have shown some promise. Golden and coworkers used DFMO in six AIDS patients who had received standard therapy and either failed to respond to or were intolerant of the agents.[36] The dosage was 6 g/m² body surface area daily divided into three doses and given for 8 weeks. All six patients had a successful outcome. Leukopenia or thrombocytopenia or both occurred in five of the patients.

McLees and associates reported on the results of DFMO in 234 patients with *P. carinii* pneumonia who were said to have failed to respond to standard treatment.[74] The dosage was 400 mg/kg/d given in 4 doses. The intended duration of intravenous administration was 14 days followed by 4 to 6 weeks of oral therapy in a dose of 75 mg/kg every 6 hours. These patients were severely ill; 45 percent were receiving mechanical ventilation. The survival rate was 36 percent (84 of 234). Reversible thrombocytopenia occurred in 43 percent and leukopenia in 11 percent.

Although both clinical trials of DFMO suggest that the agent might be useful, a prospective comparative evaluation will be necessary to determine its true effectiveness.

Trimetrexate

Trimetrexate is a newer antifolate that differs from TMP in that it does not require an active transmembrane transport process to enter cells.[3] It is several thousand times more potent an inhibitor of dihydrofolate reductase (DHFR) than TMP and must be administered with leucovorin (preformed tetrahydrofolate) to "rescue" mammalian (host) cells.

In an open trial reported by Allegra and associates, 14 (88 percent) of 16 patients given trimetrexate plus leucovorin as initial treatment for *P. carinii* pneumonia survived, although four required additional anti-*Pneumocystis* agents.[2] In six patients relapses occurred within 3 months of completion of therapy. In a separate group of 17 patients treated with trimetrexate-leucovorin plus sulfadiazine, the survival rate was 77 percent and 71 percent required no other agents. The relapse rate was only 6 percent. Trimetrexate-leucovorin was also used as "salvage" therapy in 16 patients who either did not respond to or could not tolerate standard treatment. The survival rate was 69 percent, no patients required additional agents, and no relapses occurred. The major toxic effects in all three groups were neutropenia, thrombocytopenia, and increased hepatic enzyme levels. Trimetrexate dose reductions were required by 19 percent of the patients.

In a preliminary report by Feinberg and coworkers only 47 percent of 115 patients treated with trimetrexate-leucovorin because of intolerance to conventional therapy survived.[29] Of a second group of 40 patients treated with trimetrexate-leucovorin because of failure to respond to standard agents, only five (13 percent) survived.

Clindamycin-Primaquin

The combination of the antibacterial agent clindamycin with the DHFR inhibitor primaquin has been evaluated in at least one open clinical trial. In a group of 27 patients who had no response to standard therapy or were intolerant of it and six patients who had not been treated previously, Toma et al reported "cures" in 23.[102] Adverse reactions, predominantly skin rash, occurred in 15 patients. Clinical response seemed to occur earlier in patients treated with clindamycin-primaquin than had been observed in responding patients treated conventionally.

Treatment Strategies

A synthesis of information available concerning the treatment of *P. carinii* pneumonia leads to both general and specific recommendations. As a rule treatment should be based on a proven diagnosis, especially in institutions having the capability of making diagnoses by examining induced sputum. Because of the high incidence of adverse drug reactions, treatment without a confirmed diagnosis subjects patients to risks that might be unwarranted. Moreover, given the large number of disorders that constitute the differential diagnosis of lung disease in immunocompromised patients, establishing a precise diagnosis before undertaking treatment is sound practice.

In patients with mild to moderately severe. *P. carinii* pneumonia who can take oral medications without problems, treatment should be initiated with oral TMP 20 mg/kg/d and SMX 100 mg/kg/d. The daily dosage can be divided into two or four doses, although twice-daily administration may not be tolerated because of gastrointestinal upset. If possible, either a TMP or SMX serum concentration should be measured 90 to 120 minutes after administration of the oral or intravenous dose on day 2 or 3 of therapy. The TMP concentration should be in the range of 5 to 8 μg/ml and SMX approximately 100 to 120 μg/ml.

Both TMP-dapsone and aerosol pentamidine appear to be suitable alternative forms of outpatient therapy for patients who do not have severe *P. carinii* pneumonia. For patients being given TMP-dapsone, methemoglobin saturations should be measured at 3- to 5-day intervals. Aerosol pentamidine appears as effective as TMP-SMX and probably TMP-dapsone. Moreover, it seems not to cause systemic toxic effects, although experience is insufficient to state this with certainty.

For patients who are more severely ill or cannot take oral drugs, TMP-SMX should be given intravenously in the same doses as for oral administration at 6-hour intervals. The physician should keep in mind that administering the total amount of drug requires infusion of approximately 1 L of 5 percent dextrose in water. Patients who require fluid restriction may not tolerate this volume.

Pentamidine is the alternative for patients who have had adverse reactions to sulfa agents or specifically to TMP-SMX or who cannot be given the fluid volume required to administer TMP-SMX. The dosage of pentamidine isethionate is 3 to 4 mg/kg/d given intravenously in a single daily administration. Patients should be monitored for hypotension during and shortly after the infusion.

The median time until response to either TMP-SMX or pentamidine is approximately 4 days, and some patients worsen before they begin to improve. Response should be judged by standard indices including degree of dyspnea, fever, respiratory rate, PaO_2, and chest radiograph. Patients probably should not be considered treatment failures with either drug until after 4 days of therapy. Continued worsening after 4 days or failure to improve after 7 to 10 days is an indication to change therapy, generally from TMP-SMX to pentamidine. The role of trimetrexate in salvage therapy has not yet been established, but current data suggest that it will be useful in this regard. At present the agent should be reserved for patients who fail to respond to both TMP-SMX and pentamidine. Trimetrexate is given intravenously in a daily dose of 30 to 45 mg/m² body surface area and must be administered with leucovorin, 20 mg/m² orally or intravenously. Sulfadiazine 1 g orally four times a day seems to decrease the frequency of relapse but does not have a demonstrated role in the initial response.

All patients should be observed carefully for adverse reactions throughout therapy, especially in the second week. At the time treatment is initiated, baseline tests of hepatic and renal function, a complete blood cell count with a differential count, and a platelet count should be obtained. Blood glucose should be measured in patients being given pentamidine. These tests should be repeated at 3-day intervals at least through day 14 of treatment. Adverse reactions that necessitate changing treatment include neutropenia (polymorphonuclear leukocytes <750/µl), thrombocytopenia (platelets >40,000/µl), elevation of serum creatinine level to more than 3 mg/d, aspartate or alanine aminotransferase increased to more than five times normal, and progressively worsening skin rash, especially if accompanied by mucositis or fever. If pentamidine produces hypotension or hypoglycemia, the drug should not necessarily be discontinued but should be administered with special care.

The necessary duration of therapy is not well established, but 14 to 21 days has become standard. Assessment of response to therapy should be based on clinical and radiographic grounds. Repeat examinations for *P. carinii* in AIDS patients who have been successfully treated show *P. carinii* in more than 60 percent, indicating that this is not a reliable means of determining cure.[78]

Supportive Care

Patients with *P. carinii* pneumonia characteristically have at least some degree of hypoxemia and thus commonly require supplemental oxygen. The severity of hypoxemia determines the oxygen delivery system to be used. With mild reduction in PaO₂, nasal prongs or cannulas usually provide sufficient enrichment of inspired air. As the gas exchange abnormality becomes more severe, standard masks, high-flow masks, reservoir masks, and tight-fitting anesthesia-type masks provide increasingly high inspired oxygen contents (FIO₂). Some patients require endotracheal intubation to ensure a high FIO₂ and to enable mechanical ventilation, often with the use of positive end-expiratory pressure (PEEP). The basic principles of mechanical ventilation in patients with severe *P. carinii* pneumonia are those that apply in the management of the adult respiratory distress syndrome, with generally high tidal volumes (12 to 15 ml/kg body weight) and PEEP.

P. carinii causes respiratory failure at least in part by increasing the permeability of the alveolar-capillary membrane, which in turn leads to interstitial and subsequently alveolar accumulation of fluid. For this reason administration of intravenous fluids should be monitored carefully in patients with *P. carinii* pneumonia. Overly vigorous fluid administration may increase pulmonary parenchymal fluid accumulation and further limit gas exchange.

Although many patients with *P. carinii* pneumonia are undernourished, the role of nutrition in influencing the outcome is not known. Malnutrition impairs cellular immunity, decreases respiratory muscle strength, and may increase the tendency for fluid accumulation within the lungs by decreasing plasma protein osmotic pressure. Thus ample rationale exists for attempting vigorous nutritional repletion, although benefits have not been documented. Parenteral hyperalimentation should be monitored carefully to avoid causing intravascular volume overload.

Corticosteroid Therapy

A number of anecdotal reports attest to the putative value of corticosteroid therapy in improving gas exchange in patients with severe *P. carinii* pneumonia.[32,53,69,107] For several reasons corticosteroids might improve lung function in patients with *P. carinii* pneumonia, so a benefit for this modality is plausible. However, in a prospective, randomized, double-blind study, Clement and associates were unable to show that corticosteroids improved outcome in patients with *P. carinii* pneumonia and a PaO_2 of 50 mm Hg or lower.[12] Moreover, the findings suggest that corticosteroids might increase the number of secondary infections and other steroid-associated adverse reactions. Relatively few patients were included in this study, so a small but significant difference in survival could have been present but not detected. At this point it cannot be said that corticosteroids have no value, but they do not appear to confer a major advantage.

PREVENTION

Although zidovudine and other antiretroviral drugs will probably cause the number of cases of *P. carinii* pneumonia to decrease, an estimated 40,000 to 60,000 patients will have their first episodes of this disease in 1990.[82] Moreover, without effective prophylaxis 30 to 35 percent of patients who have had one episode of *P. carinii* pneumonia will have at least one subsequent episode.[93] Given these data, effective prophylaxis for *P. carinii* pneumonia is extremely important for both individual and public health reasons.

Because of the effectiveness of TMP-SMX in preventing *P. carinii* pneumonia in children with hematologic malignancies, the disease has largely disappeared from this population. Unfortunately, preventing *P. carinii* pneumonia in AIDS patients is much more problematic, mainly because of the high incidence of adverse reactions to TMP-SMX in this group. In a study by Kaplan and coworkers, no conclusions as to the efficacy of TMP-SMX could be drawn because of the frequency of adverse reactions.[54] Fishl and associates reported both a lower frequency of adverse reactions than previously noted and a significant reduction in the incidence of *P. carinii* pneumonia when TMP-SMX was administered in a dose of 160 and 800 mg, respectively, twice a day, together with 5 mg folinic acid once a day.[31] In this study 5 (16.7 percent) of 30 patients given the drug had adverse effects that necessitated discontinuing the agent and 50 percent had minor adverse reactions. Four of the five patients in whom TMP-SMX was discontinued had subsequent development of *P. carinii* pneumonia as did 16 (53 percent) of 30 patients given placebo. Perhaps the most important observation from this study was that the median survival in the group given TMP-SMX was 20 months compared with 11 months in the control group. This observation substantiated the beneficial effect of *P. carinii* prophylaxis on the natural history of HIV infection.

As with TMP-SMX, the use of pentamidine in treating *P. carinii* pneumonia has been marked by frequent adverse reactions. Because of these reactions and the need for parenteral administration, use of the parenterally administered drug as a preventive agent has attracted little interest. However, because *P. carinii* is located predominantly within alveoli, aerosol administration of pentamidine has been investigated. It has proved to be effective and to have a low incidence of adverse effects.[28,66]

Leoung and coworkers in a prospective, randomized trial of aerosolized pentamidine demonstrated an inverse relationship between the dose of pentamidine and the incidence of *P. carinii* pneumonia.[66] The largest number of cases occurred in the subjects receiving 30 mg of pentamidine every 2 weeks; subjects receiving 150 mg every 2 weeks had an intermediate incidence of the disease; and subjects given 300 mg once a month had the lowest incidence. Only the difference in *P. carinii* incidence between the 30 mg and the 300 mg doses was statistically significant. In all three groups the aerosol was generated by a jet nebulizer that produced small particles (mean aerodynamic diameter 1.6 μm) delivered through a unidirectional breathing circuit with a small particle filter on the expiration limb of the device (Respigard II, Marquest Medical Products, Inc., Englewood, Colo.).

Investigators have noted that when *P. carinii* pneumonia developed in patients who had been given pentamidine aerosol prophylaxis, the upper lobes of the lungs were the predominant sites of disease.[68] This observation strongly suggests that the disease emerges where the pentamidine concentrations are the lowest. With normal tidal breathing little of the aerosol would be deposited in the upper lung zones, but with deeper breathing, exhaling to residual volume and then inhaling to total lung capacity, more even deposition would be achieved. Extrapulmonary pneumocystosis has also been noted in patients receiving aerosol pentamidine prophylaxis.

Adverse reactions to inhaled pentamidine aerosol have been few and generally mild. Coughing is common, especially in cigarette smokers, and bronchospasm may occur. These complications can be minimized by pretreatment with an inhaled bronchodilator such as albuterol. A few patients have had hypersensitivity reactions, but even patients who have had adverse reactions to intravenous pentamidine have generally not had difficulty with the aerosol.[84]

In the report by Leoung and associates, aerosol pentamidine and zidovudine did not have additive toxicity.[66] The two drugs did have an additive protective effect; patients who received both agents had greater levels of protection than provided by either drug alone.

Diaminodiphenylsulfone (dapsone), an antileprosy agent, has been used successfully with trimethoprim to treat *P. carinii* pneumonia. Dapsone alone appears to be useful as a preventive agent. Reports from two groups of investigators suggest that the drug is both safe and effective. Metroka et al reported substantial protective effects from dapsone given in doses of 25 mg four times a day.[76] Adverse reactions occurred in 10 percent of patients. Lang and coworkers found dapsone 50 to 100 mg/d to be effective in preventing *P. carinii* pneumonia and to have a low rate of adverse effects.[61]

Dapsone offers the advantages of being inexpensive and easily administered. However, the cost savings are offset somewhat by the need to monitor patients for adverse reactions, especially anemia. Moreover, the possible additive toxic effects of dapsone and zidovudine have not been determined.

Pyramethamine-sulfadoxine (Fansidar) has been tried in relatively small numbers of patients and seems to decrease the incidence of *P. carinii* pneumonia.[30] However, a major concern has been the drug's propensity to cause severe adverse reactions, including fatal Stevens-Johnson syndrome. For this reason its use has been limited. Given the better safety and probably at least equal efficacy of other agents, pyramethamine-sulfadoxine should not be used for preventive therapy.

Based on available data, the CDC has recommended that prophylaxis for *P. carinii* pneumonia be instituted for any HIV-infected adult who has had a previous episode of *P. carinii* pneumonia, who has a circulating CD4 + cell count of $<200/\mu$l peripheral blood, or who has a CD4 + cell count that is less than 20 percent of the total lymphocyte count.[10] The CDC has also recommended that patients with HIV infection have CD4 + cells measured at 6-month intervals or more frequently if a patient has an HIV-associated condition, such as thrush, that suggests immunocompromise. CD4 + counts may vary considerably over time, and thus rigid adherence to the 200 CD4+ cell threshold may miss some patients at risk for *P. carinii* infection. Candidates for prophylaxis should be evaluated to exclude current active pulmonary diseases, especially *Mycobacterium tuberculosis* infection. Persons with untreated active pulmonary tuberculosis who are given aerosol pentamidine may pose a particular hazard for spreading the organism.[11] Only aerosol pentamidine has been approved by the Food and Drug Administration as a prophylactic agent for *P. carinii*. The optimum regimen appears to be 300 mg given once a month with the Respigard II nebulizer. Bronchodilators given before pentamidine administration may minimize cough or bronchospasm. Patients should be instructed to inhale periodically to total lung capacity and inhale the aerosol in a recumbent position.

The use of dapsone alone as a prophylactic agent seems promising based on preliminary data.[61,76] If these findings are borne out in more rigorous studies, dapsone may prove even more useful than aerosol pentamidine because it is easily administered and inexpensive. Data currently available suggest that dapsone should be the second-line prophylaxis if aerosol pentamidine cannot be used. The usual prophylactic dosage has been 50 to 100 mg/d in single or divided doses.

REFERENCES

1. AIDS Program, Center for Infectious Diseases: AIDS Wkly Surveillance Rep, Oct 16, 1989
2. Allegra CJ, Chabner BA, Tuazon CU, et al: Trimetrexate for the treatment of *Pneumocystis carinii* pneumonia in patients with the acquired immunodeficiency syndrome. N Engl J Med 317:978, 1987
3. Allegra CJ, Kovacs JA, Drake JC, et al: Activity of antifolates against *Pneumocystis carinii* dehydrofolate reductase and identification of a potent new agent. J Exp Med 165:926, 1987
4. Beck JM, Shellito J: Effects of human immunodeficiency virus on pulmonary host defenses. Semin Respir Infect 4:75, 1989
5. Bibgy T, Margolskee D, Curtis J, et al: The usefulness of induced sputum in the diagnosis of *Pneumocystis carinii* pneumonia in patients with the acquired immunodeficiency syndrome. Am Rev Respir Dis 133:515, 1986
6. Blumenfeld W, Wagar E, Hadley WK: Use of the transbronchial biopsy for diagnosis of opportunistic pulmonary infections in the acquired immunodeficiency syndrome. Am J Clin Pathol 81:1, 1984
7. Bornstein RS, Yarbro JW: An evaluation of the mechanism of action of pentamidine isethionate. J Surg Oncol 2:393, 1970
8. Broaddus VC, Dake MD, Stulbarg MS, et al: Bronchoalveolar lavage and transbronchial biopsy for the diagnosis of pulmonary infections in patients with the acquired immunodeficiency syndrome. Ann Intern Med 102:747, 1985
9. Burke BA, Good RA: *Pneumocystis carinii*. Medicine 52:23, 1973
10. Centers for Disease Control: Guidelines for prophylaxis against *Pneumocystis carinii* pneumonia for persons infected with human immunodeficiency virus. MMWR 38(S-5):1, 1989
11. Centers for Disease Control: *Mycobacterium tuberculosis* transmission in a health clinic—Florida, 1989. MMWR 38:256, 1989
12. Clement M, Edison R, Turner J, et al: Corticosteroids as adjunctive therapy in severe *Pneumocystis carinii* pneumonia: A prospective placebo-controlled trial. Am Rev Respir Dis 139:A250, 1989

13. Cohen BA, Pomeranz S, Rabinowitz JG, et al: Pulmonary complications of AIDS: Radiologic features. AJR 143:115, 1984
14. Coleman DL, Dodek PM, Luce JM, et al: Diagnostic utility of fiberoptic bronchoscopy in patients with *Pneumocystis carinii* pneumonia and the acquired immunodeficiency syndrome. Am Rev Respir Dis 128:795, 1983
15. Coleman DL, Hattner RS, Luce JM, et al: Gallium lung scanning in patients with suspected pneumonia and the acquired immunodeficiency syndrome. Am Rev Respir Dis 130:1166, 1984
16. Coleman DL, Luce JM, Wilber JC, et al: Antibodies to the retrovirus associated with the acquired immunodeficiency syndrome (AIDS): Presence in presumably healthy San Franciscians who died unexpectedly. Arch Intern Med 146:713, 1986
17. Conte JE Jr, Hollander H, Golden JA: Inhaled pentamidine or reduced dose intravenous pentamidine for *Pneumocystis carinii* pneumonia: A pilot study. Ann Intern Med 107:495, 1987
18. Conte JE Jr, Upton RA, Phelps RT, et al: Use of a specific and sensitive assay to determine pentamidine pharmacokinetics in patients with AIDS. J Infect Dis 154:923, 1986
19. Curran JW, Morgan WM, Hardy AM, et al: The epidemiology of AIDS: Current status and future prospects. Science 229:1352, 1985
20. Curtis J, Goodman P, Hopewell PC: Noninvasive tests in the diagnostic evaluation for *P. carinii* pneumonia in patients with or suspected of having AIDS. Am Rev Respir Dis 133:A182, 1986
21. Deamer WC, Zollinger HU: Interstitial "plasma cell" pneumonia of premature and young infants. Pediatrics 12:11, 1953
22. Debs RJ, Blumenfeld W, Brunette EM, et al: Successful treatment with aerosolized pentamidine of *Pneumocystis carinii* in rats. Antimicrob Agents Chemother 31:37, 1987
23. Debs RJ, Straubinger RM, Brunette E, et al: Selective enhancement of pentamidine uptake in the lung by aerosolization and delivery in liposomes. Am Rev Respir Dis 135:731, 1987
24. Drake S, Lampasona V, Nicks HL, et al: Pentamidine isethionate in the treatment of *Pneumocystis carinii* pneumonia. Clin Pharm 4:507, 1985
25. Dutz W: *Pneumocystis carinii* pneumonia. Pathol Annu 5:309, 1970
26. Edman JC, Kovacs JA, Masur H, et al: Ribosomal RNA sequence shows *Pneumocystis carinii* to be a member of the fungi. Nature 334:519, 1988
27. Esterly JA: *Pneumocystis carinii* in lungs at autopsy. Am Rev Respir Dis 97:935, 1968
28. Feigal DW, Kandal K, Fallat R: Pentamidine aerosol prophylaxis for *Pneumocystis carinii* pneumonia (PCP): Efficacy in 211 AIDS and ARC patients (Abstract). In Program and abstracts of the Fourth International Conference on AIDS, Stockholm, Swedish Ministry of Health and Social Affairs, 1988
29. Feinberg J, Katy D, McDermott C, et al: Trimetrexate (TMX) salvage therapy of PCP in AIDS patients without any therapeutic options: Interim results of the first AIDS "treatment IND" protocol (Abstract No. TBO 28). In Program and abstracts of the Fifth International Conference on AIDS, Montreal, Canada, June 6–9, 1989, p 201
30. Fischl MA, Dickinson GM: Fansidar prophylaxis of *Pneumocystis* pneumonia in the acquired immunodeficiency syndrome. (Letter.) Ann Intern Med 105:629, 1986
31. Fischl MA, Dickinson GM, La Voie L: Safety and efficacy of sulfamethoxazole and trimethoprim chemoprophylaxis for *Pneumocystis carinii* pneumonia in AIDS. JAMA 259:1185, 1988
32. Foltzer MA, Hannan SE, Kozak AJ: *Pneumocystis* pneumonia: Response to corticosteroids. JAMA 253:979, 1985
33. Frenkel JK, Good JT, Schultz JA: Latent *Pneumocystis* infection of rats, relapse and chemotherapy. Lab Invest 15:1559, 1966
34. Gajdusek DC: *Pneumocystis carinii*—etiologic agent of interstitial plasma cell pneumonia of premature and young infants. Pediatrics 19:543, 1957
35. Golden JA, Hollander H, Stulbarg MS, et al: Bronchoalveolar lavage as the exclusive diagnostic modality for *Pneumocystis carinii* pneumonia. Chest 90:18, 1986
36. Golden JA, Sjoerdsma A, Santi DV: *Pneumocystis carinii* pneumonia treated with α difluoromethylornithine. West J Med 141:613, 1984
37. Gordin FM, Simon GL, Wofsy CR, et al: Adverse reactions to trimethoprim-sulfa-

methoxazole in patients with the acquired immunodeficiency syndrome. Ann Intern Med 100:495, 1984

38. Gottlieb MS, Schroff R, Schanker HM, et al: *Pneumocystis carinii* pneumonia and mucosal candidiasis in previously healthy homosexual men. N Engl J Med 305:1425, 1981
39. Hamlin WB: *Pneumocystis carinii*. JAMA 204:173, 1968
40. Hamperl H: *Pneumocystis* infection and cytomegaly of the lungs in the newborn and adult. Am J Pathol 32:1, 1956
41. Haverkos HW, PCP Therapy Project Group: Assessment of therapy for *Pneumocystis carinii* pneumonia. Am J Med 76:501, 1984
42. Hofmann B, Odum H, Platz P, et al: Humoral responses to *Pneumocystis carinii* in patients with the acquired immunodeficiency syndrome and in immunocompromised homosexual men. J Infect Dis 152:838, 1985
43. Hughes D: Chemoprophylaxis in chronic bronchitis. J Antimicrob Chemother 2:320, 1976
44. Hughes WT: Treatment of *Pneumocystis carinii* pneumonitis. N Engl J Med 295:726, 1976
45. Hughes WT: Natural mode of acquisition for de novo infection with *Pneumocystis carinii*. J Infect Dis 145:842, 1982
46. Hughes WT: The organism. In *Pneumocystis carinii* Pneumonitis. Boca Raton, Fla, CRC Press, 1987
47. Hughes WT, Feldman S, Chaudhary SC, et al: Comparison of pentamidine isethionate and trimethoprim-sulfamethoxazole in the treatment of *Pneumocystis carinii* pneumonia. J Pediatr 92:285, 1978
48. Hughes WT, Feldman S, Sanyal SK: Treatment of *Pneumocystis carinii* pneumonitis with trimethoprim-sulfamethoxazole. Can Med Assoc J 112:475, 1975
49. Hughes WT, Kuhn S, Chaudhary S, et al: Successful chemoprophylaxis for *Pneumocystis carinii* pneumonitis. N Engl J Med 297:1419, 1977
50. Hughes WT, McNabb PC, Makres TD, et al: Efficacy of trimethoprim and sulfamethoxazole in the prevention and treatment of *Pneumocystis carinii* pneumonitis. Antimicrob Agents Chemother 5:289, 1975
51. Hughes WT, Smith BL: Efficacy of diaminodiphenylsulfone and other drugs in murine *Pneumocystis carinii* pneumonitis. Antimicrob Agents Chemother 26:436, 1984
52 Ivady G, Paldy L, Koltay M, et al: *Pneumocystis carinii* pneumonia. Lancet 1:616, 1967
53. Jubran A, Matzke D, Pollard RB: Effects of corticosteroids on immediate survival from *Pneumocystis carinii* pneumonia (PCP) in patients with acquired immunodeficiency syndrome (Abstract). Presented at the Third International Conference on AIDS, Washington, DC, June 1–5, 1987
54. Kaplan LD, Wong R, Wofsy C, et al: Trimethoprim-sulfamethoxazole prophylaxis of *Pneumocystis carinii* pneumonia in AIDS (Abstract). In Proceedings of the Second International Conference on AIDS, 1986, p 53
55. Kirby HB, Kenamore B, Guckian JL: *Pneumocystis carinii* treated with pyramethamine and sulfadiazine. Ann Intern Med 75:505, 1971
56. Klein MC, Duncanson FP, Lennox TH, et al: Prospective randomized treatment for *Pneumocystis carinii* (PCP) in AIDS patients (Abstract). In Proceedings of the Second International Conference on AIDS, 1986, p 52
57. Kovacs JA, Allegra CJ, Beaver J, et al: Characterization of de novo folate synthesis in *Pneumocystis carinii* and *Toxoplasma gondii*: Potential utilization for screening therapeutic agents. J Infect Dis 160:312, 1989
58. Kovacs JA, Halpern JL, Swan JC, et al: Identification of antigens and antibodies specific for *Pneumocystis carinii*. J Immunol 140:2023, 1988
59. Kovacs JA, Ng VL, Masur H, et al: Diagnosis of *Pneumocystis carinii* pneumonia: Improved detection in sputum with use of monoclonal antibodies. N Engl J Med 318:589, 1988
60. Kucers A, Bennett NMcK: Trimethoprim and co-trimoxazole. In The Use of Antibiotics. London, William Heinemann Medical Books Ltd, 1979
61. Lang OS, Kessinger JM, Tucker RM, et al: Low dose dapsone prophylaxis of *Pneumocystis carinii* pneumonia (Abstract No. TRO5). In Proceedings of the Fifth International Conference on AIDS, 1989, p 196

62. Larter WE, John JT, Sieber OF, et al: Trimethoprim-sulfamethoxazole treatment of *Pneumocystis carinii* pneumonitis. J Pediatr 92:826, 1978
63. Lau WK, Young LS: Trimethoprim-sulfamethoxazole treatment of *Pneumocystis carinii* pneumonia in adults. N Engl J Med 297:1419, 1976
64. LeClair RA: Descriptive epidemiology of interstitial pneumocystic pneumonia: An analysis of 107 cases from the United States, 1955–1967. Am Rev Respir Dis 99:542, 1969
65. Leoung GS, Mills J, Hopewell PC, et al: Dapsone-trimethoprim for *Pneumocystis carinii* pneumonia in the acquired immunodeficiency syndrome. Ann Intern Med 105:45, 1986
66. Leoung GS, Montgomery AB, Abrams DA, et al: Aerosol pentamidine for *Pneumocystis carinii* (PCP) pneumonia: A randomized trial of 439 patients (Abstract). In Program and abstracts of the Fourth International Conference on AIDS, Stockholm, 1988
67. Lin J, Shi RJ, Lin ET: High performance liquid chromatographic determination of pentamidine in plasma. J Liquid Chromatog 9:2035, 1986
68. Lowry S, Fallat R, Feigel DW, et al: Changing patterns of *Pneumocystis carinii* pneumonia on pentamidine aerosol prophylaxis (Abstract). In Program and abstracts of the Fifth International Conference on AIDS, Montreal, Canada, June 6–9, 1989, p 419
69. MacFadden DK, Edelson JD, Hyland RH, et al: Corticosteroids as adjunctive therapy in treatment of *Pneumocystis carinii* pneumonia in patients with acquired immunodeficiency syndrome. Lancet 1:1477-79, 1987
70. Masur H, Jones TC: The interaction in vitro of *Pneumocystis carinii* with macrophages and L-cells. J Exp Med 147:157, 1978
71. Masur H, Michelis MA, Greene JB, et al: An outbreak of community acquired *Pneumocystis carinii* pneumonia. N Engl J Med 305:1431, 1981
72. Masur H, Ognibene FP, Yarchoan R, et al: CD4 counts as predictors of opportunistic pneumonias in human immunodeficiency virus (HIV) infection. Ann Intern Med 111:223, 1989
73. McCann PP, Bacchi CJ, Clarkson JR, et al: Further studies on difluoromethylornithine in African trypanosomes. Med Biol 59:434, 1981
74. McLees BD, Barlow JLR, Kuzma RJ, et al: Successful eflornithine (DFMO) treatment in AIDS patients failing conventional therapy. Am Rev Respir Dis 135:A167, 1987
75. Medina I, Leoung G, Mills J, et al: Oral therapy for *Pneumocystis carinii* pneumonia in AIDS: A randomized double-blind trial of trimethoprim-sulfamethoxazole versus dapsone trimethoprim for first episode *Pneumocystis carinii* pneumonia in AIDS (Abstract). In Proceedings of the Third International Conference on AIDS, 1987, p 208
76. Metroka CE, Jacobus D, Lewis N: Successful prophylaxis for *Pneumocystis* with dapsone or Bactrim (Abstract No. TRO4). In Proceedings of the Fifth International Conference on AIDS, Montreal, Canada, June 6–9, 1989, p 196
77. Meuwissen JHETh, Tauber I, Leeuwenberg ADEM, et al: Parasitologic and serologic observations of infection with *Pneumocystis* in humans. J Infect Dis 136:43, 1977
78. Michael P, Brodie H, Wharton M, et al: Significance of persistence of *P. carinii* after completion of treatment (Abstract). In Proceedings of the First International Conference on AIDS, 1985, p 23
79. Miller RF, Millar AB, Weller IVD, et al: Empirical treatment without bronchoscopy for *Pneumocystis carinii* pneumonia in the acquired immunodeficiency syndrome. Thorax 44:559, 1989
80. Milligan SA, Luce JM, Golden JA, et al: Transbronchial biopsy without fluoroscopy in patients with diffuse radiographic infiltrates and the acquired immunodeficiency syndrome. Am Rev Respir Dis 137:486, 1988
81. Mills J, Leoung G, Medina I, et al: Dapsone treatment of *Pneumocystis carinii* pneumonia in the acquired immunodeficiency syndrome. Antimicrob Agents Chemother 32:1057, 1988
82. Montgomery AB. *Pneumocystis carinii* pneumonia in patients with the acquired immunodeficiency syndrome: Pathophysiology, therapy, and prevention. Semin Respir Infect 4:102, 1989
83. Montgomery AB, Debs RC, Luce JM, et al: Selective delivery of pentamidine to the lung by aerosol. Am Rev Respir Dis 135:477, 1988

84. Montgomery AB, Debs RJ, Luce JM, et al: Aerosolized pentamidine as second-line therapy in patients with the acquired immunodeficiency syndrome and *Pneumocystis carinii* pneumonia. Chest 95:747, 1989
85. Montgomery AB, Luce JM, Turner J, et al: Aerosolized pentamidine as sole therapy for *Pneumocystis carinii* pneumonia in patients with the acquired immunodeficiency syndrome. Lancet 2:480, 1987
86. Moss AR, Bacchetti P, Osmond D, et al: Seropositivity for HIV and the development of AIDS or AIDS-related condition: Three year follow-up of the San Francisco General Hospital cohort. Br Med J 296:745, 1988
87. Murray JF, Felton CP, Garay S, et al: Pulmonary complications of the acquired immunodeficiency syndrome: Report of a National Heart, Lung and Blood Institute Workshop. N Engl J Med 310:1682, 1984
88. Ng VL, Gartner I, Weymouth LA, et al: The use of mucolysed induced sputum for the identification of pulmonary pathogens associated with human immunodeficiency virus infection. Arch Pathol Lab Med 113:488, 1989
89. Ng VL, Yajko DM, Gartner I, et al: Comparison of stains for the detection of *Pneumocystis carinii*. Am Rev Respir Dis 139:A147, 1989
90. Pesanti EL: In vitro effects of antiprotozoan drugs and immune serum on *Pneumocystis carinii*. J Infect Dis 141:775, 1980
91. Pifer LL, Hughes WT, Stagno S, et al: *Pneumocystis carinii* infection: Evidence for high prevalence in normal and immunosuppressed children. Pediatrics 61:35, 1978
92. Pitchenik AE, Ganjei P, Torres A, et al: Sputum examination for the diagnosis of *Pneumocystis carinii* in the acquired immunodeficiency syndrome. Am Rev Respir Dis 133:226, 1986
93. Rainer CA, Feigel DW, Leoung G, et al: Prognosis and natural history of *Pneumocystis carinii* pneumonia: Indicators for early and late survival (Abstract No. THP 154). In Proceedings of the Third International Conference on AIDS, Washington, DC, June 1–5, 1987, p 189
94. Sattler FR, Cowan R, Nielson DM, et al: Trimethoprim-sulfamethoxazole compared with pentamidine for treatment of *Pneumocystis carinii* pneumonia in the acquired immunodeficiency syndrome. Ann Intern Med 109:280, 1988
95. Sattler FR, Remington JS: Intravenous trimethoprim-sulfamethoxazole therapy for *Pneumocystis carinii* pneumonia. Am J Med 70:1215, 1981
96. Shellito J, Suzara VV, Blumenfeld W, et al: A new model of *Pneumocystis carinii* infection in mice selectively depleted of helper-T lymphocytes. J Clin Invest (in press), 1990
97. Sheppard V, Jameson B, Knowles GK: *Pneumocystis carinii* pneumonitis: A serological study. J Clin Pathol 32:773, 1979
98. Siegel SE, Wolff LJ, Baehner RL, et al: Treatment of *Pneumocystis carinii* pneumonitis. Am J Dis Child 138:1051, 1984
99. Singer C, Armstrong D, Rosen PP, et al: *Pneumocystis carinii* pneumonia: A cluster of eleven cases. Ann Intern Med 82:772, 1975
100. Stover DE, White DA, Romano PA, et al: Spectrum of pulmonary disease associated with the acquired immune deficiency syndrome. Am J Med 78:429, 1985
101. Stover DE, White DA, Romano PA, et al: Diagnosis of pulmonary disease in the acquired immune deficiency syndrome: Roles of bronchoscopy and bronchoalveolar lavage. Am Rev Respir Dis 131:659, 1984
102. Toma E, Fournier S, Poisson M, et al: Clindamycin-primaquin for *P. carinii* pneumonia in AIDS (Abstract No. TBO 31). In Proceedings of the Fifth International Conference on AIDS, Montreal, Canada, June 6–9, 1989, p 201
103. VonBehren LA, Pesanti EL: Uptake and degradation of *Pneumocystis carinii* by macrophages in vitro. Am Rev Respir Dis 118:1051, 1978
104. Waalkes TP, Denham C, DeVita VT: Pentamidine: Clinical pharmacological correlations in man and mice. Clin Pharmacol Ther 11:505, 1970
105. Waalkes TP, Makulu DR: Pharmacologic aspects of pentamidine. Natl Cancer Inst Monogr 43:171, 1976
106. Waldman RH, Pearce DE, Martin RA: Pentamidine isethionate levels in lungs, livers, and kidneys of rats after aerosol or intramuscular administration. Am Rev Respir Dis 108:1004, 1973

107. Walmsley S, Salit IE, Brunton J, et al: Corticosteroid therapy for *Pneumocystis* pneumonia in AIDS. In Program and abstracts of the 26th Interscience Conference on Antimicrobial Agents and Chemotherapy, Sept 28–Oct 1, 1986. Washington, DC, American Society for Microbiology, 1986

108. Walzer PD, Perl DP, Krogstad DJ, et al: *Pneumocystis carinii* pneumonia in the United States: Epidemiologic, diagnostic and clinical features. In Robbins JB, DeVita VT Jr (eds): Symposium on *Pneumocystis carinii* Infection. National Cancer Institute Monograph 43, DHEW Pub No NIH 76:930, Bethesda, Md, 1976

109. Walzer PD, Powell RD Jr, Yoneda K: Experimental *Pneumocystis carinii* pneumonia in different strains of cortisonized mice. Infect Immun 24:939, 1979

110. Walzer PD, Schnelle V, Armstrong D, et al: Nude mouse: A new experimental model for *Pneumocystis carinii* infection. Science 197:177, 1977

111. Watanabe JM, Chinchinian H, Weitz G, et al: *Pneumocystis carinii* pneumonia in a family. JAMA 193:685, 1965

112. Western KA, Perera DR, Schultz MG: Pentamidine isethionate in the treatment of *Pneumocystis carinii* pneumonia. Ann Intern Med 73:695, 1970

113. Wharton JM, Coleman DL, Wofsy CB, et al: Trimethoprim-sulfamethoxazole or pentamidine for *Pneumocystis carinii* pneumonia in the acquired immunodeficiency syndrome. Ann Intern Med 105:37, 1985

114. Winston DJ, Lau WK, Gale RP, et al: Trimethoprim-sulfamethoxazole for the treatment of *Pneumocystis carinii* pneumonia. Ann Intern Med 92:762, 1980

115. Wong H, Caughey G, Gamsu G, et al: Nonbronchoscopic catheter bronchoalveolar lavage in the diagnosis of *Pneumocystis carinii* pneumonia. Am Rev Respir Dis 131:A222, 1985

116. Young LS: Clinical aspects of pneumocystosis in man: Epidemiology, clinical manifestations, diagnostic approaches and sequelae. In Young LS (ed): *Pneumocystis carinii* Pneumonia. New York, Marcel Dekker, Inc, 1984, p 139

16

TOXOPLASMOSIS IN PATIENTS WITH AIDS

DENNIS M. ISRAELSKI, MD
BRIAN R. DANNEMANN, MD
JACK S. REMINGTON, MD

Toxoplasma gondii is among the most prevalent causes of latent infection of the central nervous system (CNS) throughout the world. Although a complete review of the biology of *Toxoplasma* is beyond the scope of this chapter, it is important to understand that *Toxoplasma* is a protozoan which exists in three forms: proliferative (tachyzoite), tissue cyst, and oocyst. Felines are the definitive host and reservoir for sporozoite production (oocysts), while only tachyzoites and cysts are found in incidental hosts (e.g., mammals). Each of these forms is potentially infectious for humans.[90] Following acute infection, cysts of *T. gondii* persist in the CNS as well as in multiple extraneural tissues. Although normal human hosts have immunity sufficient to maintain infection in a quiescent state, immunocompromised individuals may be at risk for reactivation and dissemination of chronic (latent) infection.[32,34] Defective cellular immunity in patients with AIDS results in loss of the primary arm of host defense against this parasite. Infection with HIV may lead to depletion of helper/inducer (CD4) T-cell lymphocytes and macrophage dysfunction[30] and predispose to reactivation and dissemination of latent *Toxoplasma* infection. Reactivation of latent infection in patients with AIDS may lead to clinically apparent disease (toxoplasmosis) which usually presents as a life-threatening encephalitis.[76,107] Thus, patients with AIDS who have been previously infected with *Toxoplasma* are at considerable risk for development of CNS toxoplasmosis.

Toxoplasmic encephalitis was observed early in the AIDS epidemic[62,42] and has now been recognized as a major cause of opportunistic infection of the CNS[59] and the most frequent cause of focal intracerebral lesions in patients with AIDS.[59,86,99,106] Because AIDS patients in the United States who develop toxoplasmic encephalitis are almost always chronically infected with the protozoan,[61] patients who from the outset of their AIDS (or even individuals without AIDS who have antibody to HIV and who are known to also have antibodies to *T. gondii*) should be considered at significant risk for development of toxoplasmic encephalitis. Data obtained in a retrospective study reveal that at least 30 percent of AIDS patients who are seropositive for *T. gondii* will ultimately develop toxoplasmic encephalitis.[39] Seroprevalence varies between different geographic locales and even within populations in the same locale. In major urban areas in the United States, the prevalence of *Toxoplasma* antibodies among (nonpediatric) individuals at high risk for HIV infection is approximately 11 to 16 percent (JS Remington et al, unpublished data). Thus, we estimate that by 1992 there will have been between 10,000 and 30,000 cases of toxoplasmic encephalitis in patients with AIDS. The high incidence of this opportunistic infection of the CNS in patients with AIDS makes it essential that physicians caring for such patients understand how to diagnose and manage toxoplasmic encephalitis.

CLINICAL PRESENTATION

In the United States, AIDS patients who develop toxoplasmic encephalitis generally do so after the diagnosis of AIDS has been made.[76,107] In areas where seroprevalence of *T. gondii* infection is high, toxoplasmic encephalitis frequently is the initial manifestation of AIDS.[5,13,38,56,81] Of 28,920 cases of AIDS reported between September 1987 and December 1988 to the CDC, 1070 (3.7 percent) had a definitive or presumptive diagnosis of CNS toxoplasmosis as their initial AIDS-defining illness (personal communication to DMI, by RM Selik, CDC Division HIV/AIDS, 1989). These figures considerably underestimate the prevalence of CNS toxoplasmosis in patients with AIDS, since the vast majority of cases in the United States are presumptively diagnosed after the diagnosis of AIDS has already been made and therefore are not reported to the CDC. With the advent of primary prophylaxis of *Pneumocystis carinii* pneumonia (PCP) with inhalational pentamidine, we anticipate that toxoplasmic encephalitis will be increasingly detected as the first opportunistic infection in patients with AIDS.

When taking a medical history, it is important to note the geographic origin or residence and dietary habits of the patient since these factors will reflect the relative risk of acquired *Toxoplasma* infection. *T. gondii* is a ubiquitous organism and causes infection throughout most of the developing world.[90] When infected beef, lamb, or pork is consumed raw or undercooked, as is customary in certain cultures, infection with *Toxoplasma* can result. Owing largely to their culinary habits, between 70 and 96 percent of the adult populations of Germany and France have serologic evidence of *Toxoplasma* infection.[80,90] This has resulted in the remarkable incidence rate of toxoplasmic encephalitis of at least 25 percent in AIDS patients in these countries.[80,82] Independent of category of risk for acquisition of HIV infection, AIDS-associated toxoplasmosis in the United States has been reported to occur significantly more often in Hispanic than in white patients.[7]

A review of the literature indicates that 10 to 74 percent of AIDS patients with toxoplasmic encephalitis are reported to have fever,[14,46,56,76,103,107] and 44 to 78 percent will complain of headache.[14,46,58,76] Altered mental status, manifested by confusion, lethargy, delusional behavior, frank psychosis, global cognitive impairment, anomia, or coma may be present initially in as many as 60 percent of patients.[14,46,56,76] Seizures as a cause for the patient to seek medical attention are seen in approximately one third of AIDS patients with toxoplasmic encephalitis.[14,46,58] Focal neurologic deficits will be evident on neurologic examination in approximately 60 percent.[14,46,76] Although hemiparesis is the most common focal finding,[46,76] patients may have evidence of aphasia, ataxia, visual field loss, cranial nerve palsies, dysmetria, or movement disorders.[56,76] An uncommon, rapidly fatal, panencephalitis form of cerebral toxoplasmosis has also been described[40,58]; unfortunately, neuroradiologic evaluation was unrevealing in these cases.[40]

In a few cases, toxoplasmic chorioretinitis has been reported to precede or accompany CNS disease.[79,99,104] Endocrinopathies secondary to the syndrome of inappropriate antidiuretic hormone secretion (SIADH)[29] or panhypopituitarism[71] may be the primary manifestation or a later complication of CNS toxoplasmosis. In addition, a case has been reported of a patient with transverse myelitis due to toxoplasmosis.[70] The patient had received irradiation and corticosteroids for a presumptive diagnosis of lymphoma and died of necrosis of the cervical cord.[70]

Toxoplasmic pneumonitis has been increasingly recognized as a cause of pulmonary infiltrates in patients with AIDS. This diagnosis should be considered in the appropriate clinical setting, especially in patients who are receiving prophylaxis for PCP and who present with symptoms and signs referable to the lung.[8,24,66] Autopsy series and case reports indicate that extraneurologic toxoplasmosis is not rare and should be considered in the differential diagnosis of unexplained disorders of the heart,[66,72,91] peritoneum,[48] pancreas,[66] liver,[66] colon,[66] and testes.[17,77]

AIDS patients with CNS toxoplasmosis are characteristically anergic and have a history of oral candidiasis and depressed numbers of CD4 T-lymphocytes.[4,89] HIV-infected patients with a CNS process and CD4 T-cell counts >400/mm³ are generally considered unlikely to have toxoplasmic encephalitis (unpublished observation and[89]), but no systematic study has been published which correlates occurrence of AIDS-associated toxoplasmosis with quantitation of T-cell lymphocyte subpopulations.

Abnormalities in routine clinical laboratory tests are too nonspecific to be of diagnostic utility. Commonly, AIDS patients are receiving antimicrobial agents which may cause hematopoietic, hepatic, or renal abnormalities.

Hyponatremia may occur from SIADH, presumably due to intracerebral mass lesions.[29] A case of toxoplasmic encephalitis with laboratory abnormalities of the hypothalamic–anterior pituitary–adrenal axis has been described.[71] CSF may be normal or reveal mild pleocytosis (predominantly lymphocytes and monocytes) and elevated protein while the glucose content is usually normal.[29,76,103,107] Computed tomography (CT) or magnetic resonance imaging (MRI) studies may be highly suggestive of toxoplasmic encephalitis.[20]

DIAGNOSIS

At present, the definitive diagnosis of toxoplasmic encephalitis can be made only by demonstration of the organism in brain tissue. Aside from the morbidity associated with obtaining a brain biopsy, neurosurgery is often impractical, since AIDS patients with neurologic syndromes frequently present with numerous or inaccessible intracerebral lesions.[59] The desire to avoid brain biopsy has resulted in the almost universal practice of initiation of empiric anti-*Toxoplasma* therapy in AIDS patients who have characteristic findings on neuroradiologic imaging studies. In this setting, alternative etiologies should be sought when the patient fails to respond clinically or radiologically; brain biopsy is frequently the only alternative in this situation.

Serology

Toxoplasmic encephalitis in patients with AIDS almost always represents reactivation of chronic (latent) infection.[63] In our experience only approximately 1 to 3 percent of AIDS patients with toxoplasmic encephalitis do not have detectable IgG *Toxoplasma* antibodies in their serum. Unfortunately, the demonstration of IgG antibodies cannot distinguish latent infection from active infection. In addition, disease activity does not necessarily correlate with the magnitude of the IgG antibody titer measured by standard techniques.[61] Furthermore, significant rise in antibody titer occurs too infrequently to be of routine value in establishing the diagnosis.[61,76] A recent study using a modification of the agglutination method,[101] however, has found that magnitude of antibody titers may prove valuable for the noninvasive diagnosis of AIDS-associated toxoplasmic encephalitis.[101]

In addition to their value in predicting which patients are at risk for development of toxoplasmosis, absence of IgG *Toxoplasma* antibodies in an AIDS patient with intracerebral mass lesions is strong evidence against the diagnosis of toxoplasmic encephalitis. IgM *Toxoplasma* antibodies, routinely measured to diagnose acute toxoplasmosis in non-AIDS patients,[90] are rarely present in AIDS patients with toxoplasmic encephalitis.[61,76]

**TABLE 16–1. METHODS FOR DEFINITIVE OR PRESUMPTIVE
DIAGNOSIS OF TOXOPLASMIC ENCEPHALITIS IN
PATIENTS WITH AIDS**

Brain biopsy
    Histopathologic evaluation
    Immunoperoxidase staining
    Isolation study
Demonstration of *Toxoplasma* in CSF (Wright-Giemsa stain)
Isolation of *Toxoplasma* from body fluid (blood, CSF)
Computed tomography (CT) and magnetic resonance imaging (MRI)
Antigen detection in body fluid (serum, CSF, urine)
Serology (including titer in agglutination assay, IgG, IgM*)
Intrathecal production of *Toxoplasma*-specific antibodies

*Useful mainly in areas of high seroprevalence.
CSF = Cerebrospinal fluid.

If the serologic status of the patient treated empirically for toxoplasmic encephalitis is unknown, determination of IgG antibody titers should be performed. Studies for demonstration of *Toxoplasma* antibodies can be performed by local, county, state, and reference laboratories (Table 16–1). We presently employ the Sabin-Feldman dye[93] and agglutination tests[90,101] to measure *Toxoplasma*-specific IgG antibodies, as opposed to the more widely used but frequently less reliable indirect fluorescent antibody assay (IFA).[90]

When CSF is available, measurement of intrathecal production of antibody to *T. gondii* may serve as a useful ancillary test.[84] The proportional production of *Toxoplasma* antibody in the CSF can be determined by the formula[51]:

$$\frac{\text{CSF dye test titer (reciprocal)}}{\text{Total CSF IgG}} \times \frac{\text{Total serum IgG}}{\text{Serum dye test titer (reciprocal)}}$$

A value greater than one is indicative of intrathecal *Toxoplasma* antibody formation and suggests the diagnosis of toxoplasmic encephalitis.[84]

Isolation Studies

Isolation of *T. gondii* from body fluids or, in the appropriate clinical setting, from tissue obtained from a patient with AIDS, should be considered diagnostic of active infection. Because isolation of the organism may not be evident for 6 days to 6 weeks after mice or tissue cultures are inoculated, the results are usually not helpful in initial management of the patient. Nevertheless, isolation of the organism may obviate future need for brain biopsy.

The epidemic of toxoplasmic encephalitis in patients with AIDS has renewed the interest in methods for in vitro isolation of the organism.[45] *Toxoplasma* readily forms plaques in tissue cultures of human foreskin fi-

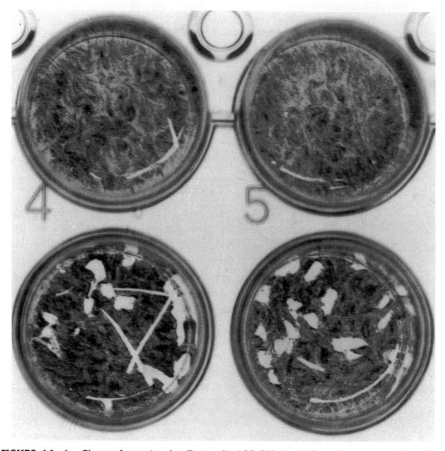

FIGURE 16–1. Plaque formation by *T. gondii*; 100 RH strain *Toxoplasma* were inoculated onto semi-confluent monolayers of human foreskin fibroblasts. Plaques (*bottom row*) were observed at 96 hr. Top row are uninfected (control) monolayers.

broblasts (Fig. 16–1) and most other cultured cells. The plaques, when stained with Wright-Giemsa and examined microscopically, are seen to consist of necrotic and heavily infected cells as well as numerous extracellular tachyzoites. As few as three organisms can cause plaque formation in a semiconfluent human fibroblast monolayer as early as 4 days after inoculation,[23] although this will vary with the virulence of the strain of *T. gondii*. Similarly, *T. gondii* may be isolated from bronchoalveolar lavage fluid in patients with toxoplasmic pneumonitis as early as 48 hours after tissue culture inoculation.[24] Any diagnostic microbiology or virology laboratory which can inoculate the buffy coat of blood or bronchoalveolar fluid into tissue culture has the capacity to isolate *T. gondii* from patients with active infection.[24,98]

Antigen Detection

Methods for detection of *Toxoplasma* antigen in serum, CSF, or other body fluid of AIDS patients are currently used as research tools to diagnose active infection. Our laboratory has employed an enzyme-linked immunosorbent assay (ELISA) to detect low concentrations of *Toxoplasma* antigen in sera, amniotic fluid, and CSF of non-AIDS patients with acute toxoplasmosis.[2] In preliminary studies using a modification of this ELISA technique, we have detected *Toxoplasma* antigens in urine samples from 5 of 20 patients with AIDS-associated toxoplasmic encephalitis.[47] The profoundly diminished capacity of the immune system of AIDS patients to both contain and kill *T. gondii* may give the organism an opportunity to replicate freely in vivo. We would expect such patients to have a relatively high parasitic burden compared to immunocompetent patients with toxoplasmosis. Thus, reliable methods for the detection of antigens of *T. gondii* in body fluids of patients with AIDS may become increasingly important for noninvasive diagnosis of toxoplasmosis.

Neuroradiologic Studies

Toxoplasmic encephalitis is the most common cause of focal intracerebral lesions in patients with AIDS (Table 16–2).[58,86,99,106] Imaging studies of the

TABLE 16–2. HISTOPATHOLOGIC DIAGNOSIS IN AIDS PATIENTS WITH FOCAL LESIONS ON COMPUTER TOMOGRAPHY

DIAGNOSIS	% PATIENTS
Toxoplasmosis	50-70
Primary CNS lymphoma	10-25
Progressive multifocal leukoencephalopathy	10-22
Nondiagnostic	10
Candida albicans abscess	3
Cryptococcoma	2
Kaposi's sarcoma	2
Mycobacterium tuberculosis abscess	1
Herpes simplex virus type 2	1

Adapted from De La Paz RL, Enzman D: Neuroradiology of acquired immunodeficiency syndrome. In Rosenblum ML, et al (eds): AIDS and the Nervous System. New York, Raven Press, 1988.

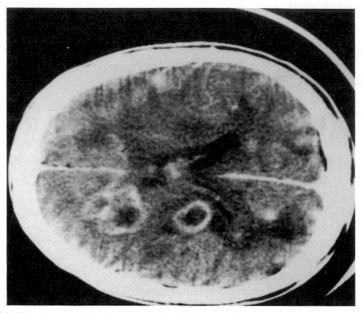

FIGURE 16–2. Computerized tomography (CT) scan of an AIDS patient with toxoplasmic encephalitis. Multiple, hypodense, ring-enhancing lesions were seen.

brain have become indispensable for diagnosis and management of these patients (Chapter 12). Typically, multiple, bilateral, hypodense, enhancing mass lesions are found on CT scan (Fig. 16–2).[25,29,76,85] Lesions have a predilection for the basal ganglia and hemispheric corticomedullary junction.[6,25,29,85] A significant degree of enhancement of intracerebral lesions is generally present on CT scan.[6,25,29,56,76,85,86,103] *Toxoplasma* abscesses may, however, fail to enhance or be solitary and located anywhere in the brain.[20]

There may be considerable variation between different scans, dependent on the dose of intravenous contrast material administered.[86] A double dose of contrast material gives maximal enhancement and demonstrates "filling in" of ring lesions on 1-hour delayed scans.[86] Thus, double-dose delayed CT scan may be preferable to single-dose nondelayed studies in that it provides more information on number, extent, and degree of enhancement of the intracerebral lesions.[20,86] CNS lymphoma, which is multicentric in at least 50 percent of cases, may also enhance on CT.[58,67] Multiple focal intracerebral lesions may also be seen in progressive multifocal leukoencephalopathy (PML). In general, the CT scan of patients with PML show areas of nonenhanced low attenuation in the hemispheric white matter conforming to the contours of the centrum ovale.[20] In conclusion, abnormalities found on CT scan are not pathognomonic for toxoplasmic encephalitis, but number, location, and degree of enhancement of the mass lesions may suggest the diagnosis.

Masses demonstrated by the more sensitive MRI may be absent on CT scan, whereas the converse does not appear to be true.[20,87] In a review of 82 AIDS patients with focal neurologic symptoms,[20] CT appeared to be as good as MRI scan in detecting focal brain lesions (70 versus 74 percent). However, in 111 AIDS patients with nonfocal neurologic symptoms, only 22 percent had CT scans that revealed focal lesions compared to 42 percent found by MRI studies.[20] As in CT scans, lesions found on MRI scans of AIDS patients with toxoplasmic encephalitis are frequently bilateral and located in the basal ganglia or cerebral corticomedullary junction.[21,87] Deep lesions, which generally range between 1 and 3 cm in diameter, may show central patterns of both low and high signal intensity, suggestive of necrosis.[20] Unlike CT, MRI scans invariably demonstrate multiple intracerebral lesions.[21,87] In fact, a single lesion on MRI scan should alert the physician to other possible etiologies for the focal neuroradiologic findings (e.g., lymphoma, fungal abscess, tuberculoma, or Kaposi's sarcoma). The finding of more than three focal lesions on MRI scan, however, is highly suggestive of toxoplasmic encephalitis.[20,21] As with results of CT scans, no MRI finding can be considered pathognomonic for toxoplasmic encephalitis.

The neuroradiologic response of toxoplasmic encephalitis to specific treatment is seen on CT scan as a reduction in mass effect, number, and extent of lesions, and enhancement. While patients who respond clinically will have evidence of improvement in their CT scan,[56,76] the time to resolution of lesions may vary from 20 days to 6 months.[60] The response of abnormalities on MRI scan to specific therapy also varies with the location and complexity of the mass lesion.[21] Peripheral lesions of uniform signal intensity on MRI scan frequently resolve after 3 to 5 weeks of therapy, whereas deeper lesions with complex central signal patterns, consistent with necrosis, take longer to resolve and leave residual lesion(s) at the site of necrosis.[20,21]

Histopathology

As alluded to earlier, despite highly suggestive neuroradiologic studies, definitive diagnosis of toxoplasmic encephalitis often requires demonstration of the organism on histopathologic sections of brain tissue obtained at biopsy. Needle brain biopsy or aspiration is limited by lack of specificity and sensitivity of the procedure to make a definitive diagnosis, since size of the specimen may be too small or there may be sampling error.[64,103] There is some evidence which demonstrates superiority of open excisional biopsy compared to needle biopsy in making the histopathologic diagnosis of toxoplasmic encephalitis.[103] Moreover, the observation of abnormal lym-

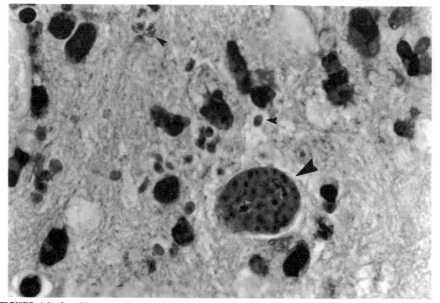

FIGURE 16–3. Hematoxylin-eosin stain of brain section of AIDS patient demonstrating necrosis and presence of *T. gondii* cysts (*broad arrowhead*) and extracellular tachyzoite forms (*narrow arrowheads*).

phocytes in areas of involvement demonstrated by needle biopsy or aspiration not infrequently has led to the erroneous diagnosis of cerebral lymphoma.

The response of the brain to *Toxoplasma* infection can vary from a granulomatous reaction with gliosis and microglial nodule formation to a severe focal or generalized necrotizing encephalitis.[29,63,76,85] Granulomatous lesions with a cellular infiltrate of abnormal lymphocytes, plasma cells, neutrophils, and monocytes may enlarge and develop central regions of necrosis.[29,63,76,85] Perivascular and intimal inflammatory cell infiltrates can lead to fibrosis or necrosis,[29,63,76,85] can result in vessel rupture or thrombosis,[63,76] and may account for the neurologic symptoms and symptoms of the patient.

The presence of numerous *Toxoplasma* cysts or tachyzoites is diagnostic (Fig. 16–3).[90] Tachyzoites, when observed, are usually found within the inflammatory reaction surrounding areas of necrosis.[29,63,76,85] Cysts or free organisms not demonstrable on routine histopathologic examination may be identified using the peroxidase-antiperoxidase method to stain *Toxoplasma* antigens and organisms in brain tissue.[15,103] This method is significantly more sensitive and no less specific in making the diagnosis of toxoplasmic encephalitis than is direct visualization of the organisms in association with cerebral inflammation and necrosis.[15,56,63] A rapid, sensitive, and specific method for diagnosis of toxoplasmic encephalitis by electron microscopy has been described.[11] Thus, when routine histopathologic studies fail to make a definitive diagnosis, appropriately fixed brain tissue should be stained by the immunoperoxidase technique or analyzed by electron microscopy in an attempt to identify *T. gondii* antigens or organisms.

Wright-Giemsa stained touch preparations should be made as immediately as is feasible from tissue obtained at brain biopsy. This can be rapidly accomplished in the clinical laboratory where stains of blood smears are performed. If organisms are demonstrated, this will enable prompt initiation of potentially life-saving therapy.[63] Similarly, when CSF can be safely obtained, Wright-Giemsa stain of a cytocentrifuge preparation of CSF may reveal the presence of tachyzoites.[22]

Differential Diagnosis

In AIDS patients with focal abnormalities on neurologic examination, multiple enhancing lesions on CT scan and a positive *Toxoplasma* antibody titer strongly suggest the diagnosis of toxoplasmic encephalitis. Regardless of results of *Toxoplasma* serology, the differential diagnosis for individuals with nonfocal symptoms and one or two lesions on CT scan includes, in addition to CNS toxoplasmosis, lymphoma, fungal abscess, mycobacterial or cytomegaloviral (CMV) disease, and Kaposi's sarcoma. Since therapy is available for each of these disorders, brain biopsy for histopathologic diagnosis may become necessary for successful management of the patient. The characteristic appearance of PML on neuroimaging studies often permits this disorder to be distinguished from other causes of intracerebral mass lesions.

Skin testing for anergy and quantitation of T-lymphocyte subsets are recommended during routine outpatient evaluation of the HIV-infected patient.[89] Results of these tests may be useful to gauge suspicion for the presence of an AIDS-related opportunistic CNS process. Thus, patients capable of delayed type hypersensitivity reactions to common antigens or who are without severely depressed CD4 cell counts may suffer from conditions unassociated with HIV infection, such as bacterial abscesses, primary or metastatic brain tumors, neurocystercycosis, arteriovenous malformations, or multiple sclerosis.

MANAGEMENT

General Principles

Since toxoplasmic encephalitis generally reflects reactivation of a latent infection, we believe all individuals with ARC or AIDS should have their sera tested for *Toxoplasma*-specific IgG antibody. Patients with positive titers are at risk for development of toxoplasmic encephalitis, and the results of the serology should be clearly available in the chart in case a patient presents with signs referable to the CNS. Head CT scan is the standard initial test for evaluation of AIDS patients suspected of having CNS toxoplasmosis. In patients with nonfocal neurologic abnormality and a negative CT scan on presentation, MRI scan should be obtained. If MRI is readily available it is preferable as the initial evaluation in such patients. Since a single lesion on MRI is uncharacteristic of *Toxoplasma* infection,[20] this should prompt biopsy of the involved area; expedient and aggressive evaluation of AIDS patients with CNS mass lesions may avert erroneous and potentially toxic treatment regimens.

AIDS patients with multiple ring enhancing intracranial lesions on neuroimaging studies should be started on therapy for presumptive toxoplasmic encephalitis. It is important to recognize that the presence of multiple simultaneous intracranial lesions is a common feature of CNS dysfunction in AIDS.[58] Focal intracranial lesions due to *Toxoplasma* may occur in association with cerebral lymphoma[60] or *M. tuberculosis*.[86] In AIDS patients with concurrent focal and diffuse CNS disease, toxoplasmosis has also been found in association with CMV encephalitis and cryptococcal meningitis.[86]

Patients who respond to empiric treatment for toxoplasmosis generally exhibit significant clinical improvement within 10 to 14 days after initiation of therapy.[56,64,76] Repeat neuroradiologic study by the same modality as originally selected should be performed 4 to 6 weeks after the initiation of therapy in patients with a satisfactory response to therapy (or earlier if response is poor). Lesions should have diminished in size and possibly in number. Change in degree of enhancement is, however, too nonspecific to be of value in the assessment of therapeutic response.[26] Progression of clinical or radiologic abnormalities after 1 week or lack of evident improvement after 2 weeks of treatment should raise the possibility of alternative or multiple etiologies. Patients with extraneurologic toxoplasmosis should be evaluated for CNS disease, since most will have intracerebral involvement as well.[66]

Corticosteroids are frequently required for management of patients with intracranial hypertension from mass effect due to *Toxoplasma* abscesses. Whether corticosteroids affect outcome in AIDS patients with toxoplasmic encephalitis is unknown. At present, therefore, AIDS patients with toxoplasmic encephalitis should be subjected to additional immunosuppression by corticosteroids only when it is neurologically contraindicated to withhold their administration. We believe whenever corticosteroids are used, the course of administration should be as brief as possible.

Whether anticonvulsant agents are necessary for prevention of seizures has not been determined, although one retrospective study has shown a negative correlation between survival and treatment with anticonvulsant medications in patients with AIDS-associated toxoplasmic encephalitis.[14] Whether this finding represents a true drug effect or it is merely that more seriously ill patients receive anticonvulsant agents is unknown. As a guideline, patients with seizures at presentation should be placed on anticonvulsant agents at least during primary treatment of the acute encephalitis.

It is important to distinguish between two forms of therapy for toxoplasmic encephalitis in patients with AIDS: primary therapy and maintenance therapy. Primary therapy is administered during what is considered the acute neurologic disease. Maintenance therapy is administered after an adequate clinical and neuroradiologic response has been observed. Maintenance therapy should be continued for life, since the rate of relapse is prohibitively high when treatment is discontinued.

Primary Therapy

At present, it is standard practice to administer the combination of pyrimethamine and sulfadiazine (or trisulfapyrimidines). This combination sequentially blocks folic acid metabolism of the proliferative form of the organism and is synergistic against *T. gondii* both in vitro[16] and in vivo.[27,28] There is no general agreement regarding dosages of pyrimethamine and sulfonamides which should be used for treatment of the acute encephalitis.[14,37,64,105] Anecdotal reports of AIDS patients with toxoplasmic encephalitis who fail to respond to 25 mg/d of pyrimethamine alone are sufficiently frequent (JS Remington, et al, unpublished observations) that we currently recommend 1 to 1.5 mg/kg/d (75 to 100 mg/d) after a 200-mg loading dose (Table 16–3). Whether toxoplasmic encephalitis can be effectively treated solely with pyrimethamine at these or even higher doses is not yet known and should be investigated.

Few data regarding the pharmacokinetics of pyrimethamine are available.[9] Serum concentrations of pyrimethamine in individuals treated with the same dose of drug have great variability.[9,54,105] This variability may in part reflect erratic absorption of pyrimethamine in patients with AIDS-associated enteropathies. Although serum concentrations cannot be predicted for a given dose[54,105] or even for a given patient on a given day, serum concentrations of pyrimethamine significantly increase with increasing dose.[54] In a recent study, several patients with AIDS-associated CNS toxoplasmosis who were treated daily with 25 or 50 mg of pyrimethamine were found to have peak or trough serum concentrations lower than or barely exceeding the concentration of pyrimethamine required in vitro for toxoplasmacidal activity.[49,54,65] In contrast, all patients who were treated daily with 100 mg of pyrimethamine had peak and trough serum concentrations well above the minimal concentration required in vitro for toxoplasmacidal activity.[49,54,65] When CSF penetration of pyrimethamine was studied in small numbers of patients with AIDS[105] and meningeal leuke-

TABLE 16–3. GUIDELINES FOR SPECIFIC THERAPY OF TOXOPLASMIC ENCEPHALITIS IN PATIENTS WITH AIDS

DRUG	DOSE, INTERVAL, ROUTE	
Primary Therapy[1]		
Pyrimethamine (Daraprim)[2]	200-mg loading dose then 1-1.5 mg/kg/d	(p.o.)
Folinic Acid (leucovorin)[3]	10-50 mg/d	
	plus	
Sulfadiazine or trisulfapyrimidines[4]	4-6 g/d	(p.o.)
	alternative (investigational)	
Clindamycin	Dosage not established[5]	
Chronic Maintenance Therapy[6]		
Pyrimethamine	25-50 mg/d	(p.o.)
Folinic acid (leucovorin)	5-20 mg/d	
	plus	
Sulfadiazine or trisulfapyrimidines	2 g/d	(p.o.)
	alternative (investigational)	
Clindamycin[7]	300-450 mg q.6-8 h.	(p.o.)

[1]Primary therapy should be continued until there is complete resolution or marked improvement in clinical and neuroradiologic abnormalities. Such response usually requires at least 4 weeks of treatment; as a guideline we recommend 6 weeks of primary therapy.

[2]Patients should have complete blood counts (CBC) with white blood cell differential performed at least once weekly.

[3]Folinic acid may be incrementally adjusted to as high as 50 mg/d, if needed to attempt to ameliorate pyrimethamine-induced bone marrow toxicity. Folinic acid should be administered in 2 to 4 divided daily doses and may be given parenterally if poor absorbtion is suspected.

[4]If a sensitivity reaction to sulfadiazine occurs, the patient may not have a cross-reaction when a trisulfa-pyridimine preparation which does not contain sulfadiazine is substituted. When mild or moderate un-toward reactions to a sulfonamide occur and the severity of the disease is significant, it is reasonable to either continue sulfadiazine or change to trisulfapyrimidines (all preparations of trisulfapyrimidines available in the United States in 1990 contain sulfadiazine in addition to sulfamethazine and sulfamerazine). If toxoplasmic encephalitis is not clinically severe, it may be reasonable to continue pyrimethamine and to wait (e.g., 24-48 h) for the presumed drug reaction to decrease and to then substitute the alternative sulfonamide preparation.

[5]Clindamycin may be used as an alternative primary therapy *in combination with pyrimethamine* in any patient who has a severe reaction to sulfonamides. No firm recommendations can be made regarding dosage or route. At this time we suggest as a guideline that clindamycin be given intravenously (900-1200 mg i.v. q.6-8 h) until marked clinical improvement is noted and thereafter to administer the oral preparation (450-600 mg q.6 h).

[6]The relapsing nature of toxoplasmic encephalitis makes lifelong chronic maintenance therapy necessary for secondary prophylaxis against recrudescence of disease.

[7]Clindamycin may be used as alternative maintenance therapy when sulfonamides cannot be tolerated. We suggest clindamycin be used *in combination with pyrimethamine*.

mia,[35,100] CSF concentration of drug was between 10 and 25 percent of the serum concentration. Whether pyrimethamine is present and active in abscess cavities in the brain is not known. Recent data, however, suggests that pyrimethamine may be concentrated in the brain.[55]

Because it is not possible to predict serum or brain concentrations of pyrimethamine in patients with AIDS and toxoplasmic encephalitis, we recommend the synergistic combination of pyrimethamine plus sulfadiazine (or trisulfapyrimidine) for the management of the acute encephalitis

(Table 16–3). Trimethoprim-sulfamethoxazole cannot be recommended for treatment of toxoplasmic encephalitis since the activity of this combination against *T. gondii* is significantly inferior to pyrimethamine-sulfadiazine both in vitro and in animal models of toxoplasmosis.[41,63]

Standard therapy is limited by the high incidence of toxicity associated with both drugs in combination. The most notable toxicity of pyrimethamine is dose-related bone marrow suppression resulting in thrombocytopenia, granulocytopenia, or megaloblastic anemia.[50,74,75] At doses of 75 to 100 mg/d, hematologic abnormalities are to be anticipated but may be difficult to disassociate from those frequently found with HIV infection per se. Patients receiving pyrimethamine should have complete blood counts, including platelets and white blood cell differential, monitored frequently (1 to 2 times per week).

Folinic acid (leucovorin calcium) may prevent or be used to treat marrow toxicity due to pyrimethamine[50,90] and is not antagonistic to the activity of pyrimethamine or sulfadiazine on *T. gondii*.[33] The oral dose of folinic acid administered to these patients is usually 10 to 20 mg/d in divided doses[78] (Table 16–3). If hematologic abnormalities develop and malabsorption of the folinic acid is suspected, folinic acid may be administered parenterally. Some investigators increase folinic acid up to 50 mg/d for suspected pyrimethamine associated hematologic toxicity.[56] Few data suggest that higher doses may prevent progression of or reverse the hematologic toxicities. *Folic acid must not be used,* since it will inhibit the anti-*Toxoplasma* activity of pyrimethamine.[33]

Although 65 to 90 percent of patients with toxoplasmic encephalitis will have an initial favorable response to pyrimethamine plus sulfadiazine,[14,56,76] untoward reactions to this combination may limit duration of therapy. Studies reveal that as many as 40 percent of AIDS patients who receive sulfadiazine and pyrimethamine for toxoplasmic encephalitis manifest signs of toxicity sufficiently severe to prompt discontinuation of the drug during the primary phase of treatment.[46,56] It is likely that the sulfonamide is discontinued prematurely in many cases in which lessening or disappearance of the rash would occur had the drug been continued. However, we recognize the concerns physicians face when confronted with this problem. Coadministration of zidovudine with pyrimethamine plus sulfonamides may increase the risk of bone marrow toxicity[53] (Chapter 8). Moreover, zidovudine has been shown in experimental models to antagonize the toxoplasmacidal activity of pyrimethamine plus sulfadiazine,[49] although the clinical relevance of these data are unknown. We currently recommend that zidovudine be withheld during the management of the acute stage of the acute encephalitis. These problems underscore the urgent need to develop safe and more effective treatment regimens.

Investigational Drugs

Clindamycin has been shown to prevent death in mice experimentally infected with *T. gondii*.[1,44,69] Anecdotal reports of AIDS patients with toxoplasmic encephalitis who have responded to clindamycin suggest a promising role for this drug during primary treatment of this disorder.[19,56,76,92] Although clindamycin has poor penetration across the normal blood-brain barrier,[94] therapeutic levels appear to enter inflamed brain.[44] Concomitant with therapeutic response, however, the resulting decrease in inflammation may prevent adequate concentrations of clindamycin from penetrating the brain, and higher daily doses may be required. Thus, definitive recommendations regarding dose, route, duration, efficacy, and toxicity of clindamycin for treatment of toxoplasmic encephalitis must await results of clinical trials (Table 16–3).

An international, randomized, prospective trial (under the auspices of the State of California Universitywide Task Force on AIDS–California Collaborative Treatment Group) that compared sulfadiazine and intravenous clindamycin in combination with pyrimethamine for primary therapy of toxoplasmic encephalitis has been recently closed to enrollment of new patients. The data are currently being analyzed.[18] The Toxoplasma Pathogen Study Group of the NIH AIDS Clinical Trials Groups has begun enrollment of patients into a multicentered pilot study of the safety and efficacy of oral clindamycin in combination with pyrimethamine for primary therapy of toxoplasmic encephalitis in patients with AIDS.

Spiramycin, which has long been used for prevention of transplacental transmission of *T. gondii*, has been reported to be ineffective for prevention, treatment, or suppression of toxoplasmic encephalitis.[57] Combined therapy with pyrimethamine, clindamycin, and spiramycin for 2 to 4 weeks followed by long-term suppression with weekly pyrimethamine (50 mg) and sulfadoxine (1000 mg) has been advocated,[81] although the role of spiramycin in the combination has never been critically evaluated. Based on available evidence, there is no justification for the use of three drugs in the primary or suppressive phase of therapy.

Recently, the new macrolide antibiotics azithromycin and roxithromycin have been shown to be highly effective in a murine model of toxoplasmosis.[3,43] While they appear promising,[64] carefully controlled clinical trials are needed before they can be recommended.

Like pyrimethamine, trimetrexate inhibits *Toxoplasma* dihydrofolate reductase, but does so far more potently.[52] Unfortunately, the reported outcome of patients with biopsy-proven toxoplasmic encephalitis treated with trimetrexate suggests that this drug used alone has only transient activity against this disorder.[83] The purine analogue arprinocid, an anticoccidial drug used in veterinary medicine, is highly active against *T. gondii* but has not been used in humans.[64]

Because AIDS patients, with their profound defect in cellular immunity, are so susceptible to uncontrolled infection with *Toxoplasma*, there is much interest in the possibility of immunologic reconstitution of these patients through the use of biologic response modifiers. Of particular interest is γ-interferon, which is known to be a major mediator of host resistance to *T. gondii*.[102] Recombinant γ-interferon (rIFNγ) can activate monocyte-derived macrophages of AIDS patients to kill *T. gondii*[73] and has significant activity in animal models of toxoplasmosis.[43,68] Further, in a murine model of toxoplasmic encephalitis, synergistic activity was observed when roxithromycin and IFNγ were combined.[43] In view of the important immunologic role of rIFNγ, future clinical trials should be designed to determine whether the use of antiretroviral agents in combination with rIFNγ may be used to improve outcome and tolerance to specific anti-*Toxoplasma* therapy. Other biologic response modifiers such as rIFNβ and recombinant interleukin 2 (rIL2) have also been shown to have anti-*Toxoplasma* activity in experimental models[95,97] but have not been used to treat AIDS-associated toxoplasmosis.

Maintenance Treatment

The unique pathogenesis of toxoplasmic encephalitis in patients with AIDS requires that intensive primary therapy be followed by a lifelong suppressive regimen. Whereas the combination pyrimethamine plus sulfadiazine is highly active against the proliferative form, it is not effective against the cyst form.[16] Relapse of toxoplasmic encephalitis after withdrawal of therapy has been attributed to the cyst form and may approach 100 percent.[14,64,87] After discontinuation of specific therapy, *Toxoplasma* cysts or cells which contain viable forms that have failed to respond to therapy may lead to recrudescence of a necrotizing encephalitis. The CT or MRI scans of patients who relapse will often demonstrate mass lesions in the same location as at initial presentation.[64] *Thus, it is essential that AIDS patients who complete a primary course and have achieved a favorable clinical and radiologic response to therapy for toxoplasmic encephalitis be maintained on lifelong anti-Toxoplasma agents* (Table 16–3).

Unfortunately, lack of published data from well-designed clinical studies has resulted in treatment recommendations based mainly on analysis of accumulated anecdotal reports. In a retrospective study by Haverkos et al, 20 of 36 patients (57 percent) who had been treated for biopsy-proven toxoplasmic encephalitis had lesions of toxoplasmic encephalitis at autopsy sufficient to be listed as the cause of death.[46] In a prospective study by Leport et al, 31 of 35 (89 percent) AIDS patients with toxoplasmic encephalitis had either a complete (N = 10) or partial (N = 21) response to 4 to 6 weeks of primary therapy[56]; 24 who responded to primary therapy were followed for a mean duration of 8 months (range 2.5 to 28 months) while on lower doses of pyrimethamine and sulfadiazine for maintenance treatment. Six (25 percent) of these patients had 10 relapses both clinically and by CT scan; of the 10 episodes of relapse, seven occurred within 5 to 7 weeks of discontinuation of primary therapy. Reinitiation of combination therapy at higher doses led to complete resolution of signs and symptoms in 8 (80 percent) of the episodes of relapse and partial response in one patient, while the other died of the relapse before therapy could be reinitiated. Four of the six patients that relapsed died; three of the deaths were unrelated to toxoplasmic encephalitis as judged by autopsy or by having had complete clinical response to therapy.[56] Nevertheless, even when postmortem examination of brains of patients who had been treated until death failed to disclose cerebral toxoplasmosis, most had immunoperoxidase stains positive for *T. gondii*.[56] The reported persistence of the proliferative form of *T. gondii* after chronic maintenance treatment and the high relapse rate of toxoplasmic encephalitis in AIDS patients after discontinuation of pyrimethamine and sulfadiazine underscores the necessity for lifelong therapy.

After successful primary therapy, drug dosages are generally decreased for lifelong maintenance therapy (Table 16–3). While the most satisfactory regimen for suppression is unknown, our colleagues in France[56] (and personal communication to JS Remington from J Vilde, November 1989) favor daily use of pyrimethamine (50 mg) with sulfadiazine.[2] Clindamycin (300 to 450 mg q.i.d. or t.i.d.) taken orally is used only in patients who cannot tolerate sulfonamides and whenever possible in combination with pyrimethamine; it should be noted, however, that patients have developed PCP while on this maintenance treatment regimen.[36]

Relapses have been observed when pyrimethamine is used alone or when a regimen is taken less frequently than daily[56] (and personal communication to JS Remington from J Vilde, 1987). Studies are needed to clarify how frequently relapses are due to a failure of the drug regimen and how often to lack of compliance on the part of the patient. In addition, clinical trials should be performed to determine whether advantage can be made of the long (5- to 7-day) half-life of pyrimethamine to define an effective and convenient maintenance regimen.

Pyrimethamine-sulfadoxine (Fansidar) may be effective as a biweekly regimen for chronic suppression of toxoplasmic encephalitis, but we are aware of a number of relapses in patients on this regimen.[4] Given the long half-life of sulfadoxine and reports of associated death(s) and life-threatening Stevens-Johnson syndrome and toxic epidermal necrolysis,[10,88] we and other physicians have been reluctant to prescribe this fixed drug combination to patients with AIDS.

When patients are placed on maintenance therapy for toxoplasmic encephalitis, we and others recommend[12] that zidovudine be added to the medical regimen. Thereafter, complete blood counts with white blood count differentials should be obtained at sufficiently frequent intervals to detect

TABLE 16—4.   METHODS FOR PREVENTION OF TOXOPLASMOSIS IN PATIENTS WITH HIV INFECTION

Individuals should take these precautions:
   Meat should be cooked $\geq 66°$ C, smoked, or cured in brine.
   Avoid touching mucous membranes of mouth and eyes while handling raw meat.
   Wash hands thoroughly after handling raw meat.
   Wash kitchen surfaces that come into contact with raw meat.
   Wash fruits and vegetables before consumption.
   Prevent access of flies, cockroaches, etc. to fruits and vegetables.
   Avoid contact with materials that are potentially contaminated with cat feces, e.g., cat
      litter boxes, or wear gloves when handling such materials or when gardening.
   Disinfect cat litter box for 5 minutes with nearly boiling water.

Adapted from Remington JS, Desmonts G: Toxoplasmosis. In Remington JS, Klein JO (eds): Infectious Diseases of the Fetus and Newborn Infant. Philadelphia, W.B. Saunders Co., 1990.

adverse drug reactions and allow for timely modifications of dosages of drugs. Close attention to results of hematologic studies may avert significant complications of drug therapy and increase the ability of patients to be maintained on a chronic regimen in addition to specific antiviral treatment.

Prevention

Serologic testing for *Toxoplasma* antibodies will distinguish those HIV-infected individuals who are at risk for reactivation of infection from those at risk for acquisition of newly acquired infection. Whether chemoprophylaxis of patients with chronic *Toxoplasma* infection and AIDS or ARC can prevent the development of toxoplasmic encephalitis is an important issue to resolve. At present, there are no experimental or clinical data regarding safety or efficacy of potential chemoprophylactic agents. Therefore, outside a properly designed clinical trial, primary prophylaxis of toxoplasmosis in patients with HIV infection cannot be recommended.

All patients who are seronegative for *Toxoplasma* antibodies and who have evidence of deficient cellular immunity should be educated regarding appropriate precautions that should be taken to prevent acquisition of *Toxoplasma* infection (Table 16—4).

SUMMARY

Toxoplasmic encephalitis is recognized as a major CNS complication in patients with AIDS and is the most frequent cause of focal intracerebral lesions in these patients. This complication of AIDS is almost always observed in patients who have a chronic (latent) infection with *Toxoplasma gondii.* Therefore, patients who from outset of their HIV infection or AIDS are known to have antibodies to *T. gondii* should be considered at risk for development of toxoplasmic encephalitis. Although serologic tests cannot distinguish active from latent infection, a patient who is seronegative for *Toxoplasma* antibodies is unlikely to have toxoplasmic encephalitis. Neuroradiologic studies may be highly suggestive of toxoplasmic encephalitis, but at present the definitive diagnosis can be made only by demonstration of *Toxoplasma* in brain tissue. The unique pathogenesis of toxoplasmic encephalitis in patients with AIDS makes necessary intensive primary therapy followed by a lifelong maintenance regimen. We recommend pyrimethamine plus sulfadiazine (or trisulfapyrimidines) for the treatment of acute disease. Clindamycin plus pyrimethamine should be used in those patients who cannot tolerate sulfonamides. Treatment should be continued until complete resolution or marked improvement of clinical and neuroradiologic abnormalities is observed. Thereafter the dose of drugs may be reduced for chronic maintenance against relapse of encephalitis. Because most patients will respond to primary therapy, those who fail to improve clinically within 14 days should be evaluated for additional or alternative causes for their intracerebral pathology. This will often necessitate brain biopsy.

REFERENCES

1. Araujo FG, Remington JS: Effect of clindamycin on acute and chronic toxoplasmosis in mice. Antimicrob Agents Chemother 5:647-651, 1974
2. Araujo FG, Remington JS: Antigenemia in recently acquired acute toxoplasmosis. J Infect Dis 141:144-150, 1980
3. Araujo FG, Remington JS: Azithromycin: A macrolide antibiotic with potent activity against *Toxoplasma gondii.* Antimicrob Agents Chemother 32:755-757, 1988
4. Balzer T, Rolfs A, Hoffken G, Depperman KM, et al: The value of pyrimethamine/ sulfadoxin (Fansidar) in the prevention of CNS-toxoplasmosis in AIDS patients. V International Conference AIDS (Abstract #WBP33), Montreal, June 1989
5. Blaser MJ, Cohn DL: Opportunistic infections in patients with AIDS: Clues to the epidemiology of AIDS and the relative virulence of pathogens. Rev Infect Dis 8:21-30, 1986
6. Bursztyn EM, Lee BCP, Bauman J: CT of acquired immunodeficiency syndrome. AJNR 5:711-714, 1984
7. Castro KG, Selik RM, Jaffe HW, et al: Frequency of opportunistic diseases in patients by race/ethnicity and HIV transmission categories—United States. Presented at Interscience Conference on Antimicrobial Agents and Chemotherapy (Abstract #570), Los Angeles, October 1988
8. Catterall JR, Hofflin JM, Remington JS: Pulmonary toxoplasmosis. Am Rev Respir Dis 133:704-705, 1986
9. Cavallito JC, Nichol CA, Brenckman WD Jr, et al: Lipid-soluble inhibitors of dihydrofolate reductase. I. Kinetics, tissue distribution, and extent of metabolism of pyrimethamine, metroprine, and etoprine in the rat, dog, and man. Drug Metab Dispos 6:329-337, 1978
10. Centers for Disease Control: Revised recommendations for preventing malaria in travellers to areas with chloroquine-resistant *Plasmodium falciparum.* MMWR 34:185-190, 1985

11. Cerezo L, Alvarez M, Price G. Electron microscopic diagnosis of cerebral toxoplasmosis. J Neurosurg 630:470-472, 1985
12. Clumeck N, DeWit S, Hermans P et al: The benefit of zidovudine on the long-term survival of AIDS patients with CNS toxoplasmosis. Presented at the 28th Interscience Conference on Antimicrobial Agents and Chemotherapy (Abstract #1474), Los Angeles, October 1988
13. Clumeck N, Sonnet J, Taelman H, et al: Acquired immunodeficiency syndrome in African patients. N Engl J Med 310:492, 1984
14. Cohn JA, McMeeking A, Cohen W, et al: Evaluation of the policy of empiric treatment of suspected toxoplasma encephalitis in patients with the acquired immunodeficiency syndrome. Am J Med 86:521-527, 1989
15. Conley FK, Jenkins KA, Remington JS: *Toxoplasma gondii* infection of the central nervous system. Use of the peroxidase-antiperoxidase method to demonstrate Toxoplasma in formalin fixed, parafin embedded tissue sections. Hum Pathol 12:690-698, 1981
16. Cook MK, Jacobs L: In vitro investigations on the action of pyrimethamine against *Toxoplasma gondii*. J Parasitol 44(3):280-288, 1958
17. Crider SR, Horstman WG, Massy GS. Toxoplasma orchitis: Report of a case and a review of the literature. Am J Med 85:421-424, 1988
18. Dannemann BR, Israelski DM, McCutchan JA, et al: Treatment of toxoplasmic encephalitis (TE) in patients with AIDS: Preliminary report of the California Collaborative Treatment Group randomized trial of pyrimethamine (P) plus sulfonamides (S) versus pyrimethamine plus clindamycin (C). International Congress Antimicrobial Agents and Chemotherapy (Abstract #562), Los Angeles, 1988
19. Dannemann BR, Israelski DM, Remington JS: Treatment of toxoplasmic encephalitis with intravenous clindamycin. Arch Intern Med 148:2477-2482, 1988
20. De La Paz RL, Enzman D: Neuroradiology of acquired immunodeficiency syndrome. In Rosenblum ML, et al (eds): AIDS and the nervous system. New York, Raven Press, 1988
21. De La Paz RL, Floris R, Brant-Zawadzki M, et al: MRI of CNS complications of acquired immunodeficiency syndrome (AIDS). AJNR In press
22. Dement SH, Cox MC, Gupta PK: Diagnosis of central nervous system *Toxoplasma gondii* from the cerebrospinal fluid in a patient with acquired immunodeficiency syndrome. Diagn Cytopathol 3(2):148 151, 1987
23. Derouin F, Mazeron MC, Garin YJF: Comparative study of tissue culture and mouse inoculation methods for demonstration of *Toxoplasma gondii*. J Clin Micro 25(9):1597-1600, 1987
24. Derouin F, Sarafti C, Beauvais B, et al: Laboratory diagnosis of pulmonary toxoplasmosis in patients with acquired immunodeficiency syndrome. J Clin Micro 27:1661-1663, 1989
25. Elkin CM, Leon E, Grenell SL, et al: Intracranial lesions in the acquired immunodeficiency syndrome: Radiological (CT) features. JAMA 253:393-396, 1985
26. Enzman DR: Imaging of infections and inflammations of the central nervous system: Computed Tomography, Ultrasound, and Nuclear Magnetic Resonance. New York, Raven Press, 1984
27. Eyles DE, Coleman N: An evaluation of the curative effects of pyrimethamine and sulfadiazine alone and in combination, on experimental mouse toxoplasmosis. Antibiot Chemother 5:529-539, 1955
28. Eyles DE, Coleman N: Synergistic effect of sulfadiazine and Daraprim against experimental toxoplasmosis in the mouse. Antibiot Chemother 3:483-490, 1953
29. Farkash AE, Maccabbee PJ, Sher JH: CNS toxoplasmosis in acquired immune deficiency syndrome: A clinical-pathological-radiological review of 12 cases. J Neurol Neurosurg Psychiatry 49:744-748, 1986
30. Fauci AS: The human immunodeficiency virus: Infectivity and mechanisms of pathogenesis. Science 239:617-622, 1988
31. Feldman HA: Effects of trimethoprim and sulfisoxazole alone and in combination on murine toxoplasmosis. J Infect Dis 128S:774, 1973
32. Frenkel JK: Effect of cortisone, total body irradiation and nitrogen mustard on chronic latent toxoplasmosis. Am J Pathol 33:618, 1957

33. Frenkel JK, Hitchings GH: Relative reversal by vitamins (p-aminobenzoic, folic and folinic acids) of the effects of sulfadiazine and pyrimethamine on Toxoplasma, mouse and man. Antibiot Chemother 7(12):630-638, 1957
34. Frenkel JK, Nelson BM, Arias-Stella J: Immunosuppression and toxoplasmic encephalitis. Hum Pathol 6:97, 1975
35. Geils GF, Scott CW Jr, Baugh CM, Butterworth CE Jr: Treatment of meningeal leukemia with pyrimethamine. Blood 38:131-137, 1971
36. Girard PM, Lepretre A, Detruchis P, et al: Failure of pyrimethamine-clindamycin combination for prophylaxis of Pneumocystis carinii pneumonia. Lancet 1:1459, 1989
37. Glatt AE, Chirgwin K, Landesman SH: Treatment of infections associated with human immunodeficiency virus. N Engl J Med 318:1439-1448, 1988
38. Glauser MP, Francioli P: Clinical and epidemiological survey of acquired immune deficiency in Europe. Eur J Clin Microbiol 3(1):55-58, 1984
39. Grant IH, Gold JMW, Armstrong D: Risk of C.N.S. toxoplasmosis in patients with A.I.D.S. Presented at the 26th Interscience Conference on Antimicrobial Agents and Chemotherapy. New Orleans, September-October 1986
40. Gray F, Gherard R, Wingate E, et al: Diffuse "encephalitic" cerebral toxoplasmosis in AIDS. Report of four cases. J Neurol [West Germany] 236:273-274, 1989
41. Grossman PL, Remington JS: The effect of trimethoprim and sulfamethoxazole on Toxoplasma gondii in vitro and in vivo. Am J Trop Med Hyg 28:445-455, 1979
42. Hauser WE, Luft BJ, Conley BK, et al: Central nervous system toxoplasmosis in homosexual and heterosexual adults. N Engl J Med 307:498-499, 1982
43. Hofflin JM, Remington JS: In vivo synergism of roxithromycin (RU 965) and interferon against Toxoplasma gondii. Antimicrob Agents Chemother 31:346:348, 1987
44. Hofflin JM, Remington JS: Clindamycin in a murine model of toxoplasmic encephalitis. Antimicrob Agents Chemother 31:492-496, 1986
45. Hofflin JM, Remington JS: Tissue culture isolation of Toxoplasma from blood of a patient with AIDS. Arch Intern Med 145:925-926, 1985
46. Haverkos HW: Assessment of therapy for Toxoplasma encephalitis. Am J Med 82:907, 1987
47. Huskinson J, Stepick-Biek P, Remington JS. Detection of antigens in urine during acute toxoplasmosis. J Clin Micro 27:1099-1101, 1989
48. Israelski DM, Skowren G, Leventhal JP, et al: Toxoplasma peritonitis in a patient with acquired innunodeficiency syndrome. Arch Intern Med 148:1655-1657, 1988
49. Israelski DM, Tom C, Remington JS: Zidovudine antagonizes the action of pyrimethamine in experimental infection with Toxoplasma gondii. Antimicrob Agents Chemother 33:30-34, 1989
50. Kaufman HE, Geisler PH: The hematologic toxicity of pyrimethamine (Daraprim) in man. Arch Ophthalmol 64:140-146, 1960
51. Kennedy CR, Robinson RO, Valman HB, et al. A major role for viruses in acute childhood encephalopathy. Lancet (1):989-991, 1986
52. Kovacs JA, Allergra CJ, Chabner BA, et al: Potent effect of Trimetrexate, a lipid-soluble antifolate, on Toxoplasma gondii. J Infect Dis 155:1027-1032, 1987
53. Leport C, Chakroun M, Matheron S, et al: Efficacite et tolerance de la zidovudine chez 32 malades atteints de toxoplasmose cerebrale au cours du syndrome d'immunodeficit acquis. La Presse Medicale 17:1813-1814, 1988
54. Leport C, Meulemans A, Dameron G et al: Levels of pyrimethamine in serum of AIDS patients treated for toxoplasmic encephalitis. Presented at the 4th European Congress of Clinical Microbiology (Abstract #843), pp 43. Nice, April 1989
55. Leport C, Meulemans A, Robine D, et al: Penetration of pyrimethamine into human brain tissue after a single dose administration. Presented at the 29th Interscience Conference on Antimicrobial Agents and Chemotherapy (Abstract #248), Houston, September 1989
56. Leport C, Raffi F, Katlama C, et al: Treatment of central nervous system toxoplasmosis with pyrimethamine/sulfadiazine combination in 35 patients with the acquired immunodeficiency syndrome. Am J Med 84:94-100, 1988
57. Leport C, Vilde JL, Katlama C, et al: Failure of spiramycin to prevent neurotoxoplasmosis in immunosuppressed patients. JAMA 255:2290, 1987
58. Levy RM, Bredesen DE: Central nervous system dysfunction in acquired immunodeficiency syndrome. J AIDS 1:41-64, 1988

59. Levy RM, Bredesen DE, Rosenblum ML: Neurological manifestations of the acquired immunodeficiency syndrome (AIDS): Experience at UCSF and review of the literature. J Neurosurg 62:475-495, 1985
60. Levy RM, Rosenbloom S, Perrett LV: Neuroradiological findings in the acquired immunodeficiency syndrome (AIDS): A review of 200 cases. AJNR 7:833-839, 1986
61. Luft BJ, Brooks RG, Conley FK, et al: Toxoplasmic encephalitis in patients with AIDS. JAMA 252:913, 1984
62. Luft BJ, Conley FK, Remington JS: Outbreak of central-nervous system toxoplasmosis in Western Europe and North America. Lancet (1):781-784, 1983
63. Luft BJ, Remington JS: Toxoplasmosis of the central nervous system. In Remington JS, Swartz MN, (eds): Current Topics in Infectious Disease, vol 6. New York, McGraw-Hill Book Co, 1985
64. Luft BJ, Remington JS: Toxoplasmic encephalitis. J Infect Dis 157:1-6, 1988
65. Mack DG, McLeod R: New micromethod to study the effect of antimicrobial agents on Toxoplasma gondii: Comparison of sulfadoxine and sulfadiazine individually and in combination with pyrimethamine and study of clindamycin, metronidazole, and cyclosporin A. Antimicrob Agents Chemother 26:26-30, 1984
66. Marche C, Mayorga R, Trophilme D, Wolff M, Frottier J, Coulaud JP: Pathological study of extraneurological toxoplasmosis (ENT) in AIDS. IV International Conference on AIDS (Abstract #7074), Stockholm, June 1988
67. McArthur JC: Neurologic manifestations of AIDS. Medicine 66:407-437, 1987
68. McCabe RE, Luft BJ, Remington JS: Effect of murine interferon gamma on murine toxoplasmosis. J Infect Dis 150:961-962, 1984
69. McMaster PRB, Powers KG, Finerty JF, Lunde MN: The effect of two chlorinated lincomycin analogues against acute toxoplasmosis in mice. Am J Trop Med Hyg 22(1):14-17, 1973
70. Mehren M, Burns PJ, Mamani MD, et al: Toxoplasmic myelitis mimicking intramedullary cord tumor. Neurology 38:1648-1650, 1988
71. Milligan SA, Katz MS, Craven PC: Toxoplasmosis presenting as panhypopituitarism in a patient with the acquired immune deficiency syndrome. Am J Med 77:760-764, 1984
72. Moskowitz L, Hensley GT, Chan JC, Adams: Immediate cause of death in acquired immunodeficiency syndrome. Arch Pathol Lab Med 109:735-738, 1985
73. Murray HW, Scavuzzo D, Jacobs JL, et al: In vitro and in vivo activation of human mononuclear phagocytes by interferon-γ. J Immunol 138:2457-2462, 1987
74. Myatt AV, Coatney GR, Hernandez T, et al: A further study of the toxicity of pyrimethamine (Daraprim) in man. Am J Trop Med 2:1000-1001, 1953
75. Myatt AV, Hernandez T, Coatney GR: Studies in human malaria. Am J Trop Med 2:788-795, 1953
76. Navia BA, Petito CK, Gold JWM, et al: Cerebral toxoplasmosis complicating the acquired immune deficiency syndrome: Clinical and neuropathological findings in 27 patients. Ann Neurol 19:224-238, 1986
77. Nistal M, Santana A, Paniaqua R, et al: Testicular toxoplasmosis in two men with the acquired immunodeficiency syndrome. Arch Pathol Lab Med 110-746, 1986
78. Nixon PF, Bertino JR: Effective absorption and utilization of oral formyl-tetrahydrofolate in man. N Engl J Med 286:175-179, 1972
79. Parke DW, Font RL: Diffuse toxoplasmic retinochoroiditis in a patient with AIDS. Arch Ophthalmol 104:571-575, 1986
80. Pohle HD, Eichenlaub D: Toxoplasmosis of the CNS in AIDS patient. Symposium on HIV and the Nervous System, Berlin, February 1987
81. Pohle HD, Eichenlaub D: CNS toxoplasmosis in patients with AIDS. AIDS-Forschung (AIFO) 3:122-135, 1987
82. Pohle HD, Ruf B, Eichenlaub D, et al: CNS-toxoplasmosis in AIDS patients incidence and results of treatment with pyrimethamine and macrolide antibiotics. Presented at the IV International Conference on AIDS (Abstract #7076), Stockholm, June 1988
83. Polis MA, Masur H, Tuazon C, et al: Salvage therapy of trimetrexate-leucovorin for treatment of cerebral toxoplasmosis in AIDS patients. Clin Res 37:437A, 1989
84. Potasman I, Resnick L, Luft BJ, Remington JS: Intrathecal production of antibodies against T. gondii in patients with toxoplasmic encephalitis and AIDS. Ann Intern Med 108:49-51, 1988

85. Post MJD, Chan JC, Hensley GT, et al: Toxoplasma encephalitis in Haitian adults with acquired immunodeficiency syndrome: A clinical-pathologic-CT correlation. AJNR 140:861-868, 1983
86. Post MJD, Kursunoglu SJ, Hensley GT, et al: Cranial CT in acquired immunodeficiency syndrome: Spectrum of diseases and optimal contrast enhancement technique. AJNR 6:743-754, 1984
87. Post MJD, Sheldon JJ, Hensley GT, Tobias JA, Chan JC, Quencer RM, Moskowitz LB: Central nervous system disease in acquired immunodeficiency syndrome: Prospective correlation using CT, MR imaging and pathologic studies. Radiology 158 (1):141-148, 1986
88. Raviglione MC, et al: Fatal toxic epidermal necrolysis during prophylaxis with pyrimethamine and sulfadoxine in a human immunodeficiency virus-infected person. Arch Intern Med 148:2683-5, 1988
89. Redfield RR, Wright DC, Tramont EC. The Walter Reed staging classification for HTLV-II/LAV infection. N Engl J Med 314:131-132, 1986
90. Remington JS, Desmonts G: Toxoplasmosis. In Remington JS, Klein JO (eds): Infectious Diseases of the Fetus and Newborn Infant. Philadelphia, WB Saunders Co. 1990
91. Roldan EO, Moskowitz L, Hensley GT: Pathology of the heart in acquired immunodeficiency syndrome. Arch Pathol Lab Med 111:943-946, 1987
92. Rolston K, Hoy J: Role of clindamycin in the treatment of central nervous system toxoplasmosis. Am J Med 83:551-554, 1987
93. Sabin AB, Feldman HA: Dyes as microchemical indicators of a new immunity phenomenon affecting a protozoon parasite (Toxoplasma). Science 108:660-663, 1948
94. Sande MA, Mandell GL: Anticrobial Agents. In Gilman AG, Goodman LS, Rall TW, Murad F (eds): Goodman and Gilman's The Pharmacological Basis of Therapeutics, 7th ed. New York, Macmillan Publishing Co., 1985
95. Schmitz JL, Carlin JM, Borden EC, et al: Beta interferon inhibits *Toxoplasma gondii* growth in human monocyte-derived macrophages. Infect Immun 57:3254-3256, 1989
96. Selik RM, Starcher ET, Curran JW: Opportunistic diseases reported in AIDS patients: Frequencies, associations, and trends. AIDS 1:175-182, 1987
97. Sharma SD, Hofflin JM, Remington JS: In vivo recombinant interleukin 2 administration enhances survival against a lethal challenge with *Toxoplasma gondii*. J Immunol 135:4160-4163, 1985
98. Shepp DH, Hackman RC, Conley FK, et al: *Toxoplasma gondii* reactivation identified by detection of parasitemia in tissue culture. Ann Intern Med 103:218-221, 1985
99. Snider WD, Simpson DM, Nielson S: Neurological complications of AIDS: Analysis of 50 patients. Ann Neurol 14:403, 1983
100. Stickney DR, Simmons WS, DeAngelis RL, Rundles RW, Nichol CA: Pharmacokinetics of pyrimethamine (PRM) and 2,4-diamino -5-(3′,4′-dichlorophenyl) -6-methylpyrimidine (DMP) relevant to meningeal leukemia. Proc Am Assoc Cancer Res 14:52, 1973
101. Suzuki Y, Israelski DM, Dannemann BR, et al: Diagnosis of toxoplasmic encephalitis in patients with acquired immunodeficiency syndrome by using a new serologic method. J Clin Micro 26:2541-2543, 1988
102. Suzuki Y, Orellana MA, Schreiber RD et al: Interferon-γ: The major mediator of resistance against *Toxoplasma gondii*. Science 240:516-518, 1988
103. Wanke CH, Tuazon CU, Kovaks A, et al: Toxoplasma encephalitis in patients with acquired immune deficiency syndrome. Am J Trop Med Hyg 36:509-516, 1987
104. Weiss A, Margo CE, Ledford DK, et al: Toxoplasmic retinochoroiditis as an initial manifestation of the acquired immune deficiency syndrome. Am J Ophthalmol 101(2):248-249, 1986
105. Weiss LM, Harris C, Berger M, et al: Pyrimethamine concentrations in serum and cerebrospinal fluid during treatment of acute toxoplasma encephalitis in patients with AIDS. J Infect Dis 157:580-583, 1988
106. Whelan MA, Kricheff II, Handler M, et al: A.I.D.S.: Cerebral computed tomographic manifestations. Radiology 149:477, 1983
107. Wong B, Gold JWM, Brown AE, et al: Central nervous system toxoplasmosis in homosexual men and parenteral drug abusers. Ann Intern Med 100:36-42, 1984

17

CRYPTOCOCCAL MENINGITIS IN AIDS

LORI A. PANTHER, MD
MERLE A. SANDE, MD

Cryptococcus neoformans is the most common deep-seated fungal infection in patients with AIDS. Cryptococcal meningitis is the most frequently observed syndrome in these patients. Though clinical and laboratory examinations may be nonspecific, the diagnosis is confirmed by culture and serologic testing. Therapy with antifungal agents is rapidly changing as newer orally administered, less toxic drugs come into use. Epidemiology, clinical presentation, laboratory characteristics, and therapy of cryptococcal meningitis in AIDS patients will be reviewed.

EPIDEMIOLOGY

Cryptococcus is found worldwide; the most common sites of isolation are soil and pigeon droppings. The fungus causes disease by primary respiratory tract infection via inhalation of viable organisms. There is no evidence for animal-person or person-person transmission. Despite evidence for primary infection via the aerosol route, cryptococcal infection does not occur in clusters because clinical disease usually does not occur in immunocompetent patients but in patients immunocompromised by corticosteroid therapy, malignancies, or HIV infection.[8]

Cryptococcal infection is the fourth most common infection found in AIDS patients after *Pneumocystis carinii*, cytomegalovirus, and mycobacterial infections.[8] Cryptococcosis is the initial manifestation of AIDS in 40 to 45 percent of such patients.[7,11]

Cryptococcal infection of the central nervous system (CNS) is one of the four most common neurologic complications of AIDS, along with toxoplasmosis (Chapter 16), progressive multifocal leukocencephalopathy (Chapter 12), and primary CNS lymphoma[23] (Chapter 22). Cryptococcal meningitis is the most frequently seen clinical presentation, occurring in 66 to 84 percent of AIDS patients with cryptococcal infections.[7,19,33] In one large series, cryptococcal meningitis occurred in 12.8 percent of all patients with neurologic complications of AIDS.[22] In a CDC study, cryptococcal meningitis occurred in 5.4 percent of 23,307 reported AIDS cases in the United States and was the only manifestation of AIDS in 3.6 percent.[23]

In the CDC study mentioned above, the prevalence of cryptococcal meningitis in AIDS patients was highest in intravenous drug abusers and Haitians (8.8 percent in both groups). In addition, the incidence among blacks was twice that of whites. Geographic variations in prevalence did occur, with New Jersey having the most cases (7.8 percent), probably related to a higher proportion of Haitian, black, and intravenous drug-abusing AIDS patients in that area.

CLINICAL PRESENTATION

Though cryptococcal meningitis is often the index diagnosis in AIDS, its clinical presentation is usually indolent and nonspecific. Symptoms and signs usually do not localize to the CNS (Table 17-1). Progressive malaise, fatigue, and loss of appetite may accompany a mild headache and intermittent fevers. Patients uncommonly present with neck stiffness, seizures, or focal neurologic symptoms. Physical examination is usually unrevealing. Thus the diagnosis of cryptococcal meningitis must always be entertained in the patient at risk for HIV infection who presents with a nonspecific, vague, slowly progressive illness. Mean duration of symptoms before diagnosis was 31 days in one series of 22 patients, with three having no symptoms or signs referable to the CNS.[33] Fever is found in approximately 60 to 80 percent and classically occurs in an exaggerated diurnal pattern.[7,8,33] Headache was the most common presenting symptom, found in at least 70 percent of patients[7,10,19,33]; it is classically bifrontal but can be diffuse or one-sided. Although headache is a common complaint in many

TABLE 17–1.   CLINICAL PRESENTATION OF CRYPTOCOCCAL MENINGITIS IN AIDS

Fever (60–80%)
Headache (>70%)
Stiff neck (20–30%)
Photophobia (20%)
Nausea, vomiting, malaise (40–70%)
Altered mental status (19–28%)
Seizures (4–8%)

HIV-positive patients without CNS infection, a new or progressively severe headache warrants investigation. Complaints of a stiff neck occur in only 20 to 30 percent.[7,33] Approximately one fifth report photophobia.[7,33] Other nonspecific symptoms such as nausea, vomiting, and malaise are common, occurring in 40 to 70 percent.[7,19,33] Altered mental status occurs in 19 to 28 percent, seizures in 4 to 8 percent, and focal deficits in 6 to 11 percent.[7,19,33] Holtzman et al[17] found that 13 percent of 100 HIV-positive patients presenting with new onset seizures had cryptococcal meningitis. Nonspecific neurologic symptoms such as irritability, somnolence, impaired memory, and behavior changes are frequently reported.[8]

Extraneural cryptococcosis occurs often in AIDS patients with cryptococcal meningitis. One study[13] found that 50 percent of AIDS patients with cryptococcal meningitis had disseminated disease, compared to 12.5 percent of non-AIDS patients. Dismukes et al[11] and Chuck and Sande[7] found that two thirds of AIDS patients with cryptococcal meningitis also had infection outside the CNS. The most common sites of extraneural cryptococcosis are the lungs, genitourinary tract, bone marrow, and blood.[10,19] Painless umbilicated skin papules resembling molluscum contagiosum have been reported. Concomitant opportunistic infections may also occur; 13 percent of cases in a recent review of 89 patients were also diagnosed with *P. carinii* pneumonia.[7]

Physical signs of cryptococcal meningitis are also remarkably nonspecific. Temperature over 38.4° C was found in 56 percent of patients in one study.[7] Only 25 to 30 percent of patients have meningismus on physical examination.[7,33] Altered mental status, dementia, or focal neurologic findings occur in less than 20 percent.[7,19,33] Occasionally, cranial nerve palsies or lateralizing signs are found on neurologic examination. Papilledema on fundoscopic examination is rare. Late recrudescence of any neurologic symptom or sign may reflect obstructive hydrocephalus.[8]

LABORATORY STUDIES (Table 17-2)

Routine blood and cerebrospinal fluid (CSF) studies are usually not helpful in the diagnosis of cryptococcal meningitis. Testing for cryptococcal antigen (CRAG) is the most sensitive and specific test and is usually positive in both serum and CSF. Identifying the fungus on India ink examination and culturing *C. neoformans* from the CSF confirms the diagnosis.

Peripheral Blood Findings

Routine peripheral blood findings in AIDS patients with cryptococcal meningitis are of little diagnostic value. Most patients have a white blood cell count (WBC) of less than 4000/mm³, but it ranges from 1300 to 27,900

TABLE 17–2.   LABORATORY FINDINGS OF CRYPTOCOCCAL MENINGITIS IN AIDS

Peripheral Blood Findings
WBC usually <4000/mm³; range 1300–27,900/mm³
Serum CRAG +; 99% sensitivity
CSF Findings
High opening pressure in 60%
WBC low; <20/mm³ in >60%; differential shows lymphocytosis
Glucose normal in >70%
Protein >40 mg/dl in >50%
CRAG + and lower than serum CRAG; 91% sensitivity
India ink + in >70%
Abnormal head CT in 29%

WBC/mm³.[7,19] In one retrospective series the only serum test found to correlate with a significantly decreased survival was a serum sodium of less than 135 mg/dl found in 22 percent of patients.

Measurement of the serum CRAG is highly sensitive in predicting cryptococcal infection. Agglutination of antibody-coated latex beads detected CRAG in 99 percent of patients with cryptococcal meningitis.[7] Though false positive results are rare, a positive test for CRAG should be confirmed by positive culture for the yeast. Cross-reactivity with rheumatoid factor or *Trichosporon beigelii* can lead to a false positive test for serum CRAG. Rheumatoid factor cross-reactivity can be eliminated by pretreating the sample with reducing agents or by enzymatic digestion. Anticryptococcal antibody and skin tests are measurable but not specific for active infection, but they may be useful for epidemiologic studies.[8]

The serum CRAG titer is usually very high in AIDS patients with cryptococcal meningitis. Serum CRAG is positive in 75 to 99 percent of patients in titers ranging from 1:2 to 1:2,000,000,[7,13,19,33] tending to be greater than CSF CRAG titers.[15,19,33] A serum CRAG titer of greater than 1:8 correlates with isolation of organisms by culture from the CSF or an extrameningeal source.[15]

The significance of a persistently positive serum CRAG despite appropriate therapy remains unknown. Chuck et al[7] found serum CRAG to be elevated or unchanged in 26 percent of patients at the end of primary therapy; the 74 percent of patients on follow-up with a serum CRAG of greater than 1:8 had no difference in survival compared to those patients with lower titers. Eng et al[13] suggested that a persistently positive serum CRAG titer despite negative cultures during appropriate therapy may be due to a defect in the clearance of cryptococcal antigen from the serum or continued release of CRAG from dead and dying yeast.

Fungal cultures of blood and other sites such as suspicious-looking skin lesions, bronchial washings, liver, bone marrow, and urine are often positive. Of AIDS patients with cryptococcal meningitis 36 to 68 percent had the organism isolated from extraneural sites.[7,13,19,33] Chuck et al[7] found that disseminated disease correlated with shorter survival.

Cerebrospinal Fluid Findings

Cryptococcal meningitis is definitely established by identifying the organism in the CSF. The CSF typically reveals an unremarkable cell count and chemistry examination but is usually positive on India ink examination and has a high CRAG titer and a positive fungal culture.

Opening pressures measured at the time of lumbar puncture may be elevated. An opening pressure of more than 200 mm Hg was found in 62 to 66 percent of cases with a range from 80 to 555 mm Hg.[7,33]

The CSF WBC count usually exhibits a minimal lymphocytosis. A WBC of less than 20/mm^3 was found in 69 to 79 percent of patients[7,33]; one study found a CSF WBC count of less than 5 cells/mm^3 in 64 percent.[19] Rarely does the CSF show an eosinophilic pleocytosis[8] or hemorrhage. In AIDS patients, no correlation has been found between CSF WBC count and survival.[7,33]

CSF glucose and protein levels are not predictive of active cryptococcal infection. Glucose is usually normal or near normal. Glucose levels of less than 40 mg/dl occurred in only 24 to 31 percent of patients,[7,15,19] ranging from 7 to 114 mg/dl in one study,[7] though in another series 65 percent of patients had glucose of less than 50 mg/dl.[33] CSF protein levels exhibit a wide range of values. Several series have shown that 48 to 68 percent of patients have a CSF protein level of at least 40 mg/dl[7,15,19,33]; Chuck et al[7] found CSF protein levels to range between 14 and 300 mg/dl.

CSF cell counts and chemistries can be misleading in the diagnosis of cryptococcal meningitis; it is not unusual to find a completely normal CSF.[19] However, even in the face of normal or near-normal CSF findings, direct examination of the CSF, measurement of CSF CRAG, and CSF fungal culture usually leads to the diagnosis.

The CSF CRAG titer is usually lower than serum CRAG in cryptococcal meningitis. Kovacs et al[19] found a mean CSF CRAG of 1:294 with a mean serum CRAG of 1:373; similarly Eng et al[13] found mean CSF and serum CRAG titers to be 1:256 and 1:512, respectively. Chuck et al[7] found 9 percent of patients to have a negative CSF CRAG.

Direct examination of the CSF using India ink can provide an immediate diagnosis of cryptococcal meningitis. Since mononuclear leukocytes can look like cryptococci, strict criteria for the identification of the fungus in the CSF should be used: the yeast cells should have a double refractile cell wall, refractile cytoplasmic inclusions, and a distinctly outlined capsule and should exhibit narrow-based budding (Fig. 17-1). Poorly encapsulated cryp-

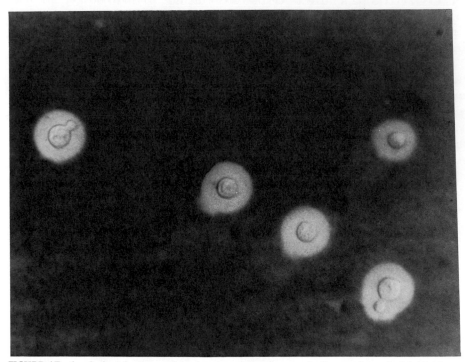

FIGURE 17–1. India ink preparation showing *C. neoformans* in the cerebrospinal fluid. Note budding forms. (Courtesy Keith W. Hadley, M.D., Ph.D.)

tococci have been reported on CSF examination in some AIDS patients.[5] Gram stain of the CSF is not reliable; stains such as Mayer's mucicarmine, methenamine silver, and PAS will easily reveal the organisms in tissue.[8]

In several series, 72 to 82 percent of AIDS patients with cryptococcal meningitis have been found to have positive results on India ink preparation.[7,11,15,19,33] Gal et al[15] found that India ink examination had an 84 percent sensitivity and a 53 percent specificity in predicting CSF culture results. Zuger et al[33] showed that a positive India ink examination was associated with a high (47 percent) mortality; no patients died in the period of follow-up who had a negative India ink examination on repeat lumbar puncture. Chuck et al[7] found that of 39 patients who had lumbar punctures on follow-up after primary therapy, seven had positive India ink examinations and of these, five had positive cultures.

A positive CSF culture is the gold standard in establishing a diagnosis of cryptococcal meningitis. A false negative CSF culture in cryptococcosis of the CNS may be secondary to low yeast load, and if cryptococcal infection is suspected, repeat CSF cultures could be done in an attempt to recover the organism. The only two cases of negative CSF fungal cultures in one series were those patients who had cryptococcoma of the CNS.[33]

Because of the nonspecific presentation of cryptococcal meningitis in AIDS patients, it may be prudent to image the brain to rule out mass lesions before lumbar puncture is done, especially if there is a focal neurologic examination. Space-occupying lesions such as cryptococcoma, toxoplasmosis, lymphoma, and other less common infectious and noninfectious etiologies may produce a clinical picture similar to cryptococcal meningitis. In 13 HIV-positive patients with first-time seizures who were eventually diagnosed with cryptococcal meningitis, none showed mass lesions on computer tomography (CT) scans of the head.[17] In other studies, Chuck et al[7] found 17 of 58 patients (29 percent) with cryptococcal meningitis had an abnormal head CT; 10 of these (58 percent) had cerebral atrophy, 6 (35 percent) had focal abnormalities, and 1 had meningeal enhancement. Zuger et al[33] found 4 of 13 patients with abnormal head CT scans, 3 of whom had focal lesions. In non-AIDS patients with cryptococcal meningitis and CNS mass lesions, 20 percent had no symptoms or signs of CNS disease.[14]

MICROBIOLOGY

In culture, *C. neoformans* grows in the yeast phase on solid culture media, appearing as smooth, convex, tan colonies. In contrast to most nonpathogenic *Cryptococcus* spp, *C. neoformans* can grow at 37° C but grows more rapidly at 30° C. Microscopically, the yeast cell is round to oval, 4 to 6 μm in diameter, with narrow-based budding. The surrounding capsule may vary in size, but this does not seem to be related to virulence, although cryptococci that totally lack a capsule may have decreased virulence.[6,8]

The capsule of *C. neoformans* is made of largely unbranched α-1-3 linked mannose residues. Differences in side-chain substitutions on the residues, growth requirements, and DNA homologies divide the species into four main serotypes designated A, B, C, and D. Serotypes A, D, and the variant AD have been found to be similar and thus classified as *C. neoformans* var *neoformans;* serotypes B and C have been similarly classified into the group *C. neoformans* var *gattii.*

Serotypes A and D (var *neoformans*) have been isolated worldwide from typical environmental sources such as pigeon droppings, but serotypes B and C (var *gattii*) have not been isolated from the environment. Of the isolates in the United States (except southern California), Canada, and Japan, 90 percent are var *neoformans;* 86 percent of these are serotype A. Serotype D is most common in Europe. Serotypes of the var *gattii* tend to occur in tropical and subtropical climates, most of which is serotype B and is located in Hawaii, Australia, southeast Asia, southern Africa, and southern California. Serotype C is rare; 88 percent of isolates have been from southern California.[20]

No correlation has been observed between serotype and susceptibility to amphotericin B or flucytosine. Observations in humans and animals suggest that serotypes B and C (var *gattii*) require more prolonged treatment, possibly because of their slower growth and their propensity to infect patients with weaker host defenses.[4] However, in 14 AIDS patients studied in San Francisco, all were serotypes A, D, or AD (var *neoformans*).[27]

TREATMENT (Table 17-3)

The mainstay of treatment for cryptococcal meningitis in AIDS patients is amphotericin B, though newer drugs may offer some advantages over amphotericin in both primary and maintenance therapy. Type and total amount of primary and maintenance therapies remain controversial aspects of caring for AIDS patients with cryptococcal meningitis. Comparative trials of antifungal agents are ongoing with respect to efficacy, ease of administration, and significant side effects.

Primary Therapy: Amphotericin B and Flucytosine

Amphotericin B is a polyene antibiotic produced by *Streptomyces* spp and is fungistatic to *C. neoformans*. It acts by binding to yeast membrane sterols causing abnormal permeability and cell death. It is 95 percent bound to plasma lipoproteins and thus is poorly soluble in water, causing it to pen-

**TABLE 17–3.   MANAGEMENT OF SUSPECTED
CRYPTOCOCCAL MENINGITIS**

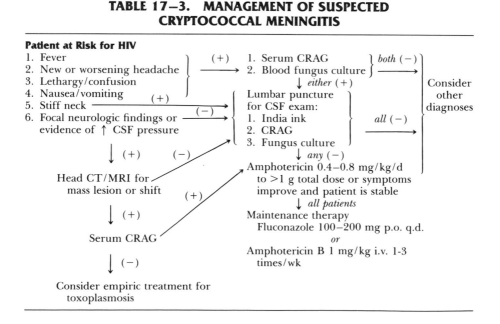

etrate poorly into the CSF. The minimum inhibitory concentration of amphotericin B for *C. neoformans* ranges from 0.03 to 0.6 μg/ml, although this may not correlate with clinical efficacy; with usual doses, serum concentrations of the drug range from 0.21 to 1.15 μg/ml. It is given intravenously; because chemical phlebitis is such a common complication, a central line should be used. Side effects that occur during or immediately after administration include fever, rigors, nausea, and vomiting; these can be reduced in severity by administering acetaminophen 650 mg p.o. and diphenhydramine 25 to 50 mg i.v. 30 to 60 minutes before the amphotericin is given. Rigors can sometimes be ameliorated with administration of meperidine 25 to 50 mg i.m. Phlebitis and systemic side effects can be reduced by the administration of 25 mg of hydrocortisone with the amphotericin B solution; concomitant administration of heparin has not been shown to reduce this complication. Other side effects include anemia, thrombocytopenia, renal tubular acidosis, hypokalemia, and hypomagnesemia. Dose-related impairment of renal function occurs in the majority of patients and is usually reversible when the daily dose is lowered or withheld. Patients receiving total doses over 3.5 to 4.0 g may have some residual impairment of renal function.[12,24,29]

Total effective amphotericin dose in primary therapy of cryptococcal meningitis remains unknown and in fact probably varies from patient to patient. Single doses range from 0.4 to 0.8 mg/kg/d. In most studies, total doses have usually exceeded 1 g and sometimes approach 4 g, and daily treatment has usually continued as long as cultures of CSF or any other extraneural site remained positive. Other observations have shown good results with decreasing frequency of administration to 2 to 5 times weekly after the patient's clinical situation improves or stabilizes with daily amphotericin administration. A case can be made for treating these patients with daily amphotericin until symptoms improve or resolve, then changing to amphotericin 0.4 to 0.8 mg i.v. 2 to 3 times weekly or fluconazole 100 to 200 mg p.o. daily (see Maintenance Therapy). If symptoms reappear, reinstitution of daily amphotericin may be necessary. Intrathecal therapy has been ineffective in a small number of cases and reliably causes chemical arachnoiditis.[10,19,33] The total amount of amphotericin B dose does not appear predictive of relapse.

Flucytosine is a fluorinated pyrimidine which is metabolized to fluorouracil once it is given; it is fungistatic to *C. neoformans* by inhibiting thymidylate synthetase and thus preventing nucleic acid synthesis. It is well absorbed by the oral route, has minimal serum protein binding, and is thus dialyzed to a significant extent. Minimal inhibitory concentrations for *C. neoformans* range from 0.5 to 4.0 μg/ml; because toxic side effects are associated with serum levels of more than 100 μg/ml, serum levels should be monitored and kept in a range of 25 to 50 μg/ml. Resistance to the drug is known to occur when flucytosine is used as sole therapy in cryptococcosis and thus is always used in combination with amphotericin B.

Significant side effects of flucytosine are anemia, leukopenia, thrombocytopenia, nausea, vomiting, and enterocolitis; these are more common in those patients with preexisting renal impairment or with high serum levels of the drug.[16,29]

Although combination amphotericin B and flucytosine in non-AIDS patients has been shown to be superior to amphotericin B alone[3] in AIDS patients, several series show that addition of flucytosine does not increase survival or decrease toxicity or side effects of amphotericin. Zuger et al[33] found that mortality was unchanged (approximately 30 percent) in patients treated with amphotericin B alone versus amphotericin B plus flucytosine, and 36 percent of patients had to discontinue flucytosine because of toxic side effects. No difference in improvement in either group was also observed by Kovacs et al[19] with similar findings with respect to toxicity of flucytosine. Chuck et al[7] found no difference in survival between patients treated with amphotericin B and those treated with combination therapy and found that 53 percent of patients on flucytosine discontinued the drug due to toxicity.

Primary Therapy: Antifungal Azoles

Newer agents in the treatment of systemic mycoses are the imidazoles and triazoles. Both classes of drugs act by inhibiting cellular cytochrome P450 pathways, thereby interfering with membrane sterol synthesis.

Ketoconazole is an imidazole derivative metabolized by the liver to inactive compounds and is 90 percent protein-bound and therefore not dialyzable. Its half-life is approximately 8 hours, and liver or renal dysfunction does not have an appreciable effect on serum concentrations of the drug. Oral absorption is variable and is decreased by antacids or H_2 receptor blocker. Usual dosage is 400 mg/d; penetration into the CSF is less than 10 percent. Most common side effects include dose-related anorexia, nausea, and vomiting; rash and asymptomatic elevations in liver function tests have also been observed. Dose-dependent side effects include decreased levels of serum testosterone causing impotence or menstrual irregularities and a decrease in ACTH-stimulated cortisol response.[8,26,28]

Ketoconazole has not been an effective alternative for primary treatment of cryptococcal meningitis in AIDS patients,[25] though it was effective in prolonging life when used as suppressive therapy.[7,18] Currently, ketoconazole is not recommended as first-line therapy in AIDS patients with active cryptococcal meningitis.

Itraconazole, a triazole derivative, has a much longer half-life than ketoconazole (17 hours). Like ketoconazole, it is metabolized in the liver to inactive substances, is 99 percent protein-bound, and is poorly dialyzed. Penetration into the CSF is also poor. Usual dosage is 200 to 400 mg/d. Side effects are few: nausea, asymptomatic elevation in liver enzymes in 5 percent of patients, hypokalemia, transient pedal edema, and rarely headache and hypertension.

There is limited experience with itraconazole as primary therapy for cryptococcal meningitis in AIDS patients. At doses of 100 to 200 mg/d, one series of 16 patients showed cure or improvement in 44 percent.[10]

Fluconazole, another triazole derivative, differs markedly in pharmacokinetic profile compared to the previously discussed azole compounds. The drug is fungistatic to *C. neoformans*. It is metabolically stable, with 90 percent of the dose excreted unchanged in the urine, and the half-life is approximately 22 hours. Absorption from the gastrointestinal tract is good. It is only 11 percent bound to serum proteins and is thus water-soluble and significantly dialyzed. The drug has good penetration into the CSF, with CSF concentrations 60 to 80 percent that of serum concentrations in the presence of noninflamed and inflamed meninges, respectively. Minimal inhibitory concentrations against *C. neoformans* range from 3.12 to 6.25 $\mu g/$ ml. Side effects are minimal with nausea and bloating being the most common, asymptomatic elevation in liver function tests in a small percentage of patients, and rash. Unlike ketoconazole, inhibition of testosterone and corticosteroid synthesis is minimal.[1,2,28]

Studies of fluconazole are underway to evaluate its efficacy in primary treatment of cryptococcal meningitis in AIDS patients because of its attractiveness as an easily administered drug, its excellent penetration into the CSF, and its minimal side effects. At doses of 50 to 200 mg/d, one study showed four out of five patients with active meningitis had clinical and microbiologic improvement.[30] In a 10-week trial, Larsen and Leal[21] compared 17 patients treated with 400 mg/d of fluconazole to nine patients receiving amphotericin B plus flucytosine at the usual doses and found less improvement in the fluconazole group (42 versus 100 percent), more deaths (29 versus 0 percent), and longer duration of positive CSF cultures (39 versus 18 days). A larger study by Dismukes and the NIAID Mycoses Study Group[11] compared 91 patients treated with fluconazole and 39 patients treated with amphotericin B. Half of the patients in both groups improved, though there were more early deaths in the fluconazole group. The overall mortality rate was the same in both groups, but conversion to negative cultures was more rapid with amphotericin B.[11] Though fluconazole shows promise, it appears to be less effective than amphotericin as initial primary therapy and should probably be used predominantly for maintenance therapy, as discussed below.

Maintenance Therapy

Studies of AIDS patients with cryptococcal meningitis demonstrate that chronic suppressive therapy is associated with decreased incidence of relapse and longer survival. Observations with several of the major antifungal agents will be briefly reviewed.

Amphotericin B has been used as maintenance therapy to prevent relapse of cryptococcal meningitis in AIDS patients. At 0.5 to 1.44 mg/kg/wk given in one to three divided doses, survival was increased in a group of patients receiving amphotericin B maintenance as compared to those patients receiving no maintenance therapy.[7] Similarly, Zuger et al[33] noted 0 percent versus 50 percent relapse in similar groups at 13 weeks, but when follow-up was extended there were no relapses in six patients in whom maintenance therapy was stopped.[34] Kovacs et al[19] found a 60 percent relapse rate after cessation of treatment. Flucytosine has not been used in suppressive therapy. Chuck et al[7] found cumulative survival to be significantly longer in patients treated with ketoconazole in doses of 800 to 1000 mg/d (238 days) or amphotericin B (280 days), and both were better than no suppressive treatment at all (141 days). However, 21 percent of patients on ketoconazole suppression had to be changed to amphotericin B because of toxicity. Itraconazole has had limited study in suppressive therapy; three patients with negative CSF cultures on a 200 mg/d dose showed clinical improvement, although India ink examination remained positive in two patients.[32] At doses of 30 to 200 mg/d of fluconazole, Sugar and Saunders[31] showed only 3 of 19 patients relapsed or died of active disease; the majority of patients had minor side effects, but only one had to discontinue the drug due to thrombocytopenia. Another study showed that only 1 in 14 patients on doses similar to those above had recrudescence of cryptococcal meningitis.[30] While studies are ongoing to evaluate its efficacy, fluconazole shows outstanding promise as maintenance therapy at a daily dose of 100 to 200 mg p.o.

PROGNOSTIC INDICATORS

Although several prognostic indicators have emerged from the mentioned clinical trials above, there does not seem to be consistency between studies. Before the AIDS epidemic, it was noted that patients with cryptococcal meningitis who died tended to have high opening pressures on lumbar puncture, low CSF glucose concentration, CSF WBC less than 20/mm³, positive India ink examination, and CRAG titers greater than 1:32 in the CSF.[9] However, these prognostic parameters do not appear to apply to AIDS patients.

Only a few serum laboratory studies appear to have prognostic value in AIDS patients. A serum sodium of less than 135 mg/dl correlated with decreased survival in one retrospective analysis.[7] A CSF CRAG of greater than 1:2 has been shown to correlate with a positive CSF fungal culture.[15] Several studies have found that height of the serum CRAG titer was not predictive of survival or relapse[7,15,19,30]; however, Zuger et al[33] found a 50 percent mortality in patients with a serum CRAG titer of more than 1:10,000 and 100 percent mortality rate with a CSF CRAG of greater than 1:10,000. Zuger et al[33] also demonstrated that a CSF CRAG of greater than 1:8 at the end of primary therapy predicted clinical relapse, while Stern et al[30] found CSF CRAG titers unchanged during treatment and not predictive of relapse. Chuck et al[7] reported that 74 percent of patients had a serum CRAG of more than 1:8 following treatment but no difference in survival compared to patients with lower titers.

Some CSF findings have been inconsistent predictors of poor outcome in AIDS patients. No correlation has been found between CSF WBC count and survival.[7,33] Though one study[33] found a CSF CRAG of more than 1:10,000 to correlate with a 100 percent mortality rate, others have found no correlation between level of CSF CRAG titer and survival.[7,15] Zuger et al[33] showed that a positive India ink examination was associated with a 47 percent mortality rate; no patients died in the period of follow-up who had a negative India ink examination. Chuck et al[7] found that a positive culture for *Cryptococcus* from an extrameningeal source correlated with a shorter survival.

SUMMARY

In summary, cryptococcal meningitis does not usually present as a fulminant disease in AIDS patients. HIV-positive patients at risk for cryptococcal meningitis are blacks, Haitians, and intravenous drug abusers. Clinical presentation is usually nonspecific; other common CNS abnormalities should always be entertained in the differential diagnosis. Laboratory findings are usually minimally abnormal and may be misleading. Amphotericin B remains the mainstay of therapy, though other less toxic oral drugs are being studied. Maintenance therapy probably decreases the incidence of relapse and increases survival.

REFERENCES

1. Arndt CAS, Walsh TJ, Lester McCully C, Balis FM, Pizzo PA, Poplack DG: Fluconazole penetration into cerebrospinal fluid: Implications for treating fungal infections of the central nervous system. J Infect Dis 157:178-180, 1988
2. Bennett JE: Antifungal agents: In Mandel GL, Douglas RG, Bennett JE (eds). Principles and Practice of Infectious Diseases. New York, Churchill Livingstone, 1990, pp 361-370
3. Bennett JE, Dismukes WE, Duma RJ: A comparison of amphotericin B alone and combined with flucytosine in the treatment of cryptococcal meningitis. N Engl J Med 310:126-131, 1979
4. Bhattacharjee AK, Bennett JE, Glaudemans CPJ: Capsular polysaccharides of *Cryptococcus neoformans*. Rev Infect Dis 6:619-624, 1984
5. Bottoni EJ, Toma M, Johansson BE, Wormser GP: Capsule-deficient *Cryptococcus neoformans* in AIDS patients (Letter). Lancet 1:400, 1985

6. Bulmer GS, Sans MD, Gunn CM: Cryptococcus neoformans: I. Nonencapsulated mutants. J Bacteriol 94:1475-1479, 1967

7. Chuck SL, Sande MA: Infections with *Cryptococcus neoformans* in the acquired immunodeficiency syndrome. N Engl J Med 321:794-799, 1989

8. Diamond RD: Cryptococcus neoformans. In Mandel GL, Douglas RG, Bennett JE (eds). Principles and Practice of Infectious Diseases. New York, Churchill Livingstone, 1990, pp 1980-1989

9. Diamond RD, Bennett JE: Prognostic factors in cryptococcal meningitis: A study in 111 cases. Ann Intern Med 80:176-181, 1974

10. Dismukes WE: Cryptococcal meningitis in patients with AIDS. J Infect Dis 157:624-628, 1988

11. Dismukes W, Cloud G, Thompson S, et al: Fluconazole versus amphotericin B therapy of acute cryptococcal meningitis. In Programs and Abstracts of the Twenty-Ninth Interscience Conference on Antimicrobial Agents and Chemotherapy. Houston, American Society for Microbiology, 1989, p 82

12. Dugoni BM, Guglielmo J, Hollander H: Amphotericin B concentration in cerebrospinal fluid of patients with AIDS and cryptococcal meningitis. Clin Pharm 8:220-221, 1989

13. Eng RHK, Bishburg E, Smith SM: Cryptococcal infections in patients with acquired immune deficiency syndrome. Am J Med 81:19-23, 1986

14. Fujita NK, Reynard M, Sapico FL, Guze LB, Edwards JE Jr: Cryptococcal intracerebral mass lesions: The role of computed tomography and nonsurgical management. Ann Intern Med 94:382-388, 1981

15. Gal AA, Evans S, Meyer PR: The clinical and laboratory evaluation of cryptococcal infections in the acquired immunodeficiency syndrome. Diagn Microbiol Infect Dis 7:249-254, 1987

16. Grant IH, Armstrong D: Fungal infections in AIDS: Cryptococcosis. In Sande MA, Volberding PA (eds). The Medical Management of AIDS. Philadelphia, WB Saunders, 1988, pp 225-233

17. Holtzman DM, Kaku DA, So YT: New onset seizures associated with human immunodeficiency virus infection: Causation and clinical features in 100 cases. Am J Med 87:173-177, 1989

18. Karaffa CA, Rehm SJ, Keys TF: The acquired immunodeficiency syndrome and cryptococcosis (Letter). Ann Intern Med 104:891-892, 1986

19. Kovacs JA, Kovacs AA, Polis M, et al: Cryptococcosis in the acquired immunodeficiency syndrome. Ann Intern Med 103:533-538, 1985

20. Kwon-Chung KJ, Bennett JE: Epidemiologic differences between the two varieties of *Cryptococcus neoformans.* Am J Epidemiol 120:123-130, 1984

21. Larsen RA, Leal ME: Fluconazole compared to amphotericin B as treatment of cryptococcal meningitis. In Programs and Abstracts of the Twenty-Ninth Interscience Conference on Antimicrobial Agents and Chemotherapy. Houston, American Society for Microbiology, 1989, p 82

22. Levy RM, Bredesen DE, Rosenblum ML: Neurological manifestations of the acquired immunodeficiency syndrome (AIDS): Experience at UCSF and review of the literature. J Neurosurg 62:475-495, 1985

23. Levy RM, Janssen RS, Bush TJ, Rosenblum ML: Neuroepidemiology of acquired immunodeficiency syndrome. J AIDS 1:31-40, 1988

24. Maddux MS, Barriere SL: A review of complications of amphotericin B therapy: Recommendations for prevention and management. Drug Intell Clin Pharm 14:177-181, 1980

25. Perfect JR, Durack DT, Hamilton JD, Gallis HA: Failure of ketoconazole in cryptococcal meningitis. JAMA 247(24):3349-3351, 1982

26. Pont A, Williams PL, Loose DS, et al: Ketoconazole blocks adrenal steroid synthesis. Ann Intern Med 97:370-372, 1982

27. Rinaldi MG, Drutz DJ, Howell A, Sande MA, Wofsy CB, Hadley WK: Serotypes of *Cryptococcus neoformans* in patients with AIDS (Letter). J Infect Dis 153:642, 1986

28. Saag MS, Dismukes WE: Azole antifungal agents: Emphasis on new triazoles. Antimicrob Agents Chemother 32:1-8, 1988

29. Sande MA, Mandell GL: Antimicrobial agents: Miscellaneous antibacterial agents, antifungal and antiviral agents. In Gilman AG, Goodman LS, Gilman A (eds). Goodman and Gilman's The Pharmacologic Basis of Therapeutics. New York, Macmillan, 1980, pp 1222-1248
30. Stern JJ, Hartman BJ, Sharkey P, et al: Oral fluconazole therapy for patients with acquired immunodeficiency syndrome and cryptococcosis: Experience with 22 patients. Am J Med 85:477-480, 1988
31. Sugar AM, Saunders C: Oral fluconazole as suppressive therapy of disseminated cryptococcosis in patients with acquired immunodeficiency syndrome. Am J Med 85:481-489, 1988
32. Viviani MA, Tortorano AM, Carbonera Giani P, et al: Itraconazole for cryptococcal infection in the acquired immunodeficiency syndrome. (Letter) Ann Intern Med 106:166, 1987
33. Zuger A, Louie E, Holzman RS, Simberkoff MS, Rahal JJ: Cryptococcal disease in patients with the acquired immunodeficiency syndrome: Diagnostic features and outcome of treatment. Ann Intern Med 104:234-240, 1986
34. Zuger A, Schuster M, Simberkoff MS, Rahal JJ, Holzman, RS: Maintenance amphotericin B for cryptococcal meningitis in the acquired immunodeficiency syndrome (AIDS). Ann Intern Med 85:481-489, 1988.

18

FUNGAL INFECTIONS IN AIDS:
Histoplasmosis and Coccidioidomycosis

GRACE MINAMOTO, MD
DONALD ARMSTRONG, MD

HISTOPLASMOSIS

Disseminated histoplasmosis is increasingly recognized as an opportunistic infection associated with AIDS, as reports of AIDS have spread from New York and California cities to areas where histoplasmosis is endemic, such as the Caribbean, Central America and South America, and river valleys throughout the United States. In 1985 the CDC revised the case definition of AIDS to include disseminated histoplasmosis in the absence of other immune suppression and with evidence of HIV infection.[9] Approximately 140 patients with AIDS and disseminated histoplasmosis have been reported in the literature; of 96 patients for whom sufficient data are available, only 18 percent survived relapse-free after an average follow-up period of 5 months.[27]

Clinical Presentation (Table 18–1)

Most cases of disseminated histoplasmosis in patients with AIDS have been reported in those with a history of residence or travel in endemic areas.[5,21,23,26,37,43] Twenty-three cases have been reported in a nonendemic area,[18,32] but 20 of these patients were born in either Puerto Rico or South America, which are endemic areas, and the birthplace or travel history of the remaining three is unknown. Especially in cases in which the travel

280

TABLE 18–1. HISTOPLASMOSIS IN AIDS PATIENTS

Clinical Presentation
Nonspecific (fever, weight loss)
Pulmonary involvement common but nonspecific. Chest radiographic findings resemble
bacterial pneumonia, *Pneumocystis carinii* pneumonia, or tuberculosis
Clinical Clues
History of residence or travel in endemic area
Diagnostic Tests
Bone marrow biopsy and culture (Wright-Giemsa or methenamine silver stain)
Blood culture
Biopsy of lymph nodes, liver, or lung
Treatment
Amphotericin, 0.5–1.0 mg/kg/d, until symptoms subside (usually 6 to 8 wk)
Maintenance with ketoconazole, 400 mg/d, or amphotericin, 1 mg/kg every week

history is not fully known, the diagnosis of disseminated histoplasmosis may be easily overlooked.

The disease, which appears to result from reactivation of a latent infection, is often more severe in patients with AIDS than in other immunosuppressed persons. Clinical manifestations are not specific and usually include persistent fever and weight loss. Two reports[18,43] described a clinical syndrome resembling gram-negative sepsis, characterized by hypotension, leukopenia, disseminated intravascular coagulation, adult respiratory distress syndrome, encephalopathy, hepatic insufficiency, and renal failure. The chest radiograph may be normal or show infiltrates resembling bacterial pneumonia, *Pneumocystis carinii* pneumonia, or tuberculosis. Mediastinal widening and calcified granulomas have also been described.

Disseminated histoplasmosis in patients with AIDS can present with unusual manifestations. Petechiae secondary to thrombocytopenia as initial signs have been reported.[22] Bilateral chorioretinitis, with budding yeasts visualized in the choroid, retina, and central retinal vein, has been observed.[25] Cutaneous involvement is rare but can present as a diffuse maculopapular or papular eruption, folliculitis, erythematous plaques, papulonecrotic lesions, and indurated perianal ulcerations with a granulomatous base and brawny margins.[16,34] Gastrointestinal disease presenting as jejunal bleeding,[11] cecal[15] and rectal[8] masses, small bowel obstruction,[8] and mucosal ulceration[8,21] has been described. Histoplasmosis may also produce a meningoencephalitis,[4] brain abscesses,[3] and space-occupying central nervous system lesions.[3] Finally, systemic salmonellosis has been observed concurrently with disseminated histoplasmosis in patients with AIDS,[26] as well as in the absence of histoplasmosis; it has been suggested that blockade of the reticuloendothelial system caused by histoplasmosis predisposes to serious *Salmonella* infection.[42] The *Salmonella* infection reportedly resolved when the histoplasmosis was treated.[26]

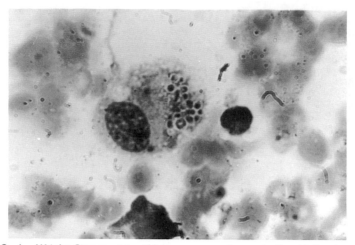

FIGURE 18—1. Wright-Giemsa stain of bone marrow demonstrating histiocytes with intracellular *Histoplasma capsulatum.*

Diagnosis

Most studies on disseminated histoplasmosis in patients with AIDS suggest that the easiest and most reliable means for establishing the diagnosis is bone marrow biopsy and culture.[5,18,22,28,43] Review of the bone marrow stained with Wright-Giemsa or Gomori's methenamine silver stain reveals histiocytes containing *Histoplasma capsulatum* (Fig. 18—1). Blood cultures are frequently positive. Occasionally, Wright-Giemsa stain of peripheral blood or buffy coat can be diagnostic.[17] Biopsies of lymph nodes, liver, and lung can be diagnostic as well and may show noncaseating or caseating granulomas.[19] *Histoplasma* serologic tests are frequently negative, although in one study,[43] five out of seven patients had demonstrable complement fixation titers to either yeast or mycelial antigen and four out of seven patients had M precipitin bands by immunodiffusion (one of these four also had an H precipitin band). *H. capsulatum* polysaccharide antigen has been detected by radioimmunoassay in both urine and serum specimens of a patient with AIDS and disseminated histoplasmosis; this appears to be a useful method for the rapid diagnosis of disseminated histoplasmosis and a means to monitor therapy efficacy.[41]

Therapy

The treatment of disseminated histoplasmosis in patients with AIDS is less effective than in other immunocompromised patients. Amphotericin B in doses of 2 to 2.5 g is successful in treating the latter[12] and does not require maintenance therapy. This regimen does not appear to be curative in AIDS patients, however. There is some efficacy, but relapse has been observed frequently with interrupted courses of amphotericin B. Ketoconazole should not be used for the initial treatment of disseminated histoplasmosis in AIDS patients, as it has been associated with treatment failures in patients with either normal host defenses[35] or immunosuppression.[33] Ketoconazole may be useful for the suppression of relapse following initial treatment with amphotericin B. Among the reported cases of disseminated histoplasmosis in AIDS, there are no significant differences in age, risk group, concomitant infections, or therapy between those patients who appeared to survive the infection and those who died from it. Three patients described[5] did not relapse while on suppressive ketoconazole therapy. However, ketoconazole, 400 mg daily, was reportedly ineffective in preventing recurrence of histoplasmosis in one patient who initially received 2 g of amphotericin B.[14] Another patient relapsed with chronic *Histoplasma* meningitis while receiving suppressive therapy with ketoconazole, 400 mg daily, while a patient receiving the same dose of ketoconazole for *H. capsulatum* isolated from sputum only developed dissemination.[40] This limited experience suggests that a full 2- to 2.5-g course of amphotericin B followed by chronic suppressive therapy with either amphotericin B or ketoconazole, 400 mg daily, may be the treatment of choice. In a recent open, nonrandomized pilot study of patients with AIDS and disseminated histoplasmosis receiving intensive initial courses (1 or 2 g) of amphotericin B followed by long-term intermittent (weekly or biweekly) amphotericin B maintenance therapy, 13 of 14 patients who did not die of other causes remained relapse-free after a median follow-up period of 14 months (range 2 to 23 months).[27]

Fluconazole and itraconazole are promising alternative antifungal agents. In an uncontrolled study of these agents in 16 patients with AIDS and disseminated histoplasmosis, 10 patients (8 receiving itraconazole, 2 receiving fluconazole) improved or went into remission after a mean duration of therapy of greater than 12 months.[13] Prospective, controlled, comparative trials are necessary to define the optimal therapy for histoplasmosis in patients with AIDS.

COCCIDIOIDOMYCOSIS

Coccidioidomycosis, caused by the dimorphic fungus *Coccidioides immitis*, is usually subclinical or associated with subacute respiratory symptoms. Disseminated disease usually occurs in immunosuppressed patients and is distinctly rare in immunocompetent persons.[2] Both the mild and disseminated forms of the disease usually occur only in persons with a history of residence or travel in endemic areas, which include Mexico, Central and South America, and the southwestern United States (Arizona, California,

Nevada, Utah, New Mexico, and western Texas). Disseminated coccidioidomycosis has been reported in patients with AIDS, all of whom had been in endemic areas, mostly Tucson, Arizona.[1,2,6,7,20,24,29,30] The first 10 cases described in the medical literature are summarized in Table 18–2. All died as a result of the infection. Recently, disseminated coccidioidomycosis was added to the list of opportunistic infections included in the CDC definition for AIDS.[10]

Disseminated coccidioidomycosis in patients with AIDS is predominantly the result of reactivation of latent infection, although some cases may be due to a primary infection. It has been pointed out that the rate of infection of disseminated coccidioidomycosis in AIDS in Tucson approximated the prevalence of positive coccidioidin skin tests in that area and that the diagnosis of coccidioidomycosis in AIDS there occurred throughout the year, not only during the expected seasonal periods.[6] On the other hand, disseminated disease has also been reported to occur in patients with AIDS shortly after moving to Tucson from nonendemic areas.[6]

Clinical Presentation (Tables 18–2 and 18–3)

The symptoms at the time of diagnosis are usually nonspecific and include malaise, fever, weight loss, cough, and fatigue. Pulmonary involvement is consistently present; unilateral or bilateral reticulonodular or nodular infiltrates are seen on chest radiograph. Central nervous system involvement manifested by meningoencephalitis[24] and brain abscess[20] has been described. Coccidioidal peritonitis has been observed.[7] Cutaneous manifestations such as abscesses, nodules, verrucous granulomas, and ulcers with sinus tracts, typical of chronic disseminated coccidioidomycosis, appear to be rare.[6] There is one report of a papulopustular eruption over the extremities, chest, and palm in a patient with AIDS and disseminated coccidioidomycosis; the involved skin lacked the typical inflammatory response of epithelial and giant-cell reaction described in coccidioidal infection.[29] Joint effusions and bone destruction, also typical lesions of dissemination, have not been reported.

Diagnosis

The diagnosis is usually made by the examination of sputum or bronchoscopically obtained specimens, which show the endosporulating spherules of *C. immitis* by periodic acid–Schiff stain (Fig. 18–2). Hematoxylin-eosin and Gomori's methenamine silver stains may also demonstrate the fungi in tissues. Bone marrow, blood, urine, lymph node, and liver cultures are frequently positive for *C. immitis*. The histologic features of tissue usually show a typical granulomatous response.[6] At autopsy, additional evidence of disseminated disease has been found in the spleen, brain, and thyroid.

Coccidioidal serologic tests are often, but not always, reactive, and the lack of a positive response does not rule out the possibility of disseminated disease in a patient with AIDS. This contrasts with the 99.7 percent positivity by complement fixation in a study of 722 patients with disseminated coccidioidomycosis with other underlying conditions.[36] Complement-fixing antibodies have been detected at serum dilutions that range from 1:2 to 1:2048. Tube-precipitating antibody, immunodiffusion, and enzyme-linked immunosorbent assay (ELISA) results may also be positive, but the experience with these is more limited. Unfortunately, serial complement fixation titers are not a reliable measure of treatment efficacy, as demonstrated by the death, from disseminated disease, of a patient whose titer had improved from 1:2048 to 1:128.[2]

Therapy

As with the treatment of disseminated histoplasmosis in AIDS patients, amphotericin B therapy for disseminated coccidioidomycosis does not appear to be curative, and lifelong treatment is indicated. Symptoms and pulmonary infiltrates often respond partially or even completely to a course

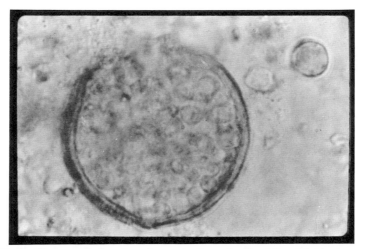

FIGURE 18–2. Wet mount of sputum demonstrating spherule of *Coccidioides immitis*. (Courtesy of Dr. Merle A. Sande.)

TABLE 18–2. CLINICAL FEATURES OF PATIENTS WITH AIDS AND DISSEMINATED COCCIDIOIDOMYCOSIS

PATIENT	AGE, RACE, SEX	SYMPTOMS	CHEST RADIOGRAPH	FUNGAL CULTURE	SEROLOGIES[a] TP	SEROLOGIES[a] CF
1[b]	32 BM	Fever, chills, weight loss	Diffuse nodular pattern	Urine Blood	−	1:2048
2[c]	39 M	Fever, cough, dyspnea, anorexia, pleuritic pain	Bilateral diffuse infiltrates	BAL Sputum	−	<1:8
3[d]	28 HM	Fever, scattered papulopustular rash	RUL infiltrate	Bone marrow Skin biopsy	ND	ND
4[e]	58 WM	Fever, weight loss, diarrhea, headache, lethargy, confusion, dyspnea	Bilateral interstitial miliary infiltrates	None (spherules seen on TBBx)	ND	ND
5[f]	30 WM	Fever, weight loss, nonproductive cough	Diffuse interstitial infilatrates	None (spherules in marrow and lung)	ND	−
6[g]	56 WM	Fatigue, fever, weight loss, sore throat, malaise	RLL nodule, mediastinal adenopathy	Blood	+	1:512
7[g]	25 WM	Right lower chest pain, cough, fever	RLL nodule	None (spherules in liver biopsy)	+	1:128
8[g]	24 WM	Fever, dyspnea, weight loss, weakness	Diffuse nodular infiltrates	Bronchial washings, TBBx, blood, urine	+	1:2
9[g]	26 WM	Fever, anorexia, cough, fatigue	Diffuse interstitial and nodular infiltrates	Bronchial washings	−	−
10[g]	35 WM	Fever, malaise	Diffuse nodular infiltrates, lingular cavitation, left hilar nodes	Bronchial washings, TBBx	−	−

Abbreviations: BAL—bronchoalveolar lavage, CF—complement fixation, CIE—counterimmunoelectropho Kaposi's sarcoma, MAI—*Mycobacterium avium-intracellulare*, ND—not done or not available, PCP—*Pneumocystis* precipitins.
[a] Only or highest titers
[b] Ampel et al[2]
[c] Roberts[30]
[d] Prichard et al.[29]
[e] Macher et al[24]
[f] Abrams et al[1]
[g] Bronniman et al[6]

SEROLOGIES				
CIE	ELISA	ID	THERAPY	OUTCOME
ND	ND	ND	2.5 g Amphotericin B then ketoconazole 400 mg/d	Died. Autopsy: Spherules in lungs, liver, spleen, kidneys. PCP in lungs, CMV in adrenals and large bowel
IgG(−)	IgG 1:400	IgM weak	Amphotericin B	Died. No autopsy
ND	ND	ND	Ketoconazole 800 mg/d then ampho-tericin B	Died. No autopsy
ND	ND	ND	Amphotericin B	Died. Autopsy: Cultures of lungs, brain, lymph node, liver, spleen, kid-ney, and thyroid posi-tive. PCP in lungs, CMV in lungs and liver
ND	ND	weak +	Amphotericin B	Died. Autopsy: Spherules in lungs, liver, spleen, lymph node
ND	ND	ND	Ketoconazole 200-400 mg/d then ampho-tericin 930 mg, then ketoconazole 200 mg/d	Developed PCP and MAI, then died. No autopsy
ND	ND	ND	Amphotericin B 1 g then ketoconazole 400 mg/d	Recurrent nodular infil-trates while off keto-conazole. Died. Au-topsy: Spherules in lungs and periaortic lymph nodes
ND	ND	ND	Amphotericin B >1.6 g	Died. No autopsy
ND	ND	ND	Amphotericin B 30 mg	Died. Autopsy: Spherules in lungs, liver, spleen, KS in lungs
ND	ND	ND	Amphotericin B 1.1 g	Died. Autopsy: Spherules in lungs, liver, spleen, kidneys, heart; dissem-inated lymphoma and CMV; *Aspergillus* pneu-monia

resis, CMV—cytomegalovirus, ELISA—enzyme-linked immunosorbent assay, ID—immunodiffusion, KS—
carinii pneumonia, RLL—right lower lobe, RUL—right upper lobe, TBBx—transbronchial biopsy, TP—tube

TABLE 18–3. COCCIDIOIDOMYCOSIS IN AIDS PATIENTS

Clinical Presentation
  Nonspecific (fever, weight loss, cough)
  Pulmonary involvement consistently present. Chest radiographs show unilateral or
    bilateral nodular or reticulonodular infiltrates
Clinical Clues
  History of residence or travel in endemic area
Diagnostic Tests
  Sputum, bronchoalveolar lavage (periodic acid–Schiff stain)
  Bone marrow biopsy and culture
  Blood and urine cultures
  Biopsy of liver, lung
Treatment
  Amphotericin, 0.5–1.0 mg/kg/d, until symptoms subside (usually 6 to 8 wk)
  Maintenance with ketoconazole, 400 mg/d, or amphotericin, 1 mg/kg every week

of amphotericin B, but relapses occur even after only brief interruptions of therapy.[6] Treatment should probably include at least a cumulative dose of 2 to 2.5 g amphotericin B followed by suppressive therapy with ketoconazole, 400 mg daily, and may require chronic amphotericin B, since one patient has been reported to have relapsed while on ketoconazole, 400 mg daily, after receiving 2.5 g amphotericin B.[2]

Several studies of the treatment of coccidioidomycosis with fluconazole or itraconazole have been published. Of 30 patients without AIDS with coccidioidomycosis receiving fluconazole, 23 showed improvement.[31] In another study, eight patients with coccidioidomycosis, of whom one had AIDS, were treated with fluconazole; five responded, including the patient with AIDS.[39] Four out of five patients without AIDS who had coccidioidal meningitis refractory to standard therapy responded to intraconazole.[38] Further trials in patients with AIDS are warranted.

SUMMARY

Histoplasma capsulatum and *Coccidioides immitis* are two fungi that are regional in occurrence and cause opportunistic fungal infections in patients with AIDS. Many cases of histoplasmosis have been reported in patients months or years after they have been in an endemic area. These are obviously cases of reactivation of latent infections. With coccidioidomycosis, the cases have been reported from endemic areas, but some also appear to be reactivation infections, and we should anticipate such cases in nonendemic areas just as with histoplasmosis. The clinical presentations may be atypical, even mimicking acute bacterial sepsis. The diagnosis should be sought in any HIV-infected patient with an unexplained infection and residence or travel in an endemic area, even in the remote past. Studies should include bone marrow examinations for histoplasmosis as well as skin biopsies with special stains and cultures for fungi for both infections. Sputum or bronchoscopy specimens have often been the source of a diagnosis in coccidioidomycosis.

Serologic tests for antibody in both diseases yield inconsistently positive results in AIDS patients. Treatment of the acute infection should be with amphotericin B followed by maintenance suppressive therapy with ketoconazole or amphotericin B.

REFERENCES

1. Abrams DI, Robia M, Blumenfeld W, et al: Disseminated coccidioidomycosis in AIDS (Letter). N Engl J Med 310:986-987, 1984
2. Ampel NM, Ryan KJ, Carry PJ, et al: Fungemia due to Coccidioides immitis: An analysis of 16 episodes in 15 patients and a review of the literature. Medicine 65:312-321, 1986
3. Anassie E, Fainstein V, Samo T, Bodey GP, Sarosi GA: Central nervous system histoplasmosis: An unappreciated complication of the acquired immunodeficiency syndrome. Am J Med 84:215-217, 1988
4. Anders KH, Guerra WF, Tomiyasu U, et al: The neuropathology of AIDS: UCLA experience and review. Am J Pathol 124:537-558, 1986
5. Bonner JR, Alexander WJ, Dismukes WE, et al: Disseminated histoplasmosis in patients with the acquired immune deficiency syndrome. Arch Intern Med 144:2178-2181, 1984
6. Bronnimann DA, Adam RD, Galgiani JN, et al: Coccidioidomycosis in the acquired immunodeficiency syndrome. Ann Intern Med 106:372-379, 1987
7. Byrne WR, Dietrich RA: Disseminated coccidioidomycosis with peritonitis in a patient with acquired immunodeficiency syndrome: Prolonged survival associated with positive skin test reactivity to coccidioidin. Arch Intern Med 149:947-948, 1989
8. Cappell MS, Mandell W, Grimes MM, Neu HC: Gastrointestinal histoplasmosis. Dig Dis Sci 33:353-360, 1988
9. Centers for Disease Control: Revision of the case definition of acquired immune deficiency syndrome for national reporting — United States. MMWR 34:373-375, 1985
10. Centers for Disease Control: Revision of the CDC surveillance case definition for acquired immunodeficiency syndrome. MMWR 36:1S-15S, 1987
11. Gerstein HC, Fanning MM, Read SE, Shepherd FA, Glynn MFX: AIDS in a patient with hemophilia receiving mainly cryoprecipitate. Can Med Assoc J 131:45-47, 1984
12. Goodwin RA, Shapiro JL, Thurman GH et al: Disseminated histoplasmosis: Clinical and pathologic correlations. Medicine 59:1-33, 1980
13. Graybill JR. Histoplasmosis and AIDS. J Infect Dis 158:623-626, 1988
14. Gustafson PR, Henson A: Ketoconazole therapy for AIDS patients with disseminated histoplasmosis (Letter). Arch Intern Med 145:2272, 1985
15. Haggerty CM, Britton MC, Dorman JM, et al: Gastrointestinal histoplasmosis in the acquired immune deficiency syndrome. West J Med 143:244-246, 1985
16. Hazelhurst JA, Vismer HF: Histoplasmosis presenting with unusual skin lesions in acquired immunodeficiency syndrome (AIDS). Br J Dermatol 113:345-348, 1985
17. Henochowicz S, Sahovic E, Pistole M, et al: Histoplasmosis diagnosed on peripheral blood smear from a patient with AIDS. JAMA 253:3148, 1985
18. Huang CT, McGarry T, Cooper S, et al: Disseminated histoplasmosis in the acquired immunodeficiency syndrome: Report of five cases from a nonendemic area. Arch Intern Med 147:1181-1184, 1987
19. Jagadha V, Andavolu RH, Huang CT: Granulomatous inflammation in the acquired immune deficiency syndrome. Am J Clin Pathol 84:598-602, 1985
20. Jarvik JG, Hesselink JR, Wiley C, Mercer S, Robbins B, Higginbottom P: Coccidioidomycotic brain abscess in an HIV-infected man. West J Med 149:83-86, 1988
21. Johnson PC, Khardori N, Najjar AF, Butt F, Mansell PW, Sarosi GA: Progressive disseminated histoplasmosis in patients with acquired immunodeficiency syndrome. Am J Med 85:152-158, 1988

22. Johnson PC, Sarosi GA, Septimus EJ, et al: Progressive disseminated histoplasmosis in patients with the acquired immune deficiency syndrome: A report of 12 cases and a literature review. Semin Respir Infect 1:1-8, 1986
23. Jones PG, Cohen RL, Batts DH, et al: Disseminated histoplasmosis, invasive pulmonary aspergillosis, and other opportunistic infections in a homosexual patient with acquired immune deficiency syndrome. Sex Transm Dis 10:202-204, 1983
24. Macher AM, DeVinatea ML, Koch Y, et al: Case for diagnosis: AIDS. Milit Med 151: M57-64, 1986
25. Macher A, Rodrigues MM, Kaplan W, et al: Disseminated bilateral chorioretinitis due to Histoplasma capsulatum in a patient with the acquired immunodeficiency syndrome. Ophthalmology 92:1159-1164, 1985
26. Mandell W, Goldberg DM, Neu HC: Histoplasmosis in patients with the acquired immune deficiency syndrome. Am J Med 81:974-978, 1986
27. McKinsey DS, Gupta MR, Riddler SA, Driks MR, Smith DL, Kurtin PJ: Long-term amphotericin B therapy for disseminated histoplasmosis in patients with the acquired immunodeficiency syndrome (AIDS). Ann Intern Med 111:655-659, 1989
28. Pasternak J, Bolivar R: Histoplasmosis in acquired immunodeficiency syndrome (AIDS): Diagnosis by bone marrow examination (Letter). Arch Intern Med 143:2024, 1983
29. Prichard JG, Sorotzkin RA, James RE III: Cutaneous manifestations of disseminated coccidioidomycosis in the acquired immunodeficiency syndrome. Cutis 39:203-205, 1987
30. Roberts CJ: Coccidioidomycosis in acquired immune deficiency syndrome: Depressed humoral as well as cellular immunity. Am J Med 76:734-736, 1984
31. Robinson PA, Knirsch AK, Joseph JA: Fluconazole for life-threatening fungal infections in patients who cannot be treated with conventional antifungal agents. Rev Infect Dis 12 (supple 3):S349-363, 1990
32. Salzman SH, Smith RL, Aranda CP: Histoplasmosis in patients at risk for the acquired immunodeficiency syndrome in a nonendemic setting. Chest 93:916-921, 1988
33. Sathapatayavongs B, Batteiger BE, Wheat J, et al: Clinical and laboratory features of disseminated histoplasmosis during two large urban outbreaks. Medicine 62:263-270, 1983
34. Sindrup JH, Lisby G, Weismann K, et al: Skin manifestations in AIDS, HIV infection, and AIDS-related complex. Int J Dermatol 26:267-272, 1987
35. Slama TG: Treatment of disseminated and progressive cavitary histoplasmosis with ketoconazole. Am J Med 74(1B):70-73, 1983
36. Smith CE, Saito MT, Simons SA: Pattern of 39,500 serologic tests in coccidioidomycosis. JAMA 160:546-552, 1956
37. Taylor MN, Baddour LM, Alexander JR: Disseminated histoplasmosis associated with the acquired immune deficiency syndrome. Am J Med 77:579-580, 1984
38. Tucker RM, Denning DW, Dupont B, Stevens DA: Intraconazole therapy for chronic coccidioidal meningitis. Ann Intern Med 112:108-112, 1990
39. Tucker RM, Galgiani JN, Denning DW, et al: Treatment of coccidioidal meningitis with fluconazole. Rev. Infect Dis 12 (supple 3):S380-389, 1990
40. Wheat LJ: Ketoconazole therapy for AIDS patients with disseminated histoplasmosis (Letter). Arch Intern Med 145:2272, 1985
41. Wheat LJ, Connolly-Stringfield P, Kohler RB, Frame PT, Gupta MR: Histoplasma capsulatum polysaccharide antigen detection in diagnosis and management of disseminated histoplasmosis in patients with acquired immunodeficiency syndrome. Am J Med 87:396-400, 1989
42. Wheat LJ, Rubin RH, Harris NL, et al: Systemic salmonellosis in patients with disseminated histoplasmosis: Case for "macrophage blockade" caused by Histoplasma capsulatum. Arch Intern Med 147:561-564, 1987
43. Wheat LJ, Slama TG, Zeckel ML: Histoplasmosis in the acquired immune deficiency syndrome. Am J Med 78:203-210, 1985

19

MYCOBACTERIAL DISEASES:
Tuberculosis and *Mycobacterium avium* Complex

MARK A. JACOBSON, MD

MYCOBACTERIUM TUBERCULOSIS INFECTION IN AIDS AND ARC

Epidemiology and Pathogenesis

Since the beginning of the AIDS epidemic, an increasing association of *M. tuberculosis* infection with AIDS or HIV infection has been noted. Nationwide, matching the first 53,395 AIDS cases with 144,123 concurrent tuberculosis cases, 3.8 percent of AIDS cases had tuberculosis, and 1.4 percent of tuberculosis cases had AIDS.[11]

Between 1978 and 1985, the yearly rate of tuberculosis more than doubled at one New York City hospital, and this increase was almost completely attributable to cases among patients with AIDS or ARC.[16] During the same time period, the incidence of tuberculosis increased from 15.4 per 100,000 to 105.5 per 100,000 among inmates of the New York State prison system, and a majority of inmates with tuberculosis reported in 1985 and 1986 had AIDS or HIV infection.[5] Nationally, from 1980 to 1984, tuberculosis decreased by 7 percent each year, but from 1985 to 1987 it increased by 1.4 percent.[11] In New York, California, Florida, and New Jersey (the states reporting the most cases of AIDS), extrapulmonary tuberculosis increased by 12 to 64 percent and tuberculosis among 25- to 44-year-olds increased by 14 to 34 percent from 1985 to 1987.[11] This suggests that HIV infection is an important factor in the changing epidemiology of tuberculosis.

Tuberculosis has been reported in 2 to 10 percent of AIDS patients studied in large retrospective series from New York, New Jersey, and Florida.[7,30,31] In San Francisco, 12 percent of 287 consecutive cases of tuberculosis in non—Asian-born males, 15 to 60 years old, also had AIDS.[7] Patients with AIDS and tuberculosis in these series were more likely to be Haitian, black, Hispanic, or intravenous drug users than white and homosexual.[7,31]

Since host resistance to M. tuberculosis is mediated by cellular immunity, it is not surprising that tuberculosis has been associated with HIV infection.[8] Epidemiologic data suggest that most cases of AIDS- or ARC-associated tuberculosis represent reactivation of latent M. tuberculosis infection acquired in the past rather than progression from recently acquired infection.[30,41] A recent prospective study of New York City intravenous drug users tested for HIV seropositivity and purified protein derivative (PPD) skin-test reactivity demonstrated that while prevalence and incidence of tuberculosis infection were similar for both HIV-seropositive and -seronegative intravenous drug users, risk of developing *active* tuberculosis was elevated for the HIV-seropositive individuals.[41]

The retrospective studies are remarkably consistent in that tuberculosis preceded the diagnosis of AIDS in half of AIDS-associated tuberculosis and occurred concurrently or following diagnosis of AIDS in the other half.[7,30] However, these retrospective studies, performed by matching tuberculosis and AIDS registries in a given hospital or community, could underestimate the full spectrum of tuberculous disease associated with HIV immune deficiency. A prospective study in Miami addressed this issue by prospectively screening tuberculosis patients for HIV antibody.[37] Thirty-one percent of 71 consecutive patients with confirmed tuberculosis were seropositive for HIV. At the time of tuberculosis diagnosis, only 27 percent of these HIV-seropositive patients had clinical evidence of AIDS or ARC. Thus, the number and incidence of tuberculosis cases related to HIV-induced immunosuppression may be considerably larger than indicated by retrospective studies.

Clinical Manifestations

While the pathogenesis of most HIV-associated tuberculosis appears to involve reactivation of latent M. tuberculosis infection, the clinical presentation is generally typical of reactivation tuberculosis only for those patients whose immune function is still relatively intact, while that of patients with AIDS or ARC tends to be much more typical of progressive primary tuberculosis. Only one third to one half of AIDS- and ARC-associated tuberculosis is confined to the lungs. The most frequent radiographic manifestations of pulmonary tuberculosis in patients with AIDS and ARC are given in Table 19—1. Pulmonary cavitation is rarely seen,[7,38,45] and the classic radiographic picture of apical infiltrates in the absence of hilar or mediastinal adenopathy has been reported in less than 10 percent of AIDS- or ARC-associated cases.[9,38,45]

One half to two thirds of AIDS- or ARC-related tuberculosis involves

TABLE 19—1.   CLINICAL FEATURES OF AIDS- OR ARC-ASSOCIATED TUBERCULOSIS

1. Radiographic features of pulmonary tuberculosis
   A. Common
      1. Hilar or mediastinal adenopathy or both
      2. Lower and middle lung-field localized infiltrate
   B. Rare
      1. Cavitation   2. Apical infiltrate
2. Extrapulmonary sites are involved in more than half of cases
   A. Peripheral lymph nodes and bone marrow are sites most likely to be positive
   B. Other extrapulmonary sites of infection: urine, blood, bone, joint, liver, spleen, cerebrospinal fluid, skin, gastrointestinal mucosa, ascites
   C. Important unusual syndromes: central nervous system mass lesion (tuberculoma), *M. tuberculosis* bacteremia

extrapulmonary sites (with or without pulmonary involvement).[7,38,45] Sites frequently positive for *M. tuberculosis* are given in Table 19—1. Granulomas are observed in about 50 percent of extrapulmonary biopsies but rarely in pulmonary biopsies.[45] Two extrapulmonary tuberculosis syndromes described in AIDS or ARC patients are of particular interest: *M. tuberculosis* bacteremia and central nervous system mass lesions. Bacteremia due to *M. tuberculosis,* rarely documented prior to AIDS (even among patients with miliary tuberculosis) has been reported as a frequent occurrence in AIDS patients with tuberculosis in Spain.[28] Fever and lymphadenitis has been the most common presentation, and chest radiographs frequently show no parenchymal abnormalities. Also, central nervous system mass lesions caused by *M. tuberculosis* were reported in a series of eight intravenous drug users with ARC.[1] These mass lesions caused a wide range of clinical manifestations and radiographic appearances on computed tomographic scans of the brain. The diagnosis was confirmed only by brain biopsy.

On the other hand, tuberculosis in patients with otherwise asymptomatic HIV infection tends to be clinically similar to tuberculosis in immunocompetent hosts.[8] Chaisson et al compared clinical findings in 17 HIV-seropositive and 40 HIV-seronegative non-Asian-born men with tuberculosis newly diagnosed at the San Francisco General Hospital TB Clinic.[9] There were no significant differences in PPD reactivity or chest radiograph findings. The median CD4+ lymphocyte count in the HIV-seropositive individuals was 350/μl, substantially higher than that generally observed in individuals with advanced ARC or AIDS. Narciso et al, in Italy, similarly reported a significant difference in mean CD4 counts among HIV-infected individuals with miliary tuberculosis (101/μl) and nonmiliary tuberculosis (312/μl).[33]

Diagnosis

Anergy is frequent in AIDS and ARC, and only 10 to 40 percent of such patients have a positive tuberculin skin test at the time of tuberculosis diagnosis[7,45] (Fig. 19 1). Nevertheless, tuberculin skin tests should be administered when tuberculosis is suspected in an AIDS or ARC patient. However, since false negative results are common, the absence of skin-test reactivity certainly does not rule out the diagnosis. Individuals with earlier stage HIV disease and tuberculosis are more likely to react to tuberculin antigen. Seventy-nine percent of such patients had a positive PPD result in one study.[9] However, because of the increasing incidence of anergy among HIV-infected individuals, a greater than 5-mm reaction to PPD should be considered evidence of tuberculosis infection.[32]

Appropriate specimens to culture for confirmation of tuberculosis include sputum, urine, blood, lymph node material, bone marrow, and liver. In the presence of pulmonary infiltrates, induced sputum or respiratory secretion obtained by bronchoscopy is the optimal specimen. Up to half of negative acid-fast bacteria (AFB) smears of respiratory or extrapulmonary specimens later are proven to be positive by culture.[8,25,45] Hence the decision to institute empiric antituberculous therapy must often be made before microbiologic confirmation of the diagnosis.

Therapy

Although tuberculosis is a more rapidly progressive and widely disseminated disease in AIDS and ARC patients than in controls without HIV infection, the response rate of AIDS and ARC patients to antituberculous therapy is generally as favorable as in non-AIDS/ARC historical controls. Treatment failures with standard two-, three-, or four-drug regimens have been uncommon in retrospective series, and drug-resistant strains of *M. tuberculosis* rarely have been isolated. Small et al recently reviewed results

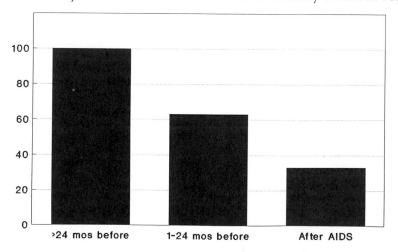

FIGURE 19—1. The percentage of HIV-infected patients with tuberculosis who have a positive tuberculin skin test progressively decreases with decreased time interval between the diagnosis of tuberculosis and the diagnosis of AIDS.[32]

of therapy of 125 AIDS patients treated for tuberculosis.[43] Only 3 (5 percent) of 61 patients who completed an adequate therapeutic regimen (isoniazid and rifampin for 9 months or isoniazid, rifampin, and pyrazinamide for 6 months) subsequently relapsed during a median 11-month follow-up period. All failures occurred in noncompliant patients. Drug toxicity required modification of the treatment regimen in 17 percent of patients (three times that of HIV-seronegative individuals in previously reported studies). Although AIDS and ARC patients with tuberculosis have had a higher rate of abnormal liver function test results associated with antituberculous therapy compared to control tuberculosis patients, serious antituberculous drug reactions requiring discontinuation of any effective regimen have been rare.

When less efficacious antituberculous regimens are used, HIV infection may have a more negative effect upon response to therapy. In a large prospective Central African study, tuberculosis was treated with 2 months of isoniazid, amithiazole, and streptomycin, followed by 10 months of isoniazid and amithiazole (a static, nonmycobactericidal agent).[36] At 6 months of therapy there was no difference in recurrence rates between HIV-seropositive and -seronegative patients. However, at 12 months of treatment, recurrence rates were 18.6 percent in HIV-seropositive versus 7 percent in seronegative patients.

The Center for Disease Control recommends initiating antituberculous chemotherapy whenever AFB are found in a specimen from a patient with HIV infection and clinical evidence of mycobacterial disease.[32] Since it is difficult to distinguish tuberculosis from disseminated *M. avium* complex infection, therapy should continue until culture results are final (usually 6 to 8 weeks). The recommended regimen for adults (Table 19–2) includes isoniazid 300 mg/d, rifampin 600 mg/d (450 mg/d for patients weighing less than 50 kg), and pyrazinamide 25 mg/kg/d for the first 2 months. Ethambutol 25 mg/kg/d should be added if extrapulmonary tuberculosis or isoniazid resistance is suspected. Subsequently, isoniazid and rifampin alone should be continued. The appropriate duration of treatment for

TABLE 19–2. EMPIRIC REGIMEN FOR HIV-ASSOCIATED TUBERCULOSIS*

First 2 Months	Additional 7 Months
1. Isoniazid 300 mg/d	1. Isoniazid 300 mg/d
2. Rifampin 600 mg/d†	2. Rifampin 600 mg/d†
3. Pyrazinamide 25 mg/kg/d	
4. Ethambutol 25 mg/kg/d if extrapulmonary disease or isoniazid resistance suspected	

*Whenever acid-fast bacteria are demonstrated in a specimen from a patient with HIV infection and clinical evidence of mycobacterial disease.
†Use 450 mg/d if weight < 50 kg.

HIV-associated tuberculosis is unknown, but a minimum duration of 9 months or at least 6 months after culture conversion seems reasonable. For patients who either cannot tolerate isoniazid or rifampin or have bone or joint disease, therapy should probably continue for 18 months.

Clinicians treating AIDS and ARC patients with isoniazid and rifampin need to be aware of a pharmacokinetic interaction between these drugs and ketoconazole (also commonly administered to AIDS and ARC patients for superficial or systemic opportunistic fungal infections) which can lead to subtherapeutic levels of both rifampin and ketoconazole.[13] This drug interaction has been associated with therapeutic failure of both antifungal and antituberculous treatment.

While response to antituberculous therapy has been good in retrospective studies, the survival rate among AIDS patients with tuberculosis has been low, similar to that for other AIDS patients followed for similar periods of time.

Prevention

Since antituberculous prophylactic therapy appears to be effective in HIV-infected populations with *M. tuberculosis* infection, CDC recommends that all asymptomatic HIV-seropositive individuals be given a skin test with five tuberculin units of PPD and all symptomatic HIV-infected patients receive both a skin test and a screening chest radiograph because of the higher probability of a false negative skin-test result.[32] Any HIV-infected patient, whatever age, with a tuberculin reaction greater than 5 mm or a history of positive skin-test reactivity should receive preventive isoniazid therapy for at least 12 months after sputum cultures have been obtained to exclude active pulmonary tuberculosis (Table 19–3).

The efficacy of prophylactic isoniazid has been highlighted recently by a prospective study of HIV-infected intravenous drug users in which none of 13 subjects with positive PPD tests who received isoniazid developed tuberculosis during follow-up compared to 7 of 36 who did not receive

TABLE 19–3. SCREENING FOR TUBERCULOSIS IN HIV-INFECTED PATIENTS

1. Screening skin test (5 tuberculin units of PPD) should be administered to all asymptomatic HIV-infected patients. Induration > 5 mm indicates tuberculous infection.
2. Skin test and chest radiograph should be administered to all symptomatic HIV-infected patients.
3. All HIV-infected patients with a positive tuberculin skin test or a history of positive tuberculin skin test should receive a minimum of 6 months prophylactic isoniazid. (Sputum mycobacterial cultures should be obtained before instituting isoniazid.)

prophylaxis.[41] Shorter courses of rifampin or rifampin plus pyrazinamide are possible alternative prophylactic regimens for isoniazid-intolerant patients, but the efficacy of such regimens has not been established.

Although risk of developing active tuberculosis is increased by concomitant HIV infection, risk of spreading tuberculosis to contacts does not appear to be greater than that observed with non-HIV-infected tuberculosis cases.[27]

DISSEMINATED *MYCOBACTERIUM AVIUM* COMPLEX INFECTION IN AIDS

Epidemiology and Pathogenesis

The association of disseminated *M. avium* complex (MAC) infection with AIDS was recognized early in the HIV epidemic.[15,26] Disseminated MAC infection has been reported only rarely in patients without AIDS.[19] According to recent CDC statistics, disseminated MAC was reported in 5.3 percent of AIDS cases between 1981 and 1987.[18] In a large retrospective series involving 366 AIDS patients, this opportunistic infection was diagnosed during the course of illness in 18 percent of AIDS patients; however, the attack rate may have been even higher, since 53 percent of 79 autopsies in this series showed evidence of disseminated MAC.[17] In another retrospective series from Miami, the frequency of atypical mycobacteriosis was 8.3 percent for non-Haitians and 11.3 percent for Haitians with AIDS.[39]

MAC is a ubiquitous soil and water saprophyte. The source of MAC invasion in AIDS patients may be gastrointestinal or respiratory. The presence of large clusters of mycobacteria within macrophages of the small bowel lamina propria suggests that the bowel might be the portal of entry. However, respiratory isolation of MAC preceded evidence of disseminated infection in 23 of 30 patients in one series, suggesting MAC infection begins in the lungs.[17]

In AIDS, the key host defect allowing dissemination of MAC may be macrophage dysfunction. MAC is able to survive within macrophages unless intracellular killing mechanisms (defective in AIDS) are activated. Also, lymphokines present in abnormal levels in AIDS, such as tumor necrosis factor, γ-interferon, and interleukin-2, may play an important role in host defense against MAC.

In AIDS, MAC causes high-grade, widely disseminated infection. Virtually all AIDS patients with invasive MAC infection (as opposed to stool, urine, or respiratory secretion colonization) have had positive mycobacterial blood cultures.[17] In the majority of those autopsied, MAC also could be isolated from spleen, lymph nodes, liver, lung, adrenals, colon, kidney, and bone marrow. The magnitude of mycobacteremia usually ranges from 10^1 to 10^4 cfu/ml of blood.[46] At autopsy, spleen, lymph nodes, and liver have yielded up to 10^{10} cfu/g of tissue.[46] Histopathologic studies of involved organs typically have shown absent or poorly formed granulomas and AFB within macrophages[15] (Color Plate ID).

Clinical Manifestations

Since most AIDS patients with disseminated MAC infection have other concomitant infections or neoplasms, and since MAC appears to cause little histopathologic evidence of inflammatory response or tissue destruction, the relationship between constitutional symptoms, organ dysfunction, and MAC infection has been uncertain.

Nevertheless, several large retrospective studies suggest a negative effect of disseminated MAC infection on mortality and morbidity in AIDS. Horsburgh and Selik compared survival of 1101 AIDS patients with disseminated nontuberculous mycobacterial infection (96 percent of cases due to MAC) to 33,808 AIDS patients without disseminated nontuberculous mycobacterial infection.[18] Median survival of patients with an index AIDS diagnosis of disseminated nontuberculous mycobacterial infection was 7.4 months compared with 13.1 or 10.5 months for patients with an index AIDS diagnosis of *Pneumocystis carinii* pneumonia or another AIDS-defining opportunistic infection. This analysis was methodologically flawed by the passive collection of data, resulting in substantial loss to follow-up and by the investigator's use of the date of laboratory confirmation of diagnosis as the date of AIDS diagnosis.[6] For patients with disseminated MAC infection, the longer time to culture confirmation of the diagnosis (typically 4 to 6 weeks compared to less than 1 week for most other key opportunistic pathogens) would bias toward shorter survival.[6]

At San Francisco General Hospital, we have examined the association between disseminated MAC infection and blood transfusion requirements.[23] Between July 1, 1987, and June 30, 1988, blood specimens from 574 patients were submitted to our mycobacteriology laboratory for culture. Among the AIDS/ARC patients transfused during the same time period, patients with a positive blood culture for MAC had a relative risk of 5.23 ($P < .001$) for receiving packed red blood cell (PRBC) transfusions compared to patients whose blood submitted for mycobacterial culture was negative. This would suggest that disseminated MAC infection is associated with increased morbidity in AIDS.

An alternative hypothesis is that patients with disseminated MAC infection are more immunosuppressed than those with other AIDS diagnoses and thus more susceptible to MAC infection, that is, that underlying immunosuppression rather than MAC infection is responsible for shorter survival. However, Horsburgh and Selik demonstrated that helper/suppressor lymphocyte ratios (a crude measure of immune function) were equivalent in AIDS patients with and without disseminated nontuberculous mycobacterial infection.[18]

TABLE 19–4. CLINICAL SYNDROMES ASSOCIATED WITH DISSEMINATED MAC INFECTION IN AIDS[17]

1. Systemic
   Fever   Weight loss, often associated with anemia
   Malaise   Neutropenia
2. Gastrointestinal
   a. Chronic diarrhea and abdominal pain (MAC invasion of colon often observed at autopsy)
   b. Chronic malabsorption (histopathologic changes in small intestine similar to Whipple's disease often observed at autopsy)
   c. Extrabiliary obstructive jaundice secondary to periportal lymphadenopathy

There are four clinical syndromes, often overlapping, that have been associated with disseminated MAC infection. The characteristics of these syndromes are summarized in Table 19–4.

Since 1987, there have been increasing numbers of cases in which AIDS patients receiving antiretroviral therapy with zidovudine (AZT) have developed *localized* visceral or cutaneous MAC abscesses without mycobacteremia.[2,35] Unlike disseminated infection (see below), these lesions have responded remarkably well to drainage and antimycobacterial therapy. These case series have led to speculation that improved immune function resulting from AZT therapy was responsible for localization of infection.

Diagnosis

Recent studies have demonstrated that special blood culture techniques for isolating mycobacteria, such as the Bactec system or Dupont isolator, are the most sensitive methods to diagnose disseminated MAC infection,[49] with sensitivity approaching 100 percent. Time to culture positivity ranges from 5 to 51 days. It is uncommon for blood cultures to be negative in the presence of positive histology from lymph node, liver, or bone marrow biopsies. However, one advantage to biopsied specimens is that stains may demonstrate AFB or granuloma weeks before blood cultures turn positive. At one center, stool AFB smear and culture positivity correlated well with true MAC bacteremia.[17] However, in other studies, stool cultures were positive in only half of mycobacteremias, and only two thirds of positive stools correlated with true disseminated infection. The importance of MAC isolation from sputum is uncertain.

Therapy

MAC is resistant to all standard antituberculous drugs (except ethambutol) at concentrations achievable in plasma. Yet, half or more of MAC strains can be inhibited by achievable concentrations of ansamycin (rifabutine), rifampin, clofazimine, cycloserine, amikacin, ethionamide, ethambutol, azithromycin, and ciprofloxacin[14,21,47-49] (Table 19–5). Unfortunately,

TABLE 19–5. DRUGS CAPABLE OF INHIBITING MOST MAC STRAINS AT CONCENTRATIONS ACHIEVABLE IN PLASMA

Ansamycin (rifabutine)	Ethambutol	Amikacin
Cycloserine	Azithromycin	Ciprofloxacin
Rifampin	Clofazamine	Ethionamide

drug levels necessary to kill MAC in vitro (minimum bactericidal concentration) have been 8 to more than 32 times that of inhibitory levels.[47] While combinations of antimycobacterial agents have shown in vitro inhibitory synergism, bactericidal synergism has been more difficult to demonstrate.[47,48] In addition, for in vivo killing, drugs must penetrate macrophages as well as the MAC cell wall. Nevertheless, in animal models of disseminated MAC infection, both single and combination antimycobacterial regimens have reduced mycobacterial colony counts by several logs and improved survival.[20,24]

In AIDS patients with MAC bloodstream infection, results of uncontrolled, combination antimycobacterial drug trials have been inconclusive. Ansamycin, provided by CDC under an Investigation New Drug (IND) application has been given in combination with other antimycobacterial drugs to over 600 AIDS patients with disseminated MAC infection.[34] Limited follow-up data has shown that eradication of MAC infection was uncommon, and the CDC subsequently terminated its IND program because of lack of evidence of efficacy. Among 13 patients treated at the National Institutes of Health with ansamycin and clofazimine, only three had persistently negative cultures while on therapy, and only one had apparent clinical improvement.[29] Similarly, at Memorial Sloan-Kettering Cancer Center, only three of 15 AIDS patients with disseminated MAC infection had decreased colony-forming-unit counts detected during therapy by sequential cultures.[17]

Two more recent uncontrolled clinical trials suggest a more beneficial effect of combination antimycobacterial therapy.[1,10] Agins et al reported that 5 of 7 AIDS patients with disseminated MAC infection treated with ethambutol, clofazimine, ansamycin, and isoniazid remained abacteremic for 3 to 6 months during which time fever, weight loss, and night sweats resolved.[1] In a California Collaborative Treatment Group study, 10 patients who received amikacin (7.5 mg/kg/d) for 4 weeks and ciprofloxacin, ethambutol, and rifampin for 12 weeks had a mean 1.2 log decrease in blood mycobacterial counts and a marked reduction in fever and night sweats.[10]

As mentioned above, in several small case series of AIDS patients with localized MAC infection, combination antimycobacterial therapy has been quite effective.[2,35]

In HIV-infected patients, it may be difficult to distinguish tuberculosis from MAC disease. Therefore, an antituberculous regimen should be instituted whenever AFB are demonstrated in a specimen from a patient with HIV infection and clinical evidence of mycobacterial disease.[32] If the AFB are later shown to be MAC, the antituberculous regimen should be discontinued.

Based on in vitro studies, a number of experimental drugs appear to have improved bactericidal activity against MAC. These promising new agents include liposome-encapsulated amphotericin, roxithromycin, and tumor necrosis factor.[3,44]

OTHER ATYPICAL MYCOBACTERIAL INFECTIONS IN AIDS

Disseminated infections caused by *M. kansasii*, *M. gordonae*, *M. fortuitum*, *M. chelonei*, *M. haemophilum*, and *M. xenopi* also have been reported in patients with AIDS.[12,18,40] These cases generally have had clinical presentations similar to that of MAC infection and pathologic evidence of pulmonary, intestinal, liver, and bone marrow involvement. In vitro sensitivity of isolates to standard antituberculous drugs has been variable.[12,22,40] *M. kansasii* has been the most frequently reported of these atypical mycobacteria, with disseminated infection present at the time of index AIDS diagnosis in 0.2 percent of patients.[18] Response to antimycobacterial therapy was poor in one small series of AIDS patients with disseminated *M. kansasii* infection.[42] However, we observed complete clinical resolution of disseminated pulmonary *M. kansasii* infection in an AIDS patient treated with isoniazid, rifampin, and ethambutol.[22] This patient's isolate was sensitive to rifampin and ethambutol and resistant to isoniazid. Given the frequent sensitivity of other atypical mycobacteria to one or more standard antituberculous drugs, multidrug therapy tailored to in vitro sensitivities is indicated for AIDS patients with non-MAC atypical mycobacterial infection.

REFERENCES

1. Agins BD, Berman DS, Spicehandler D, et al: Effect of combined therapy with ansamycin, clofazimine, ethambutol, and isoniazid for mycobacterium avium infection in patients with AIDS. J Infect Dis 159:784-787, 1989
2. Barbaro DJ, Orcutt VL, Coldiron BM: Mycobacterium avium–mycobacterium intracellulare infection limited to the skin and lymph nodes in patients with AIDS. Rev Infect Dis 11:625-628, 1989
3. Bermudez LEM, Young LS: Activities of amikacin, roxithromycin, and azithromycin alone or in combination with tumor necrosis factor against mycobacterium avium complex. Antimicrob Agents Chemother 32:1149-1153, 1988
4. Bishburg E, Sunderam G, Reichman LB, et al: Central nervous system tuberculosis with the acquired immunodeficiency syndrome and its related complex. Ann Intern Med 105:210-213, 1986
5. Braun MM, Truman BI, Maguire B, DiFerdinando GT, et al: Increasing incidence of tuberculosis in a prison inmate population. JAMA 261:393-397, 1989
6. Chaisson RE, Hopewell PC: Mycobacteria and AIDS mortality. Am Rev Respir Dis 139: 1-3, 1989
7. Chaisson RE, Schecter GF, Theuer CP, et al: Tuberculosis in patients with the acquired immunodeficiency syndrome. Am Rev Respir Dis 136:570-574, 1987

8. Chaisson RE, Slutkin G: Tuberculosis and human immunodeficiency virus infection. J Infect Dis 159:96-100, 1989

9. Chaisson RE, Theurer D, Elias D, et al: HIV seroprevalence in patients with tuberculosis. Presented at the 28th International Conference on Antimicrobial Agents and Chemotherapy (Abstract #571), Los Angeles, 1988

10. Chiu J, Nussbaum J, Bozzette S, et al: Treatment of disseminated *Mycobacterium avium* with ciprofloxacin, ethambutol, rifampin and amikacin. Presented at the V International Conference on AIDS (Abstract #M.B.P.300.), Montreal, 1989

11. Ciesielski CA, Bloch AB, Dooley SW, CDC, Atlanta: Assessing the impact of human immunodeficiency virus (HIV) on tuberculosis morbidity in the United States. Presented at the 29th International Conference on Antimicrobial Agents and Chemotherapy (Abstract #269.), Houston, 1989

12. Eng RHK, Forrester C, Smith SM, et al: Mycobacterium xenopi infection in a patient with acquired immunodeficiency syndrome. Chest 86:145-147, 1984

13. Engelhard D, Stutman HR, Marks MI: Interaction of ketoconazole with rifampin and isoniazid. N Engl J Med 311:1681-1683, 1984

14. Gangadharam PRJ, Kesavalu L, Rao PNR, Perumal VK, Iseman MD: Activity of amikacin against *Mycobacterium avium* complex under simulated in vivo conditions. Antimicrob Agents Chemother 32:886-889, 1988

15. Greene JB, Sidhu GS, Lewin S, et al: Mycobacterium avium-intracellulare: A cause of disseminated life-threatening infection in homosexuals and drug abusers. Ann Intern Med 97:539-546, 1982

16. Handwerger S, Mildvan D, Senie R, McKinley FW: Tuberculosis and the acquired immunodeficiency syndrome at a New York City Hospital: 1978-1985. Chest 91:176-180, 1987

17. Hawkins CC, Gold JWM, Whimbey E, et al: Mycobacterium avium complex infections in patients with the acquired immundeficiency syndrome. Ann Intern Med 105:184-188, 1986

18. Horsburgh CR, Selik RM: The epidemiology of disseminated nontuberculosis mycobacterial infection in the acquired immunodeficiency syndrome (AIDS). Am Rev Respir Dis 139:4-7, 1989

19. Horsburgh CR, Mason UG, Farhi DC, et al: Disseminated infection with mycobacterium avium-intracellulare. Medicine 64:36-48, 1985

20. Inderlied CB, Kolonoski PT, Wu M, et al: Amikacin, ciprofloxacin, and imipenem treatment for disseminated mycobacterium avium complex infection of beige mice. Antimicrob Agents Chemother 33:176-180, 1989

21. Inderlied CB, Kolonoski PT, Wu M, et al: In vitro and in vivo activity of azithromycin (CP 62,993) against the mycobacterium avium complex. J Infect Dis 159:994-997, 1989

22. Jacobson MA, Isenberg WM: Mycobacterium kansasii diffuse pulmonary infection in a patient with acquired immune deficiency syndrome. Am J Clin Pathol 91:236-238, 1989

23. Jacobson MA, Peiperl L, Volberding PA, et al: Red blood cell transfusion therapy for anemia in patients with AIDS and ARC: Incidence associated factors, and outcome. Transfusion 30:133-137, 1990

24. Kolonoski PT, Wu M, Petrofsky ML, et al: Combination of amikacin, azithromycin and clofazimine for the treatment of disseminated *Mycobacterium avium* complex infection in beige mice. Presented at the 29th International Conference on Antimicrobial Agents and Chemotherapy, (Abstract #1323), Houston, 1989

25. Louie E, Rice LB, Holzman RS: Tuberculosis in non-Haitian patients with acquired immunodeficiency syndrome. Chest 90:542-545, 1986

26. Macher AM, Kovacs JA, Gill V, et al: Bacteremia due to mycobacterium avium-intracellulare in the acquired immunodeficiency syndrome. Ann Intern Med 99:782-785, 1983

27. Manoff SB, Cauthen GM, Stoneburner RL: TB patients with AIDS: Are they more likely to spread TB? Presented at the IV International Conference on AIDS. (Abstract #4621), Stockholm, 1988

28. Martin-Scapa C, Cosin J, Gomez-Rodrigo J, et al: Mycobacteremia in AIDS patients. Presented at the IV International Conference on AIDS (Abstract #7539), Stockholm, 1988

29. Masur H, Tuazon C, Gill V, et al: Effect of combined clofazimine and ansamycin therapy on Mycobacterium avium–Mycobacterium intracellulare bacteremia in patients with AIDS. J Infect Dis 155:127-129, 1987

30. Morbidity and Mortality Weekly Report: Tuberculosis and acquired immunodeficiency syndrome—New York. 36:5785-5795, 1987

31. Morbidity and Mortality Weekly Report. Tuberculosis and acquired immunodeficiency syndrome—Florida. 35:587-590, 1987

32. Morbidity and Mortality Weekly Report: Tuberculosis and human immunodeficiency virus infection: Recommendations of the Advisory Committee for the elimination of tuberculosis (ACET). 38:236-250, 1989

33. Narciso P, Leoni GC, Sette P, et al: Clinical immunological and prognostic aspects of tuberculosis in HIV patients. V International Conference on AIDS (Abstract #Th.B.P. 56), Montreal, 1989

34. O'Brien RJ, Lyle MA, Snider DE: Rifabutin (Ansamycin LM 427): A new rifamycin-S derivative for the treatment of mycobacterial diseases. Rev Infect Dis 6:519-530, 1987

35. Packer SJ, Cesario T, Williams JH: Mycobacterium avium complex infection presenting as endobronchial lesions in immunosuppressed patients. Ann Intern Med 109:389-393, 1988

36. Perriens J, Karahunga C, Williame JC, et al: Mortality, treatment results and relapse rates of pulmonary tuberculosis in African HIV(+) and HIV(−) patients. Presented at the V International Conference on AIDS (Abstract#M.B.O.38), Montreal, 1989

37. Pitchenik AE, Burr J, Suarez M, et al: Human T-cell lymphotropic virus-III (HTLV-III) seropositivity and related disease among 71 consecutive patients in whom tuberculosis was diagnosed. Am Rev Respir Dis 135:875-879, 1987

38. Pitchenik AE, Rubinson HA: The radiographic appearance of tuberculosis in patients with the acquired immune deficiency syndrome (AIDS) and pre-AIDS. Am Rev Respir Dis 131:393-396, 1985

39. Pitchenik AE, Cole C, Russell BW, et al: Tuberculosis, atypical mycobacteriosis, and the acquired immunodeficiency syndrome among Haitian and non-Haitian patients in South Florida. Ann Intern Med 101:641-645, 1984

40. Rogers PL, Walker RE, Lane HC, et al: Disseminated mycobacterium haemophilum infection in two patients with the acquired immunodeficiency syndrome. Am J Med 84:640-642, 1988

41. Selwyn PA, Hartel D, Lewis VA, et al: A prospective study of the risk of tuberculosis among intravenous drug users with human immunodeficiency virus infection. N Engl J Med 320:545-550, 1989

42. Sherer R, Sable R, Sonnenberg M, et al: Disseminated infection with *mycobacterium kansasii* in the acquired immunodeficiency syndrome. Ann Intern Med 105:710-712, 1986

43. Small PM, Schecter GF, Sande MA, Hopewell PC: Response to tuberculosis therapy in patients with AIDS. Presented at the 29th International Conference on Antimicrobial Agents and Chemotherapy (Abstract #1066), Houston, 1989

44. Squires KE, Murphy WF, Madoff LC, et al: Interferon-gamma and mycobacterium avium-intracellulare infection. J Infect Dis 159:599-600, 1989

45. Sunderam G, McDonald RJ, Maniatis T, et al: Tuberculosis as a manifestation of the acquired immundeficiency syndrome (AIDS). JAMA 256:362-366, 1986

46. Wong B, Edwards FF, Kiehn TE, et al: Continuous high-grade mycobacterium avium-intracellulare bacteremia in patients with the acquired immune deficiency syndrome. Am J Med 78:35-40, 1985

47. Yajko DM, Nassos PS, Hadley WK: Therapeutic implications of inhibition versus killing of mycobacterium avium complex by antimicrobial agents. Antimicrob Agents Chemother 31:117-120, 1987

48. Yajko DM, Kirihara J, Sanders C, et al: Antimicrobial synergism against mycobacterium avium complex strains isolated from patients with acquired immune deficiency syndrome. Antimicrob Agents Chemother 32:1392-1395, 1988

49. Young LS. Mycobacterium avium complex infection. J Infect Dis 157:863-867, 1988

20

INFECTIONS DUE TO ENCAPSULATED BACTERIA, *SALMONELLA*, *SHIGELLA*, AND *CAMPYLOBACTER*

RICHARD E. CHAISSON, MD

Although the majority of serious infections in patients with HIV infection are due to protozoa, fungi, or viruses, bacterial infections are also important in this population. Disseminated atypical mycobacterial infections were recognized early in the epidemic,[12] and a growing list of bacterial complications of AIDS has been observed over time (Table 20-1). The frequency of serious infections with *Streptococcus pneumoniae*, *Haemophilus influenzae*, and *Salmonella* species has been shown to be increased in HIV-infected and AIDS patients compared with control populations.[8,43] These infections are characterized by atypical presentations, high rates of bacteremia, and frequent relapses despite appropriate therapy. Other bacteria may also cause disease more often in HIV-infected patients than in normal hosts, although this has not been firmly established. This article reviews the pathophysiology, epidemiology, clinical features, and management of infections with encapsulated and enteric bacteria in HIV infection and AIDS.

PATHOPHYSIOLOGY

A number of bacterial pathogens are able to evade host defense mechanisms in HIV-infected individuals. Table 20-1 lists organisms by the immune derangement that permits them to cause disease in AIDS. T-cell

TABLE 20–1. HIV-RELATED BACTERIAL INFECTIONS

Organisms Associated with T-Cell Defects
Mycobacterium avium complex
Mycobacterium tuberculosis
Salmonella
Listeria
Organisms Associated with B-Cell Defects
Steptococcus pneumoniae
Haemophilus influenzae
Branhamella catarrhalis
Campylobacter jejuni
Campylobacter-like organisms
Shigella

abnormalities, primarily of the CD4+ (helper) lymphocytes, result in infection and disease with a number of bacterial agents that require intact cell-mediated immunity (CMI) for control. Quantitative loss of CD4+ cells, impairment in clonal proliferation of CD4+ cells, and a decline in the production of γ-interferon all contribute to infections with organisms that require a CMI response.[6,24] *Mycobacterium, Salmonella,* and *Listeria* are thought to cause disease in AIDS because of impaired cellular immunity.

Derangements of cellular immunity have recently been demonstrated in the gut of patients with AIDS and ARC.[40] In addition to the loss of CD4+ lymphocytes and reversal of the CD4+:CD8+ ratio that occurs systemically, the intestinal mucosa of patients infected with HIV likewise has abnormally low numbers of T cells, especially CD4+ cells, and reversal of the CD4+:CD8+ ratio. Generalized increases in mucosal mononuclear cells and CD8+ lymphocytes are also seen.[40] Alterations in the production of mucosal IgA have been reported in AIDS and HIV-seropositive patients. These defects in cellular and humoral immunity in the gut of patients with advanced HIV disease may explain the increased frequency of enteric infections as well as the high rate of their systemic spread, as local defenses are unable to contain pathogens and prevent access to the bloodstream.

A number of B-cell abnormalities have been described in association with HIV infection and AIDS (Table 20-2), and these are associated with infectious complications with bacteria that require intact humoral immunity for control.[2,21,25,32] HIV infection frequently results in a nonspecific polyclonal increase in IgG secretion.[25] Coinfection with Epstein-Barr virus or cytomegalovirus (CMV) may potentiate this effect, and B cells may also undergo spontaneous proliferation. The polyclonal gammopathy of AIDS is often associated with increases in circulating immune complexes, which may have a variety of clinical consequences.[6]

The most serious change in humoral immunity seen in patients with AIDS is a lack of response to a variety of de novo antigenic stimuli.[2,25,32] Paradoxically, in spite of generalized increases in immunoglobulin synthe-

TABLE 20–2. B-CELL DEFECTS ASSOCIATED WITH HIV INFECTION

Spontaneous B-cell proliferation
Nonspecific polyclonal IgG secretion
Circulating immune complexes
Decreased response to pokeweed mitogen, staphylococcal protein A, pneumococcal
   polysaccharide

sis, the HIV-infected individual may be unable to mount a humoral immune response to new antigens from infectious agents such as encapsulated bacteria. B cells in AIDS patients respond poorly to keyhole limpet hemocyanin, pokeweed mitogen, and staphylococcal protein A.[2,25,32] In addition, response to a soluble recall antigen, tetanus toxoid, is impaired, as is responsiveness to T cell–independent antigens, such as polyvalent pneumococcal vaccine.[2,32] The relatively greater frequency of infections with encapsulated organisms seen in children with AIDS may be the result of lack of differentiated B cells producing specific antibodies to these agents, whereas adults with previous exposure presumably are more likely to maintain effective antibodies to these pathogens.[3,31]

Impairment of macrophage function may also result in infections with pyogenic bacteria in AIDS patients.[6] HIV infects monocytes and macrophages directly and results in qualitative functional defects. Moreover, decreased production of γ-interferon by T cells is associated with diminished phagocytic activity of macrophages. Loss of phagocytic function by macrophages, coupled with B-cell defects, is probably a factor in the high frequency of bacteremic pyogenic infections in advanced HIV disease.

Granulocytes from patients with HIV infection may show decreased chemotaxis, impaired phagocytosis, and reduced bacterial killing.[10] Moreover an increasing frequency of infections associated with granulocytopenia is being seen in AIDS patients as a result of therapy with myelotoxic drugs. In particular, the antiviral agents azidothymidine (AZT, zidovudine)[39] and ganciclovir (DHPG) cause severe reductions in granulocytes and may result in opportunistic infection with *Staphylococcus aureus*, *Klebsiella pneumoniae*, *Escherichia coli*, *Pseudomonas aeruginosa*, and other Enterobacteriaceae. Antitumor therapy for Kaposi's sarcoma is often associated with granulocytopenia, and myelosuppression secondary to severe mycobacterial disease is not uncommon in AIDS.

EPIDEMIOLOGY

Encapsulated Bacteria

Pneumonia due to pyogenic bacteria has been noted in patients with AIDS since early in the epidemic[28] (Table 20-3). Simberkoff and coworkers

TABLE 20–3. INCIDENCE OF BACTERIAL PNEUMONIAS IN PATIENTS WITH HIV INFECTION OR AIDS

AUTHOR	POPULATION	NUMBER OF CASES/ TOTAL PATIENTS
Simberkoff et al[44]	Hospitalized AIDS patients	5
Polsky et al[34]	Hospitalized AIDS patients	13/336
Gerberding et al[14]	Hospitalized AIDS patients	22
Witt et al[49]	Hospitalized AIDS patients	21/59
Selwyn et al[43]	IV drug users	14/159*

*Seronegative control rate, 6/277 ($P < 0.05$).

in 1984 reported four cases of community-acquired pneumococcal pneumonia, two with bacteremia, in AIDS patients from New York.[44] An additional patient had hospital-acquired pneumococcal pneumonia despite having received pneumococcal vaccine against the specific serotype of S. pneumoniae that caused his illness.

Polsky and colleagues found that 10 percent of cases of pneumonia in AIDS patients at Memorial Sloan-Kettering Cancer Center were due to community-acquired bacteria, with an annual attack rate of 17.9 per 1000 AIDS patients.[34] Eight of 18 episodes were due to pneumococcus and another eight were caused by H. influenzae. Four of 13 patients had recurrences 2 to 6 months following the initial episode. Antibody titers failed to rise appropriately after infection with the pneumococcus in the three patients tested. Gerberding and associates in San Francisco noted 17 patients with AIDS or ARC who had pneumonia caused by encapsulated organisms, including 10 relapses following appropriate therapy.[14] Seventy-five percent of episodes were bacteremic. Witt and colleagues reported community-acquired pneumonias in 21 of 59 AIDS and ARC patients from Boston City Hospital.[49] The incidence of pneumonia appeared to be higher among intravenous drug users and Caribbean-born heterosexuals (58 and 53 percent, respectively) than in homosexual or bisexual men (14 percent). One third of the patients had recurrent bacterial pneumonia despite appropriate therapy. Agents responsible for infection included the pneumococcus, H. influenzae, other Haemophilus species,[5] Branhamella catarrhalis, group B streptococci, S. aureus, Legionella, and Mycoplasma pneumoniae. Schlamm and Yancovitz found a high rate of H. influenzae pneumonia in young adults with AIDS, ARC, or risk factors for HIV infection.[42]

Compelling evidence that the incidence of bacterial pneumonias is increased in HIV-seropositive individuals comes from Selwyn and coworkers in New York.[43] In a 12-month prospective study of HIV infection in heroin addicts, 14 of 159 (9 percent) HIV-seropositive patients developed bacterial pneumonias, primarily due to H. influenzae and pneumococcus, compared with 6 of 277 (2 percent) seronogative controls (P < 0.05). Data from the death registry in New York show a more than twelvefold increase in mortality from community-acquired pneumonias in intravenous drug users since the beginning of the AIDS epidemic, possibly the result of HIV-induced immunosuppression.[45]

Bacteremia with a variety of organisms, some associated with pneumonias, has been reported in AIDS patients from several institutions.[11,14,23,44,48,49] In a study of 10 San Francisco hospitals, Redd et al found that 25 percent of patients with pneumococcal bacteremia had symptomatic HIV infection.[38] The incidence of pneumococcal bacteremia in AIDS patients, 9.4 cases per 1000 persons per year, was a hundredfold higher than previously reported. Bacteremia is often associated with a localized site of infection, such as an abscess or pneumonia.

Yamaguchi et al at Johns Hopkins Hospital observed a 46 percent prevalence of bacteremia in HIV-seropositive patients with pneumococcal pneumonia.[50] The proportion of pneumococcal disease occurring in HIV-seropositive patients increased from 2 percent in 1985 to 9 percent in 1989.[50]

Enteric Pathogens

Multiple case reports of nontyphoidal salmonellosis in patients with AIDS have been published.[5,13,15,18,29,35,46] Case series from Jacobs and associates[18] and Glaser and coworkers[15] include high rates of *Salmonella* bacteremia and frequent relapses despite appropriate antimicrobial therapy. Occurrence of salmonellosis prior to the diagnosis of AIDS was noted in a substantial proportion of cases. Fischl and coworkers[13] reported that at the University of Miami Hospital 6 of 14 blood cultures yielding nontyphoidal *Salmonella* in a 2½-year period were from AIDS patients, and in three patients this was the initial AIDS-related opportunistic infection.

The incidence of salmonellosis in San Francisco AIDS patients was found by Celum and associates to be 20 times greater than in age- and sex-matched controls.[8] Using population-based disease registries for both AIDS and *Salmonella* infections, these investigators found a significantly higher incidence of bacteremia in AIDS patients than in controls (45 percent versus 9 percent) and noted that one third of *Salmonella* infections occurred prior to the diagnosis of AIDS. An association of salmonellosis and raw milk consumption was seen.

Sexually transmitted enteric infections with *Shigella*, *Campylobacter*, and *Campylobacter*-like organisms (*C. cinaedi* and *C. fennellae*) are prevalent in homosexual men and are associated with risk of HIV infection.[27,36,37] Clinical experience with patients with ARC and AIDS suggests that infections with *Shigella* and *Campylobacter* are more resistant to therapy and tend to recur after treatment with appropriate agents.[4,9,33] Bacteremia, particularly with *Campylobacter* species, is not unusual, although comparative studies with immunocompetent controls have not been reported.[30]

CLINICAL PRESENTATION

Pneumonia

The presentation of bacterial pneumonias in AIDS patients is similar to that seen in nonimmunosuppressed hosts and differs from the typical presentation of *Pneumocystis carinii* pneumonia.[22] The onset of symptoms is often abrupt, and their duration is generally only several days.[14,49] Fever, productive cough, and dyspnea are characteristic, and pleuritic chest pain was present in 69 percent of patients in one series.[14] Localizing findings on physical examination, such as rales, bronchial breath sounds, egophany, and dullness to percussion, are common. Laboratory studies usually show a relative leukocytosis with an increased number of band forms, elevated sedimentation rate, and arterial hypoxemia. Chest radiographs are almost always abnormal, with focal lobar or segmental consolidation more common than diffuse infiltrates (Fig. 20-1). *H. influenzae* may be more often associated with diffuse infiltrates than *S. pneumoniae*,[34] with up to one quarter of *H. influenzae* pneumonias causing diffuse, bilateral infiltrates.[42] Gram stain of the sputum reveals many neutrophils, and organisms suggestive of the causative agent may be seen. Sputum cultures are usually positive, and blood cultures are positive in 40 to 80 percent of cases.

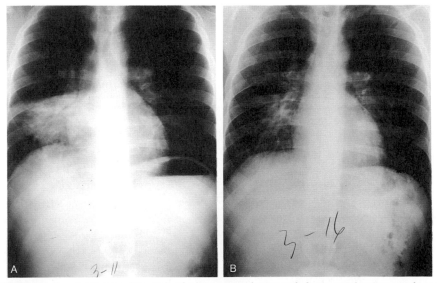

FIGURE 20–1. *A,* Chest radiograph of a homosexual man with fever, productive cough, and pleuritic chest pain. Sputum and blood cultures produced *S. pneumoniae. B,* Five days later the focal infiltrate is resolving, but symptoms persist. Giemsa-stained induced sputum revealed *P. carinii.*

Differential diagnosis includes other opportunistic infections, particularly *P. carinii* pneumonia. Patients presenting with symptoms consistent with a bacterial pneumonia whose chest radiographs show focal consolidation should have sputum Gram's stain and cultures of sputum and blood performed and should receive empiric antimicrobial therapy. In patients for whom a definitive diagnosis is not made, or in those who fail to respond to therapy, diagnostic evaluation for pneumocystosis should be performed. In several series, up to 10 percent of patients with pyogenic pneumonia have presented with concomitant *P. carinii* pneumonia.[9,42] AIDS patients with bacterial pneumonia who fail to respond to appropriate therapy may be found on subsequent evaluation to have *P. carinii* pneumonia. Patients with diffuse pulmonary infiltrates are less likely to have bacterial pneumonias than are those with focal infiltrates. Nevertheless, sputum induced for *P. carinii* examination or bronchoalveolar lavage specimens, or both, should be stained and cultured for pyogenic pathogens, particularly if purulence is noted.

Empiric treatment of suspected bacterial pneumonia should include coverage for the most common pathogens. Trimethoprim-sulfamethoxazole is an excellent agent, providing activity against the pneumococcus, *H. influenzae,* and *Branhamella* as well as *P. carinii*. Patients allergic to sulfa may be empirically treated with a second-generation cephalosporin, ampicillin (if the local incidence of β-lactamase-producing *H. influenzae* is low), or a semisynthetic penicillin and an aminoglycoside. Broad-spectrum agents such as third-generation cephalosporins and imipenem are not usually indicated.

Enterocolitis

Diarrhea is a common complaint in AIDS patients and is associated with a host of organisms (Table 20-4). Salmonellosis in AIDS and ARC patients presents with diarrhea in more than one half of cases, whereas up to 45 percent may be manifested by a febrile illness without colitis. When diarrhea is present, it is usually severe and may be associated with cramping, bloating,

TABLE 20—4.   INFECTIOUS CAUSES OF DIARRHEA IN AIDS

Enterocolitis	Proctitis
Entamoeba histolytica	*Neisseria gonorrhoeae*
Giardia lamblia	*Chlamydia trachomatis*
Cryptosporidium	Herpes simplex
Shigella flexneri	*Treponema pallidum*
Campylobacter jejuni	
Salmonella spp.	
Cytomegalovirus	

and nausea. Tenesmus and rectal pain are rare and suggest proctitis due to herpes simplex, *Neisseria gonorrhoeae, Chlamydia,* or syphilis. Fever is present in the majority of patients with salmonellosis. Blood counts and blood chemistry studies are nonspecific. Stool examination may show fecal leukocytes, but the sensitivity of this test in AIDS patients with salmonellosis is not established. Cultures of stool and blood establish the diagnosis. Stool should also be examined for ova and parasites and for *Cryptosporidium*. Flexible sigmoidoscopy may be performed in patients in whom a diagnosis is not made by noninvasive means to allow inspection for CMV lesions or Kaposi's sarcoma and for biopsies (see Chapter 11).

Shigella and *Campylobacter* infections are usually associated with severe, often bloody diarrhea, cramping, nausea, and fever. Fecal leukocytes are generally present and cultures reveal the organism. *Campylobacter*-like organisms can be cultured only in special media and are not routinely sought.

Asymptomatic enteric infections, previously reported in sexually active homosexual men,[37] also are prevalent in AIDS patients. Laughon et al found that 39 percent of 28 AIDS patients without diarrhea harbored pathogenic organisms in stool.[26] Fifty-five percent of AIDS patients with diarrhea were found to have an infectious etiology. *Shigella* and *Campylobacter* accounted for one quarter of the symptomatic infections (Table 20-5).

Therapy for enteric pathogens should be directed against specific organisms. Empiric therapy generally requires two agents, one active against *Salmonella* and *Shigella* and another against *Campylobacter*. Therapy with the quinolones norfloxacin and ciprofloxacin is usually adequate to cover all three agents.[41] *Salmonella* may be treated with ampicillin, chloramphenicol, trimethoprim-sulfamethoxazole, or a cephalosporin, depending on anti-

TABLE 20–5.   BACTERIAL AND OTHER ENTERIC INFECTIONS IN AIDS PATIENTS WITH AND WITHOUT DIARRHEA*

	NO. POSITIVE/NO. CULTURED (% +)	
	AIDS/DIARRHEA **N = 49**	**AIDS/NO DIARRHEA** **N = 28**
Shigella sp	2/41 (5%)	0/20
Campylobacter sp	5/47 (11%)	2/24 (8%)
Chlamydia trachomatis	5/44 (11%)	2/16 (12.5%)
Vibrio parahaemolyticus	2/47 (4%)	0/26
Clostridium difficile toxin	3/42 (7%)	0/19
Cryptosporidium	7/45 (16%)	0/19
Giardia lamblia	2/45 (4%)	1/19 (5%)
Isospora belli	1/45 (2%)	0/19
Herpes simplex	7/38 (18%)	
Any agent	28/49 (57%)	11/28 (39%)

*Adapted from Laughan BE, Druckman DA, Vernon A, et al: Prevalence of enteric pathogens in homosexual men with and without acquired immunodeficiency syndrome. Gastroenterology 94:984-993, 1988.

microbial sensitivities. Although nonimmunocompromised hosts are generally not treated for salmonellosis, therapy is always indicated in immunocompromised HIV-infected patients. The duration of treatment for bacteremias should be at least 10 to 14 days; AIDS patients with enteritis should receive 1 to 2 weeks of therapy. Judicious use of antimotility agents such as loperamide may decrease symptoms. Chronic suppressive antimicrobial therapy may be indicated, particularly for patients who have had one or more relapses.

Recurrent *Salmonella* Bacteremia

AIDS patients are apparently uniquely susceptible to recurrent episodes of *Salmonella* bacteremia. Patients typically present with fever and chills, usually without evidence of the septic shock syndrome (hypotension and progressive metabolic acidosis). All blood cultures are usually positive for nontyphoidal strains of *Salmonella*. Therapy with conventional antibiotics such as ampicillin and trimethoprim-sulfamethoxazole results in disappearance of symptoms and resolution of bacteremia. However, once antibiotics are discontinued, relapse of bacteremia is common. Jacobson et al reported therapeutic success with ciprofloxacin, 750 mg twice daily by mouth, both as initial therapy (with clearing of bacteremia) and as suppressive treatment.[19]

PREVENTION

Preventive measures for the control of bacterial infections in AIDS patients may reduce the incidence of disease. Three approaches—hygienic measures, prophylactic antibiotics, and immunotherapy—may be employed in selected settings. Hygienic control is particularly important for prevention of enteric infections. Avoidance of oral-anal sexual contact will reduce the transmission of pathogenic organisms. *Salmonella* infections in AIDS patients have been linked to raw milk, snake powders, pet turtles, and domestic turkeys.[8,46,47] Patients with HIV infection should avoid unsanitary water supplies, particularly in developing countries. Appropriate infection control precautions should be employed in the care of patients with enteric infections.

Antibiotic prophylaxis with trimethoprim-sulfamethoxazole is recommended for children with AIDS and adults who have had an episode of *P. carinii* pneumonia. Unfortunately, the frequency of adverse reactions to this agent limits its utility in this population.[16,20] Prophylactic penicillin may be appropriate for AIDS patients who have had relapses of pneumococcal disease, although the efficacy of this is not established. Use of prophylactic antibiotics for all adult ARC and AIDS patients is not recommended.

Passive immunotherapy with immunoglobulin can reduce the frequency of bacterial infections in children with ARC or AIDS, and monthly immunoglobulin injection is indicated for children with symptomatic HIV infection.[7] The routine use of immunoglobulin in adults is not recommended.

Active immunization with polyvalent pneumococcal vaccine is probably not effective in the majority of infected patients once they become symptomatic.[2] Responses to pneumococcal vaccine are suboptimal in the majority of AIDS and ARC patients, although HIV-seropositive persons with more than 450 CD4+ cells per μl appear to respond as well as uninfected controls.[17] Thus, immunization of asymptomatic HIV-infected individuals is a rational health maintenance approach and has been recommended by the Advisory Committee on Immunization Practices.[1] Immunization with *H. influenzae* capsular vaccine is recommended for all HIV-infected children in accordance with childhood immunization guidelines.

REFERENCES

1. Advisory Committee on Immunization Practices: Pneumococcal polysaccharide vaccine. MMWR 38:64-76, 1989
2. Ammann AS, Schiffman G, Abrams D, et al: B-cell immunodeficiency in acquired immune deficiency syndrome. JAMA 251:1447-1449, 1984
3. Bernstein LJ, Krieger BZ, Novick B, et al: Bacterial infection in the acquired immunodeficiency syndrome of children. Pediatr Infect Dis 4:472-475, 1985
4. Blaser MJ, Hale TL, Formal SB: Recurrent shigellosis complicating human immunodeficiency virus infection: Failure of pre-existing antibodies to confer protection. Am J Med 86:105-107, 1989
5. Bottone EJ, Wormser GP, Duncanson FP: Nontyphoidal Salmonella bacteremia as an early infection in acquired immunodeficiency syndrome. Diagn Microbiol Infect Dis 2:247-250, 1984
6. Bowen DL, Lane HC, Fauci AS: Immunopathogenesis of the acquired immunodeficiency syndrome. Ann Intern Med 103:704-709, 1985
7. Calvelli TA, Rubinstein AR: Intravenous gamma-globulin in infant acquired immunodeficiency syndrome. Pediatr Infect Dis 5(Suppl 3):S207-S210, 1985
8. Celum CL, Chaisson RE, Rutherford GW, et al: Incidence of salmonellosis in patients with AIDS. J Infect Dis 156:998-1002, 1987
9. Dworkin B, Wormser GP, Abdoo RH, et al: Persistence of multiply antibiotic-resistant *Campylobacter jejuni* in a patient with acquired immune deficiency syndrome. Am J Med 5:965-970, 1986
10. Ellis M, Gupta S, Galant S, et al: Impaired neutrophil function in patients with AIDS or AIDS-related complex: A comprehensive evaluation. J Infect Dis 158:1268-1276, 1988
11. Eng RH, Bishburg E, Smith SM, et al: Bacteremia and fungemia in patients with acquired immune deficiency syndrome. Am J Clin Pathol 1:105-107, 1986
12. Fainstein V, Bolivar R, Mavligit G, et al: Disseminated infection due to *Mycobacterium avium-intracellulare* in a homosexual man with Kaposi's sarcoma. Ann Intern Med 97:539-546, 1982
13. Fischl MA, Dickinson GM, Sinave C, et al: Salmonella bacteremia as manifestation of acquired immunodeficiency syndrome. Arch Intern Med 146:113-115, 1986
14. Gerberding JL, Krieger J, Sande MA: Recurrent bacteremic infection with *S. pneumoniae* in patients with AIDS virus (AV) infection (Abstract 443). Program and abstracts of the 26th Interscience Conference on Antimicrobial Agents and Chemotherapy, American Society for Microbiology, 1986, p 177

15. Glaser JB, Morton-Kute L, Berger SR, et al: *Salmonella typhimurium* bacterium associated with the acquired immunodeficiency syndrome. Ann Intern Med 102:189-193, 1985

16. Gordin FM, Simon GL, Wofsy CB, et al: Adverse reactions to trimethoprim-sulfamethoxazole in patients with the acquired immunodeficiency syndrome. Ann Intern Med 100:495-499, 1984

17. Huang K-L, Ruben FL, Rinaldo CR, et al: Antibody responses after influenza and pneumococcal immunization in HIV-infected homosexual men. JAMA 257:2047-2050, 1987

18. Jacobs JL, Gold JWM, Murray HW, et al: Salmonellosis infections in patients with the acquired immunodeficiency syndrome. Ann Intern Med 102:186-188, 1985

19. Jacobson MA, Hahn SM, Gerberding JL, Lee B, Sande MA: Ciprofloxacin for Salmonella bacteremia in the acquired immunodeficiency syndrome (AIDS). Ann Intern Med 110(12):1027-1029, 1989

20. Jaffe HS, Abrams DI, Ammann AJ, et al: Complications of cotrimoxazole in treatment of AIDS-associated *Pneumocystis carinii* pneumonia in homosexual men. Lancet 2:1109-1111, 1983

21. Katz IR, Krown SE, Safai B, et al: Antigen-specific and polyclonal B-cell responses in patients with acquired immunodeficiency disease syndrome. Clin Immunol Immunopathol 39:359-367, 1986

22. Kovacs JA, Hiemenz JW, Macher AM, et al: *Pneumocystis carinii* pneumonia: A comparison between patients with the acquired immunodeficiency syndrome and patients with other immunodeficiencies. Ann Intern Med 100:663-671, 1984

23. Krumholz HM, Sande MA, Lo B: Community-acquired bacteremia in patients with acquired immunodeficiency syndrome: Clinical presentation, bacteriology, and outcome. Am J Med 86:776-779, 1989

24. Lane HC, Depper JM, Green WC, et al: Qualitative analysis of immune function in patients with the acquired immunodeficiency syndrome: Evidence for a selective defect in soluble antigen recognition. N Engl J Med 313:79-84, 1985

25. Lane HC, Masur H, Edgar LC, et al: Abnormalities of B-cell activation and immunoregulation in patients with the acquired immunodeficiency syndrome. N Engl J Med 309:453-458, 1983

26. Laughon BE, Druckman DA, Vernon A, et al: Prevalence of enteric pathogens in homosexual men with and without acquired immunodeficiency syndrome. Gastroenterology 94:984-993, 1988

27. Moss AR, Osmond D, Bacchetti P, et al: Risk factors for AIDS and HIV seropositivity in homosexual men. Am J Epidemiol 125:1035-1047, 1987

28. Murray JF, Felton CP, Garay SM, et al: Pulmonary complications of the acquired immunodeficiency syndrome: Report of a National Heart, Lung and Blood Institute Workshop. N Engl J Med 310:1682-1688, 1984

29. Nadelman RB, Mathur-Wagh U, Yancovitz SR, et al: Salmonella bacteremia associated with the acquired immunodeficiency syndrome (AIDS). Arch Intern Med 145:1968-1971, 1985

30. Ng VL, Hadley WK, Fennell CL, et al: Successive bacteremias with *Campylobacter cinaedi* and *Campylobacter fennelliae* in a bisexual male. J Clin Microbiol 25:2008-2009, 1987

31. Oleske J, Minnefor A, Cooper R Jr, et al: Immune deficiency syndrome in children. JAMA 249:2345-2349, 1983

32. Pahwa SG, Quilop MTJ, Lange M, et al: Defective B-lymphocyte function in homosexual men in relation to the acquired immunodeficiency syndrome. Ann Intern Med 101:757-763, 1984

33. Perlman DM, Ampel NM, Schifman RB, et al: Persistent Campylobacter jejuni infections in patients with human immunodeficiency virus (HIV). Ann Intern Med 108:540-546, 1988

34. Polsky B, Gold JWM, Whimbey E, et al: Bacterial pneumonia in patients with the acquired immunodeficiency syndrome. Ann Intern Med 104:38-41, 1986

35. Profeta S, Forrester C, Eng RHK, et al: Salmonella infections in patients with the acquired immunodeficiency syndrome. Arch Intern Med 145:670-672, 1985

36. Quinn TC, Goodell SE, Fennell C, et al: Infections with *Campylobacter jejuni* and *Campylobacter*-like organisms in homosexual men. Ann Intern Med 101:187-192, 1984

37. Quinn TC, Stamm WE, Goodell SE, et al: The polymicrobial origin of intestinal infections in homosexual men. N Engl J Med 309:576-582, 1983

38. Redd SC, Rutherford GW, Sande MA, et al: Pneumococcal bacteremia in San Francisco residents with HIV infection (Abstract 56a). Program and abstracts of the 28th Interscience conference on Antimicrobial Agents and Chemotherapy, Washington, DC, American Society for Microbiology, 1988

39. Richman DD, Fischl MA, Grieco MH, et al: The toxicity of azidothymidine (AZT) in the treatment of patients with AIDS and AIDS-related complex: A double-blind, placebo-controlled trial. N Engl J Med 317:192-197, 1987

40. Rogers VD, Kagnoff MF: Gastrointestinal manifestations of the acquired immune deficiency syndrome. West J Med 146:57-67, 1987

41. Ruiz-Palacios GM: Norfloxacin in the treatment of bacterial enteric infections. Scand J Infect Dis 48(Suppl):55-63, 1986

42. Schlamm HT, Yancovitz SR: Haemophilus influenzae pneumonia in young adults with AIDS, ARC, or risk of AIDS. Am J Med 86:11-14, 1989

43. Selwyn PA, Feingold AR, Hartel D, et al: Increased risk of bacterial pneumonia in HIV-infected drug users without AIDS. AIDS 2:267-272, 1988

44. Sinberkoff MS, El Sadr W, Schiffman G, Raha JJ Jr: *Streptococcus pneumoniae* infections and bacteremia in patients with acquired immunodeficiency syndrome, with report of pneumococcal vaccine failure. Am Rev Respir Dis 130:1174-1176, 1984

45. Stoneburner RL, Guigli P, Kristal A: Increasing mortality in intravenous narcotics users in New York City and its relationship to the AIDS epidemic: Is there an unrecognized spectrum of HTLV-III/LAV-related disease? (Abstract 699). Presented at the Second International Conference on AIDS, Paris, June, 1986

46. Tauxe RV, Rigau-Perez JG, Wells JG, et al: Turtle-associated salmonellosis in Puerto Rico: Hazards of the global turtle trade. JAMA 254:237-239, 1985

47. Weber J: Gastrointestinal disease in AIDS. Clin Immunol Allergy 6:519-541, 1986

48. Whimbey E, Gold JWM, Polsky B, et al: Bacteremia and fungemia in patients with acquired immunodeficiency syndrome. Ann Intern Med 104:511-514, 1986

49. Witt DJ, Craven DE, McCabe WR: Bacterial infections in adult patients with the acquired immunodeficiency syndrome (AIDS) and AIDS-related complex. Am J Med 82:900-906, 1987

50. Yamaguchi E, Charache P, Chaisson RE: Increasing incidence of pneumococcal infection associated with HIV infection in an inner city hospital, 1985-1989 (Abstract). Am Rev Respir Dis, in press

21

MANAGEMENT OF HERPES VIRUS INFECTIONS (CMV, HSV, VZV)

W. LAWRENCE DREW, MD, PhD
WILLIAM BUHLES, PhD
RONALD J. DWORKIN, MD
KIM S. ERLICH, MD

CYTOMEGALOVIRUS

Infection with cytomegalovirus (CMV) is extremely common in patients with AIDS and can result in several clinical illnesses including chorioretinitis, pneumonia, esophagitis, colitis, encephalitis, adrenalitis, and hepatitis.[2] Autopsy and clinical studies indicate that 90 percent of AIDS patients develop active CMV infection during their illness. Up to 25 percent of these individuals may experience life- or sight-threatening infections due to this virus. Retinitis occurs in 5 to 10 percent of AIDS patients, whereas gastrointestinal disease and pneumonia occur in 5 to 10 percent and 5 percent, respectively. Not all patients with blood, urine, or tissue cultures positive for CMV have clinical illness related to the infection, and a diagnosis of disease caused by CMV should be made by tissue biopsy with histologic evidence of virus-mediated damage. Detection of CMV antigen or nucleic acid in tissue are alternative methods for establishing that CMV is actually causing tissue infection. If virus culture is positive for CMV and no other pathogen is identified in tissue, the virus may be the cause of the clinical illness and a therapeutic trial may be warranted. This section reviews these clinical syndromes and their treatment with ganciclovir (DHPG).

Kim S. Erlich was supported by Public Health Service grant 5-T32-AI07234 from the National Institutes of Health.

Chorioretinitis

Ocular disease due to CMV occurs only in patients with severe immunodeficiency and is especially common in patients with AIDS. Clinical evidence of CMV retinitis occurs in at least 5 to 10 percent of AIDS patients, and autopsy series have revealed that CMV retinitis is present in up to 30 percent of patients. Retinitis is occasionally the presenting manifestation of AIDS, but it more commonly presents months to years after the diagnosis of AIDS has been established. Retinitis usually begins unilaterally, but progression to bilateral involvement is common due to the associated viremia. Systemic CMV infection also is frequently present, and other viscera may be simultaneously diseased. Unilateral visual-field loss, decreased visual acuity, or the presence of "floaters" is often the presenting complaint. Ophthalmologic examination typically reveals large creamy to yellowish white granular areas with perivascular exudates and hemorrhages (referred to as a "cottage cheese and catsup" appearance) (Fig. 21–1). These abnormalities are usually found initially at the periphery of the fundus, but, if left untreated, the lesions often progress to involve the macula and the optic disc. Histologic examination reveals coagulation necrosis and microvascular abnormalities.[1,46]

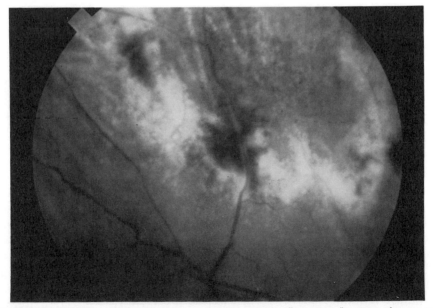

FIGURE 21–1. Funduscopic appearance of CMV retinitis, illustrating "cottage cheese and catsup" appearance resulting from perivascular exudates and hemorrhages. (Courtesy Dr. L. Schwartz, San Francisco.)

TABLE 21–1. COMPARISON OF COURSE OF CMV DISEASE IN GANCICLOVIR VERSUS UNTREATED CONTROL PATIENTS WITH AIDS

CMV SITE	NO. PATIENTS IMPROVED OR STABILIZED/TOTAL	
	GANCICLOVIR-TREATED	UNTREATED CONTROLS
Retina	208/254 (82%)	2/61 (3%)
Gastrointestinal tract/colon	33/39 (85%)	NA
Lung	18/23 (78%)	1/7 (14%)

NA = Not available.

Differentiating suspected CMV retinitis lesions from "cotton wool spots" is essential. Cotton wool spots appear as small, fluffy, white lesions with indistinct margins and are not associated with exudates or hemorrhages.[1,46] They are common in AIDS patients, are usually asymptomatic, and probably result from microvascular lesions secondary to HIV infection. These lesions do not progress and often undergo spontaneous regression.

All patients with AIDS should have a thorough ophthalmologic examination (including pupillary dilatation) at regular intervals. Patients with suspected or confirmed CMV chorioretinitis should be considered for treatment with 9-(1,3-dihydroxy-2-propoxymethyl) guanine (DHPG) or ganciclovir. Ganciclovir is effective in the treatment of CMV chorioretinitis, although lesions usually recur once therapy is discontinued.[3,21]

Initial "induction" treatment for CMV retinitis consists of 5 mg/kg twice daily or 2.5 mg/kg every 8 hours for 14 days. The optimal dosage for maintenance therapy remains under investigation but is approximately one half the induction dose, that is 5 mg/kg/d for 5 to 7 days per week or 6 mg/kg/d for 5 days per week. Initial response (improvement or stabilization in vision or opthalmoscopic appearance) occurs in approximately 80 percent of treated patients. By comparison, the disease is relentlessly progressive in 90 percent of patients if left untreated (Table 21–1). Visual-field defects present at the onset of therapy do not reverse, but a decrease in visual acuity due to edema of the macula may improve with treatment. Maintenance therapy throughout the life of the patient appears critical, because the virus is only suppressed by ganciclovir and not eliminated. Table 21–2 compares patients with CMV retinitis who received no maintenance therapy with those who received either low- or high-dose maintenance therapy. The data suggest that 25 to 35 mg/kg/wk maintenance therapy is required for sustained remission. Toxicity, however, especially neutropenia, limits the dose and duration of maintenance therapy. Even with continued maintenance therapy, progression of CMV retinitis eventually occurs. This may result from viral resistance to the drug or from the patient's continued deterioration with progression of HIV infection. Retinal detachment may occur in later stages as the necrotic retina scars and thins. Intravitreal injection has been used in certain special situations, such as

TABLE 21–2. CLINICAL RELAPSE OF CMV RETINITIS IN PATIENTS WITH AIDS

	MAINTENANCE GANCICLOVIR		
	NONE	LOW DOSE*	HIGH DOSE*
No. of patients	41	10	70
Mean cumulative induction dose (mg/kg)	162	155	167
Percent relapse-free on day 120	14%	0	58%
Median days to relapse†	37	31	145

*Low dose: 10–20 mg/kg/wk; high dose: 25–35 mg/kg/wk.
†Kaplan-Meier estimate.

patients in whom neutropenia limited the systemic use of the drug, and in one series[5] appeared effective and relatively safe. Controlled, comparative studies are underway to determine efficacy and safety.

Pneumonia

Isolation of CMV from pulmonary secretions or lung tissue in AIDS patients with pneumonia who undergo bronchoscopy is common, but a true pathogenic role of the virus in the disease process is usually not apparent. Many patients with pulmonary disease and CMV isolation from the lung have concomitant infection with other pathogens, especially *Pneumocystis carinii*. Many of the patients respond to therapy directed at *P. carinii* pneumonia (PCP) alone, raising the question of whether CMV is a true pulmonary pathogen. Patients with positive CMV cultures from lung tissue and no other pathogens identified on diagnostic bronchoscopy may have invasive CMV pneumonia. The diagnosis of CMV pneumonia is enhanced by a combination of factors, including positive CMV culture from lung tissue or pulmonary secretions, the presence of pathognomonic cells with intranuclear inclusion bodies, CMV antigen or nucleic acid in tissue, and the absence of other pathogenic organisms.

When CMV causes pulmonary disease in AIDS, the syndrome is that of an interstitial pneumonia. Patients often complain of gradually worsening shortness of breath, dyspnea on exertion, and a dry, nonproductive cough. The heart and respiratory rate are elevated, and auscultation of the lungs often reveals minimal findings with no evidence of consolidation. Chest radiograph shows diffuse interstitial infiltrates similar to those in PCP. Hypoxemia is invariably present.

Therapy with ganciclovir should be considered when a patient has documented CMV pulmonary infection as the only pathogen identified and a progressive deteriorating clinical course.[38] Ganciclovir is less effective in treating pneumonia than retinitis in patients with AIDS; only approximately 60 percent of patients with pneumonia respond to an initial course of therapy. Unlike the case with retinitis, therapy may be stopped once the pneumonia has resolved. The treatment dosage is 5 mg/kg twice daily, although higher dosage may be necessary to produce a clinical response. Recent evidence suggests that the combination of ganciclovir with high-dose intravenous immunoglobulin is more efficacious than ganciclovir alone in treating CMV pneumonia in bone marrow transplant recipients.[18a,33a] There is no data to support this combination in AIDS patients, however.

Central Nervous System Infection

Subacute encephalitis caused by CMV probably occurs in AIDS, but encephalitis in AIDS may also occur as a result of neural involvement by HIV. CMV is not a neurotropic virus, but isolation and identification of CMV in brain tissue or cerebrospinal fluid has been reported. This supports the hypothesis that CMV can, on occasion, produce central nervous system infection[14,15,24] (Chapter 12).

CMV encephalitis in AIDS appears comparable to "subacute" encephalitis from other pathogens. Personality changes, difficulty concentrating, headaches, and somnolence are frequently present. The diagnosis can be confirmed only by brain biopsy, with evidence of periventricle necrosis, giant cells, intranuclear and intracytoplasmic inclusions, and isolation or other identification of the virus, for example, by antigen or nucleic acid.[24] CMV may also cause myelitis, presenting as a spinal cord syndrome with lower extremity weakness, spasticity, and bowel and bladder symptoms. Administration of ganciclovir should be considered in AIDS patients with CMV encephalitis and myelitis, but no data on its efficacy are available.

Gastrointestinal Infection

Colitis

CMV colitis occurs in at least 5 to 10 percent of AIDS patients (Chapter 11). Diarrhea, weight loss, anorexia, and fever are frequently present. The differential diagnosis includes infection due to other gastrointestinal pathogens, including *Cryptosporidium, Giardia, Entamoeba, Mycobacterium, Shigella, Campylobacter,* and *Strongyloides stercoralis,* and involvement by lymphoma or Kaposi's sarcoma. Sigmoidoscopy reveals diffuse submucosal hemorrhages and diffuse mucosal ulcerations, although a grossly normal-appearing mucosa may be encountered in up to 10 percent of those with histologic evidence of CMV colitis (Fig. 21–2). Biopsy reveals vasculitis, neutrophilic infiltration, CMV inclusions, and nonspecific inflammation.

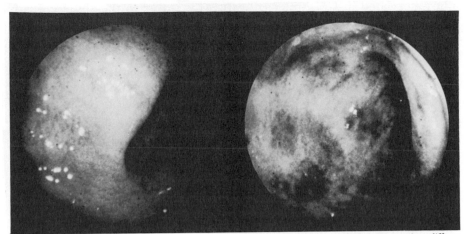

FIGURE 21—2. Sigmoidoscopic appearance of CMV colitis (two views), demonstrating diffuse submucosal hemorrhages and mucosal ulcerations. (Courtesy Dr. D. Dieterich, New York.)

Esophagitis

Clinically evident esophagitis in AIDS patients is most commonly due to either *Candida albicans* or herpes simplex virus (HSV), but CMV may also cause esophagitis. Patients with esophagitis who do not have *Candida* or HSV detected by endoscopy, histology, or culture and who have CMV detected by these methods should be treated with ganciclovir. The dosage for treating CMV colitis or esophagitis should be 5 mg/kg twice daily for 14 to 21 days (depending upon clinical response). Response rates are in the 70 to 80 percent range. Maintenance therapy is usually not necessary, although relapse or recurrences may occur.

Treatment with Ganciclovir

Since June 1989, approval has been given for marketing ganciclovir, 9-(1,3-dihydroxy-2-propoxymethyl) guanine, for the treatment of CMV retinitis in immunocompromised patients, including patients with AIDS.

Structure and Mechanism of Action

Ganciclovir (DHPG, Cytovene) is a nucleoside analogue that differs from acyclovir (Zovirax) by a single hydroxyl side chain. This structural change confers on the drug approximately 50 times more activity than acyclovir against CMV. Acyclovir has low activity against CMV since it is not well phosphorylated in CMV-infected cells. This is due to the absence of the gene for thymidine kinase (TK) in CMV. Ganciclovir, however, is active against CMV because it does not require TK for phosphorylation. Instead, a cellular kinase or a virus-induced phosphorylating enzyme is increased in CMV-infected cells, which is capable of phosphorylating ganciclovir and converting it to the monophosphate, and then cellular enzymes convert it to the active compound, ganciclovir triphosphate. Ganciclovir triphosphate acts to inhibit the viral DNA polymerase.

Pharmacology and Dosage

Intravenous ganciclovir is the only form currently available for clinical use. Individual vials contain 500 mg per vial and contain 50 mg/ml when reconstituted in 10 ml sterile water. When administered by intravenous infusion over 1 hour in the usual dosage of 5 mg/kg, peak blood levels are approximately 6 to 15 mg/ml, and the serum half-life is 2.9 hours. The drug is given two to three times daily during initial induction, whereas maintenance therapy consists of 5 to 6 mg/kg once daily or five to seven times per week. Since the drug undergoes renal excretion, the dosage must be reduced with impaired renal function. A formula for dose reduction is presented in Table 21–3. For maintenance therapy, these recommendations should be halved.

Clinical Use

Administration of ganciclovir is indicated for the treatment of acute CMV infection, but other herpes viruses, (specifically HSV-1, HSV-2, and varicella zoster virus [VZV]), are also susceptible to the drug in vitro. Since AIDS patients with severe CMV infection frequently have illnesses due to other herpes viruses, a "bonus" of ganciclovir therapy may be an associated improvement of HSV and VZV infections. Ganciclovir is probably also active against Epstein-Barr virus, but this is not certain. Some investigators have reported that adenoviruses are also susceptible to ganciclovir.

TABLE 21–3.   DOSAGE ADJUSTMENT FOR GANCICLOVIR INDUCTION TREATMENT* IN PATIENTS WITH IMPAIRED RENAL FUNCTION

LEVEL OF RENAL FUNCTION	CREATININE CLEARANCE (ml/1.73 m²/min)	GANCICLOVIR DOSAGE (mg/kg)
Normal	> 80	5.0 b.i.d.
Mild impairment	50–79	2.5 b.i.d.
Moderate impairment	25–49	2.5 once daily
Severe impairment	<25	1.25 once daily

*For maintenance therapy these recommendations should be halved.

Virologic Response to Ganciclovir

The results of CMV cultures of blood and urine in patients treated with ganciclovir are shown in Figure 21–3. Most of these patients had CMV retinitis, although AIDS patients with CMV infections of other organ systems are included. Of these patients, 87 percent had a complete virologic response (conversions of culture from positive to negative or a more than hundredfold reduction in CMV titer) in urine, and 83 percent had a complete response in blood culture. The median time until response was 8 days for both blood and urine cultures.

Resistance

We have monitored a limited number of patients for the development of resistance to ganciclovir while on long-term therapy. None of the first 10 patients we studied exhibited the development of a resistant strain even after nearly 2 years of continuous treatment. However, Erice et al have reported three Minnesota patients whose clinical course suggested the emergence of resistance and whose CMV isolates exhibited increases in the concentration of ganciclovir required to inhibit the virus in tissue culture by 90 percent (ID_{90}) over baseline determinations.[19] Subsequently, we have found similar resistant isolates from patients in San Francisco. These strains remain sensitive to Foscarnet, which may be used as alternate therapy (see Table 21–5).

Toxicity

Toxicity frequently limits therapy with ganciclovir. The following primary organs are adversely affected.

Hematopoiesis. Neutropenia, defined as an absolute neutrophil count of less than $1000/mm^3$, occurs in nearly 40 percent of ganciclovir recipients (Table 21–4). Sixteen percent of patients receiving the drug develop neutrophil counts of less than $500/mm^3$. Neutropenia usually occurs early (that is, in the period of induction or early maintenance treatment) but may occur later in therapy as well. The leukopenia is usually reversible, but at least five patients are known to have had irreversible suppression. Many AIDS patients have low white blood counts prior to beginning therapy, so the contribution of ganciclovir to leukopenia may not be entirely clear. Nonetheless, the dosage should be reduced when absolute neutrophil counts fall below $1000/mm^3$ or discontinued when severe leukopenia occurs (absolute neutrophil counts of less than $500/mm^3$). The drug may be resumed when neutrophil counts have risen to safe levels, preferably greater than $1000/mm^3$. It is not clear that neutropenia is dose-related, as many patients on high-dose maintenance therapy do not develop this adverse reaction. Nonetheless, reduction of dosage may bring about reversal of

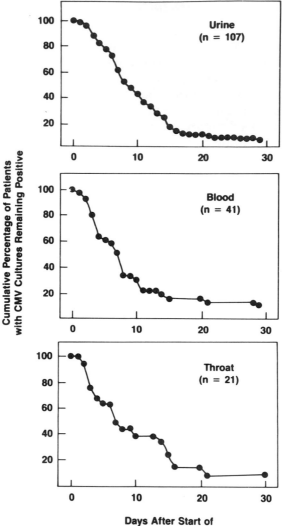

**Days After Start of
Induction Treatment**

FIGURE 21–3. Time course of conversion of cytomegalovirus (CMV) cultures of specimens of urine, blood, or throat washings from positive (before treatment) to negative (after treatment with ganciclovir). Cultures from individual patients were performed at various times after start of treatment. Numbers in parentheses are the number of patients in whom the particular body fluid or site was sequentially cultured. (From Buhles WC Jr, Mastre BJ, Tinker AJ, Strand V, Koretz SH, and the Syntex Collaborative Ganciclover Treatment Study Group: Ganciclovir treatment of life- or sight-threatening cytomegalovirus infection: Experience in 314 immunocompromised patients. Rev Infect Dis 10[suppl 3]:S495-S504, 1988.)

TABLE 21—4. COMPARISON OF NEUTROPENIA AND THROMBOCYTOPENIA IN PATIENTS WITH AIDS VERSUS THOSE WITH OTHER CAUSES OF IMMUNODEFICIENCY

HEMATOLOGIC PARAMETER	UNDERLYING AIDS	OTHER IMMUNODEFICIENCY*
Nadir of absolute neutrophil count (ANC)†		
<500	16.2%	13.3%
<500 to <1000	24.3%	10.7%
≥1000	59.5%	76.0%
Nadir of platelet count		
<20,000	5.3%	29.0%
20,000 to <50,000	8.7%	17.4%
≥50,000	86.0%	53.6%

*Percentage of patients in each category. No. = 462 patients on whom adequate hematologic data was available for neutropenia; No. = 470 for thrombocytopenia.
†Counts are number of cells per microliter.

neutropenia. Discontinuation of therapy is necessary in patients whose neutrophils do not increase during dosage reduction. Thrombocytopenia (platelet count less than 20,000/mm^3) occurs in 9 percent of patients receiving the drug and is less likely to be seen in non-AIDS patients than AIDS patients (5 percent versus 29 percent).

Other Organ Systems.   Adverse effects on the central nervous system occur in 17 percent of AIDS patients. Confusion is the most common symptom, occurring in 3 percent of patients, and 2 percent of patients experience convulsions, dizziness, headaches, or abnormal thinking. Overall, 15 percent of patients have gastrointestinal disturbances. Nausea is the most frequent complaint (5 percent), followed by vomiting (4 percent), abnormal liver function tests (3 percent), and diarrhea (2 percent).

Ganciclovir plus Azidothymidine (AZT).   Studies are in progress to determine whether the combination of AZT and ganciclovir is more toxic than either agent alone. Until these results are available, it is recommended that the two drugs not be given concurrently. Frequently the physician (and patient) must decide which drug should be discontinued. Each case must be evaluated individually, but sight-threatening disease usually mandates continuing ganciclovir. Prophylactic measures to prevent *P. carinii* infection (such as pentamidine inhalation) should be considered (Chapters 7 and 15). In addition, newer antiretroviral agents with less hematologic toxicity, such as dideoxyinosine or dideoxycytidine, may soon be available.

Gonadal Toxicity.   In preclinical animal studies, ganciclovir was determined to be a potent inhibitor of spermatogenesis. Sperm counts in humans before and during ganciclovir therapy, however, have been performed too infrequently to provide meaningful information on spermato-genesis. Follicle-stimulating hormone (FSH) and luteinizing hormone (LH) have been measured in ganciclovir-treated patients, with increases occurring in approximately 30 percent of patients. This data may suggest end-organ toxicity. Unfortunately, control patients not receiving ganciclovir must also be studied to accurately interpret these results. Nonetheless, patients wishing to reproduce should use ganciclovir only for the strongest indications.

Premature Termination of Treatment.   Approximately one third of patients must discontinue or interrupt ganciclovir treatment. The most common cause of early interruption of therapy is neutropenia (65 percent of discontinuations). Adverse CNS reactions (11 percent) and thrombocytopenia (8 percent) account for most of the remaining interruptions.

Treatment with Foscarnet

Phosphonoformic acid (PFA, Foscarnet) shows in vitro inhibitory effect against CMV and promising benefit in preliminary human trials. As with ganciclovir, PFA does not eradicate virus and therefore requires maintenance therapy to sustain the antiviral effect. Its toxicities are different from those of ganciclovir, primarily transient renal impairment. The drug is currently in trials and is not available commercially.

HERPES SIMPLEX VIRUS

Herpes simplex viruses types 1 and 2 (HSV-1, HSV-2) cause disease in both normal and immunocompromised hosts and are responsible for substantial morbidity in patients with AIDS. Since most adults with AIDS have been previously infected with HSV, they are not susceptible to primary infection. Reactivated infection and recurrent disease are common in AIDS patients, however, and may result in extensive tissue destruction with prolonged virus shedding.

The prevalence of HSV infection in homosexual AIDS patients exceeds that of the general population and likely reflects the common risk factor for transmission of both HSV and HIV (sexual contact). Serologic studies have revealed that more than 95 percent of homosexual men with AIDS have been previously infected with HSV, allowing for virus reactivation and clinical illness later in life.[31,35] AIDS subgroups other than homosexual men, such as hemophiliacs and transfusion recipients, would be expected to have lower rates of previous HSV infection.

Clinical Presentation

Because most HIV-infected patients have been infected with HSV prior to the development of AIDS, recurrent HSV is much more common than primary HSV infection. HSV infection in AIDS is often atypical compared to infection in the normal host. The severity of the illness depends on several factors, including the site of initial infection, the degree of immunosuppression, and whether the episode represents initial-primary infection (no previous exposure to either HSV type), initial-nonprimary infection (previous exposure to the heterologous HSV type), or recurrent infection.

The CDC has recently revised the diagnostic criteria for AIDS to include chronic mucocutaneous HSV infection. Large ulcerative lesions, without visceral or cutaneous dissemination, are frequent in HIV-infected patients. In an individual with no other cause of underlying immunodeficiency or who has laboratory evidence of HIV infection, ulcerative HSV infection present for longer than 1 month is diagnostic of AIDS.[34]

Orolabial Infection

Orolabial HSV infection in adults with AIDS is usually due to recurrent disease. Primary orolabial HSV infection may occur in children with AIDS, however, because HIV infection in these patients may occur prior to initial exposure to HSV.

The incubation period of primary HSV infection ranges between 2 and 12 days. In the normal host, primary orolabial infection may be asymptomatic or result in a gingivostomatitis.[12,29,43] Immunocompromised patients appear to be at greater risk than normal hosts to develop a severe clinical illness during primary HSV-1 infection, with a painful vesicular eruption occurring along the lip, tongue, pharynx, or buccal mucosa. The vesicles rapidly coalesce and rupture to form large ulcers covered by a whitish yellow necrotic film.[43,44] Fever, pharyngitis, and cervical lymphadenopathy are frequently present in adults, whereas infants may display poor feeding and persistent drooling. Orolabial recurrences (fever blisters) in AIDS may increase in frequency and severity as immunosuppression increases. Alternatively, some AIDS patients will have only infrequent, mild, self-limiting recurrences throughout their disease.[2,33] Prodromal symptoms, consisting of tingling or numbness at the site of the impending recurrence, may be present from 12 to 24 hours prior to the onset of an actual HSV recurrence.

In the normal host, orolabial herpes usually heals in 7 to 10 days. By comparison, AIDS patients often have a prolonged illness with markedly delayed lesion healing. If left untreated, chronic ulcerative lesions with persistent virus shedding may occur for several weeks.[44]

Genital Infection

Following a 2- to 12-day incubation period, local symptoms develop in the majority of individuals wtih primary genital herpes.[9] Small papules appear initially and rapidly evolve into fluid-filled vesicles which are usually painful and tender to palpation. The vesicles ulcerate rapidly and, in the normal host, heal in 3 to 4 weeks by crusting and reepithelialization. Tender inguinal adenopathy is common, and dysuria may be present even if the urethra is not infected. Systemic symptoms, such as fever, headache, myalgias, malaise, and meningismus, are also common during primary infection.[7,10]

In the normal host, recurrent genital herpes is less severe than primary infection. Compared with primary infection, recurrent herpes typically results in fewer external lesions, a shorter duration of illness, and the absence of systemic symptoms.[9,10] In AIDS patients, however, the severity and duration of recurrent genital herpes may be more severe than that seen in normal hosts. Prolonged new lesion formation with continued tissue destruction, persistent virus shedding, and severe local pain are common. As with orolabial herpes, the frequency and severity of genital recurrences may increase with increasing immunosuppression, with symptoms lasting for several weeks.[2,52]

Anorectal Infection

Chronic perianal herpes was among the first reported opportunistic infections associated with AIDS. HSV has now been recognized as the most frequent cause of nongonococcal proctitis in sexually active homosexual men.[23,41] HSV proctitis usually results from primary HSV-2 infection but may also occur due to HSV-1 infection or recurrent disease. Severe anorectal pain, perianal ulcerations, constipation, tenesmus, and neurologic symptoms in the distribution of the sacral plexus (sacral radiculopathy, impotence, and neurogenic bladder) are common findings of HSV proctitis and help differentiate it from proctitis due to other causes[23] (Fig. 21−4). Anorectal or sigmoidoscopic examination in patients with HSV proctitis typically reveals a friable mucosa, diffuse ulcerations, and occasional intact vesicular or pustular lesions.[23]

Recurrent perianal lesions due to HSV in the absence of true proctitis is also a common finding in patients with AIDS. Local pain, tenderness, itching, and pain on defecation are prominent symptoms of these lesions. Shallow ulcers in the perianal region are often visible on external examination, and ulcerative lesions frequently coalesce and extend along the gluteal crease to involve the area overlying the sacrum. These lesions are often atypical in appearance and may be confused with pressure decubiti. To prevent misdiagnosis, all perianal ulcerations and anal fissures should be cultured for HSV.

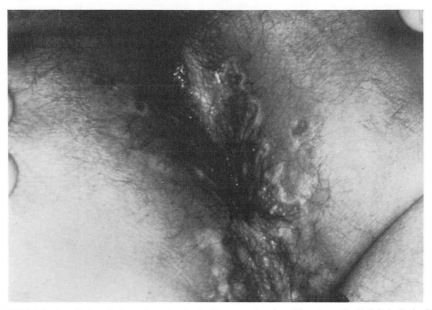

FIGURE 21—4.   Perianal ulcerations typical of herpes simplex. (Courtesy Dr. K. Erlich, Daly City, California.)

Esophagitis

Symptoms of HSV esophagitis typically include retrosternal pain and odynophagia (Chapter 11). Dysphagia may be of acute onset or chronic and may be severe enough to interfere with eating. Herpetic lesions in the oropharynx may not be present, and the clinical picture is often confused with *Candida* esophagitis. Radiographic contrast studies typically reveal a "cobblestone" appearance of the esophageal mucosa, although this finding is also present with *Candida* esophagitis. Definitive diagnosis of HSV esophagitis should be made by direct endoscopic visualization of the esophageal mucosa with positive virus culture and histopathologic evidence of invasive virus infection.

Encephalitis

HSV encephalitis occurs infrequently and is the most life-threatening complication of HSV infection in AIDS (Chapter 12). Both HSV-1 and HSV-2 have been identified in brain tissue of AIDS patients, and simultaneous brain infection with HSV and CMV have been reported.[13,16] In adults with AIDS, HSV encephalitis usually occurs as a complication of primary or reactivated orolabial HSV infection. In neonates the disease may occur as a result of primary HSV infection at the time of birth.[12]

The presentation of HSV encephalitis in adults with AIDS is often highly atypical. A subacute illness with subtle neurologic abnormalities is common in AIDS patients with HSV encephalitis, suggesting that host immune responses contribute to the clinical manifestations of the disease.[13,16] Headache, meningismus, and personality changes may develop gradually as the illness progresses. Alternatively, however, some AIDS patients may develop an acute encephalitis due to HSV infection. Abrupt onset of fever, headache, nausea, lethargy, and confusion may occur with temporal lobe abnormalities, cranial nerve defects, and focal seizures. Grand mal seizures, obtundation, coma, and death may eventually ensue.

The clinical diagnosis of HSV encephalitis may be extremely difficult, as other central nervous system infections (including HIV encephalopathy, *Cryptococcus neoformans,* and *Toxoplasma gondii*) may present in an identical fashion. Cerebrospinal fluid (CSF) usually reveals nonspecific findings, with elevated protein and a lymphocytic pleocytosis. Virus CSF cultures are usually negative.[30] Measurement of HSV antibody production in CSF has been evaluated as a means of diagnosis of HSV encephalitis but has not been evaluated in patients with AIDS.[26] Computed tomography scan, radionuclide brain scan, or electroencephalography may reveal nonspecific abnormalities and are often helpful in identifying abnormal areas for brain biopsy. Diagnosis often requires brain biopsy and the recovery of virus or demonstration of viral antigens from tissue specimens.[30] The histopathologic abnormalities typically observed in normal hosts (hemorrhagic cortical necrosis and lymphocytic infiltration) may be absent in AIDS patients.[13,16] When diagnostic brain biopsy is contraindicated or refused, a trial of empiric antiviral chemotherapy may be warranted.

TREATMENT

Acyclovir

The prompt administration of antiviral chemotherapy to AIDS patients with acute HSV infection reduces morbidity and the risk of serious complications. Acyclovir, the antiviral agent of choice for all HSV infections in AIDS, can be administered orally,[18,40,45,48] intravenously,[4,39,42,49] or topically.[11,52] The optimal route of administration, dosage, and duration of acyclovir therapy often depends on the site and severity of the acute HSV infection.

Acyclovir has a high therapeutic ratio as it undergoes selective activation (by phosphorylation) in HSV-infected cells. Acyclovir triphosphate acts by selective inhibition of viral DNA polymerase and early termination of DNA-chain synthesis. The drug has slightly higher activity against HSV-1 than HSV-2. Acyclovir distributes into all tissues, including the brain and CSF and is cleared by renal mechanisms. The serum half-life in patients with normal renal function is 2 to 3 hours, and the intravenous dose should be reduced in patients with impaired renal function.[28]

Management of HSV Infection (Table 21–5)

Most AIDS patients with primary or recurrent mucocutaneous HSV infections are not ill enough to require hospitalization and are suitable for outpatient treatment. The usual dose of acyclovir for outpatient therapy for primary infection is 200 mg five times daily. Therapy can be started while awaiting results of virus culture (if the clinical suspicion is high) or when the diagnosis has been confirmed by the appropriate laboratory techniques.[40] For mild recurrent HSV infection, 200 to 400 mg may be given three or four times a day.

Intravenous acyclovir should be reserved for patients with severe or extensive mucocutaneous HSV infection and for patients with virus dissemination, visceral organ infection (for example, brain, esophagus, eye), or neurologic complications (atonic bladder, transverse myelitis). Treatment with intravenous acyclovir may also be indicated for AIDS patients who require specific antiviral chemotherapy but are unable to tolerate or absorb oral acyclovir due to nausea, dysphagia, or protracted diarrhea. The dose of intravenous acyclovir for patients with mucocutaneous HSV infection and normal renal function is 15 mg/kg/d in three divided doses.[49] Patients with life-threatening HSV infection (encephalitis, neonatal infection, disseminated infection) or visceral organ involvement (esophagitis, proctitis) should probably receive a higher dose; usually 30 mg/kg/d in three divided doses.[12,51] Treatment should last for a minimum of 10 days, but longer therapy in AIDS patients may be necessary. As noted above, the intravenous dose should be adjusted in patients with impaired renal function. If prolonged therapy is required, oral acyclovir can be substituted for intravenous therapy when the patient is ready for hospital discharge.

Topical acyclovir is less effective than either oral or intravenous therapy, although comparative trials have not been performed. Topical acyclovir decreases the duration of virus shedding in compromised hosts with mu-

TABLE 21–5. MANAGEMENT OF HSV INFECTIONS IN AIDS

CLINICAL PRESENTATION	TREATMENT
Mucocutaneous infection, mild	Acyclovir: 200 mg p.o. 5 times daily
Mucocutaneous infection, severe	Acyclovir: 15 mg/kg/d i.v.
Visceral organ infection	Acyclovir: 30 mg/kg/d i.v.
Recurrent mucocutaneous infection	Acyclovir: 200-400 mg t.i.d. or q.i.d.
Severe infection due to acyclovir-resistant HSV	Vidarabine: 15 mg/kg/d i.v.
	Foscarnet: recommended dose not established

From Drew WL: The medical management of AIDS. Infect Dis Clin North Am. 2:505, 1988.

cocutaneous HSV infection but does not reduce new lesion formation or the risk of dissemination.[11,52] There appears to be no added benefit to the combination of topical acyclovir with either oral or intravenous acyclovir.[27] Topical acyclovir should be used only for patients with chronic ulcerative mucocutaneous HSV infection who are unable to tolerate oral medication and are not candidates for in-hospital intravenous therapy.

Treatment with acyclovir should be continued until all mucocutaneous lesions have crusted or reepithelialized. Lesions may heal slowly in AIDS patients even with optimal antiviral chemotherapy. If lesion healing does not occur while on acyclovir, repeat virus cultures should be obtained, high-dose intravenous therapy (30 mg/kg/d) should be given, and acyclovir-resistant HSV infection should be ruled out.

Suppressive Acyclovir Therapy For HSV Infection

Many AIDS patients suffer from frequently recurring HSV infection or develop new HSV recurrences shortly after antiviral chemotherapy is discontinued. These patients can often be managed with suppressive acyclovir therapy.[18,45,48] AIDS patients requiring suppressive therapy should be treated initially with oral acyclovir 200 mg q.i.d. or 400 mg b.i.d. Increase of daily dosage up to 400 mg q.i.d. may be necessary to control recurrences, but gastrointestinal tolerance to the drug may limit the amount that can be taken. "Breakthrough recurrences" which develop while on suppressive acyclovir therapy may be controlled by increasing the daily suppressive dose. Breakthrough recurrences usually do not represent the emergence of acyclovir-resistent strains.[32] Patients who demonstrate a good response to the oral regimen may attempt a reduction in the daily suppressive dose. Although suppressive acyclovir therapy is approved for no longer than 6 months, patients have been maintained on daily acyclovir for up to 48 months with no evidence of adverse reactions or cumulative toxicity. Individuals maintained on long-term suppressive therapy should be cautioned, however, that recurrences will likely develop following discontinuation of therapy and that the first recurrence may be more severe than those previously experienced.[18,45,48] Many AIDS patients receiving acyclovir may also be taking AZT. The combination of AZT and acyclovir may be synergistic against HIV, but the combination may also be more toxic than treatment with AZT alone. Ongoing studies exploring these possibilities are currently in progress.

We have reported acyclovir-resistant HSV in twelve AIDS patients with HSV infection. All these patients had been treated previously with oral or intravenous acyclovir or both, and all patients presented with chronic, localized mucocutaneous lesions. All the HSV strains were highly resistant to the acyclovir concentration required to inhibit viral plaques by 50% (ID_{50} = 7.1 to 91.4 µg/ml) in comparison to reference strains, which had

ID_{50} values ranging from 0.25 to 1.10 $\mu g/ml$. The acyclovir-resistant strains were also resistant to ganciclovir but remained susceptible to vidarabine (ID_{50} = 1.9 to 23.5 $\mu g/ml$).[20]

Since activation of vidarabine does not require viral thymidine kinase, this drug remains effective against TK($-$) acyclovir-resistant HSV. AIDS patients with severe HSV infections due to TK($-$) strains should be treated with vidarabine 15 mg/kg/d for a minimum of 10 days.[53] Foscarnet may provide a useful alternative to adenine arabinoside for the treatment of acyclovir-resistant HSV infection.[6]

VARICELLA ZOSTER VIRUS

Primary varicella zoster virus (VZV) infection is usually a childhood illness, with attack rates exceeding 90 percent in susceptible household contacts.[50] Most adults with AIDS have been previously infected with VZV and (as with HSV) are not susceptible to primary infection.[35]

AIDS patients develop recurrent VZV infection (zoster) more frequently than age-matched immunocompetent hosts. A retrospective review of 300 AIDS patients with Kaposi's sarcoma revealed that 8 percent of patients had at least one prior attack of zoster, an incidence seven times greater than expected by the age of the study group. Zoster also occurs with a higher than expected frequency in HIV-infected individuals who appear otherwise healthy. Additionally, some HIV-infected patients develop more than one episode of zoster in a relatively short period of time, an uncommon occurrence in competent hosts.[8,17,22,37,47]

Primary Infection—Varicella

Varicella in immunocompetent children is usually a benign illness. Adults, however, are more likely to develop complications during primary VZV infection; virus dissemination to visceral organs occurs in up to one third of immunocompetent adults with primary infection.[50] Although most adults with AIDS have been previously infected with VZV and are not susceptible to primary infection,[35] for those who are, a protracted and potentially life-threatening illness could follow.

Recurrent Infection—Zoster

Unlike primary VZV infection, recurrent VZV infection (zoster) is common in patients with AIDS. The illness usually begins with radicular pain and is followed by localized or segmented erythematous rash covering one to three dermatomes. Maculopapules develop in the dermatomal area, and the patient experiences increasing pain. The maculopapules progress to fluid-filled vesicles, and contiguous vesicles may become confluent with true bullae formation. In many AIDS and ARC patients, the lesions remain confined in a dermatomal distribution and heal by crusting and reepithelialization.[7,8,22,37,47] Occasionally, however, widespread cutaneous or visceral dissemination or both occur.[36] Extensive cutaneous dissemination may appear identical to primary varicella. Dissemination to lung, liver, or central nervous system may produce a life-threatening illness.

Reactivated infection involving the ophthalmic division of the trigeminal nerve often results in infection of the cornea (zoster ophthalmicus). The presence of vesicles on the tip of the nose is often associated with involvement of the eye. Although healing without sequelae may occur, untreated patients often develop anterior uveitis, corneal scarring, and permanent visual loss.[7,37]

Complications

Complications of VZV infection are common in immunocompromised patients and may cause prolonged morbidity and death.[17] Dissemination of virus to the lung, liver, and central nervous system has been associated with a mortality rate of 6 to 17 percent.

Varicella pneumonia may occur during primary VZV infection or during reactivated infection with visceral dissemination in immunocompromised patients. Symptoms are variable; many patients develop only mild respiratory symptoms, while others may suffer from severe hypoxemia and succumb to respiratory failure. Radiographic abnormalities are usually out of proportion to the clinical findings, with diffuse nodular densities on chest radiograph and occasional pleural effusions.

Encephalitis is a rare complication of VZV infection in AIDS but may occur in association with visceral dissemination (Chapter 12). The illness begins 3 to 8 days after the onset of varicella or 1 to 2 weeks after the development of zoster, but occasionally AIDS patients have developed progressive neurologic disease due to VZV up to 3 months after the onset of localized zoster.[36] Headache, vomiting, lethargy, and cerebellar findings (ataxia, tremors, dizziness) are prominent findings. Diagnosis based on clinical criteria alone can be difficult, as other central nervous system infections can present in a similar fashion.

Management of VZV Infection (Table 21–6)

Oral acyclovir in the standard dosing regimen (200 mg five times daily) does not result in serum drug levels adequate to inhibit VZV in tissue

TABLE 21–6.   MANAGEMENT OF VZV INFECTIONS IN AIDS

CLINICAL PRESENTATION	TREATMENT
Primary infection (varicella)	Acyclovir: 30 mg/kg/d i.v. or acyclovir 600-800 mg p.o. 5 times daily
Recurrent infection (localized zoster)	Acyclovir: 30 mg/kg/d i.v. or acyclovir 600-800 mg p.o. 5 times daily
Recurrent infection disseminated	Acyclovir: 30 mg/kg/d i.v.
Severe infection due to acyclovir-resistant VZV	Foscarnet?

From Drew WL: The medical management of AIDS. Infect Dis Clin North Am 2:507, 1988.

culture[28] and is not approved in the United States for the treatment of VZV infection. Higher doses of oral acyclovir (600 to 800 mg five times daily) may produce inhibiting drug levels in serum, but this regimen is sometimes poorly tolerated due to gastrointestinal side effects.

Management of primary or recurrent VZV infection in AIDS may require hospitalization and intravenous acyclovir therapy. Many AIDS patients with localized zoster will not be ill enough to require hospitalization, and the decision whether to hospitalize an individual patient must be based on several factors, including the severity of the infection, the immune status of the host, and whether visceral or cutaneous dissemination has occurred.

Immunocompromised hosts with primary or recurrent VZV infection treated with intravenous acyclovir have a reduction in the duration of virus shedding, new lesion formation, incidence of dissemination, and mortality rate.[4,39] All AIDS patients with disseminated VZV infection, either cutaneous or visceral, should be hospitalized and treated with intravenous acyclovir 30 mg/kg/d in three divided doses. Treatment should be continued for at least 7 days or until all external lesions are crusted. Oral acyclovir (600 to 800 mg five times daily) has been used for treatment of zoster in AIDS. Although no controlled studies have been performed in this population, early therapy with oral acyclovir may prevent visceral or cutaneous dissemination.

Although some studies have suggested that the use of corticosteroids reduces the incidence of postherpetic neuralgia, other studies have failed to demonstrate a beneficial effect. Corticosteroids should not be used in AIDS patients with zoster, since postherpetic neuralgia is infrequent in this population and the potential immunosuppressive effect of these drugs outweighs any possible benefits.

Treatment of Acyclovir-Resistant VZV Infection

Acyclovir-resistant VZV has been recently identified in patients with AIDS. Four strains were from patients taking long-term acyclovir for recurrent VZV or HSV infection. Acyclovir-resistant VZV strains appear to be sensitive to vidarabine or foscarnet, although clinical efficacy against these strains has not yet been documented.[25]

SUMMARY

Herpes viruses (HSV, CMV, VZV) are common in AIDS patients and often exist in a chronic or progressive form. Clinically evident CMV retinitis occurs in approximately 10 percent of AIDS patients and can be effectively treated with new nucleoside analogue, ganciclovir (DHPG). Perianal ulcers, proctitis, and other clinical syndromes caused by HSV can be effectively treated with acyclovir, which administered daily can prevent HSV recurrence. Herpes zoster in a young adult may be the first indication of immune deficiency due to HIV. Since VZV is less susceptible to acyclovir than HSV is, intravenous acyclovir or high-dose oral therapy is required to achieve inhibitory blood levels.

REFERENCES

1. Akula SK, Mansell PWA, Ruiz R: Complications of the acquired immunodeficiency syndrome. Ann Intern Med 104:726-727, 1986
2. Armstrong D, Gold JWM, Dryjanski J, et al: Treatment of infections in patients with the acquired immunodeficiency symdrome. Ann Intern Med 103:738-743, 1985
3. Bach MC, Bagwell SP, Knapp NP, Davis KM, Hedstron PS: 9-(1,3-dihydroxy-2-propoxymethyl)guanine for cytomegalovirus infections in patients with the acquired immunodeficiency syndrome. Ann Intern Med 103:381-382, 1985
4. Balfour HH, Bean B, Laskin OL, et al: Acyclovir halts progression of herpes zoster in immunocompromised patients. N Engl J Med 308:1448-1453, 1983
5. Cantrill HL, Henry K, Melroe H, et al: Treatment of cytomegalovirus retinitis with intravitreal ganciclovir. Long term results. Ophthalmology 96:367-374, 1989
6. Chatis PA, Miller CH, Schrager LE, Crumpacker CS: Successful treatment with foscarnet of an acyclovir-resistant mucocutaneous infection with herpes simplex virus in a patient with acquired immunodeficiency syndrome. N Engl J Med 320:297-300, 1989
7. Cole EL, Meisler DM, Calabrese LH, et al: Herpes zoster ophthalmicus and acquired immune deficiency syndrome. Arch Opthalmol 102:1027-1029, 1984
8. Cone LA, Schiffman MA: Herpes zoster and the acquired immunodeficiency syndrome (Letter). Ann Intern Med 100:462, 1984
9. Corey L, Adams HG, Brown ZA, et al: Genital herpes simplex virus infections: Clinical manifestations, course, and complications. Ann Intern Med 98:958-972, 1983
10. Corey L, Homes KK: Genital herpes simplex virus infections: Current concepts in diagnosis, therapy, and prevention. Ann Intern Med 98:973-983, 1983
11. Corey L, Nahmias AJ, Guinan ME, et al: A trial of topical acyclovir in genital herpes simplex virus infections. N Engl J Med 306:1313-1319, 1982
12. Corey L, Spear PG: Infections with herpes simplex viruses (parts 1 and 2). N Engl J Med 314:686-691, 749-757, 1986
13. Dix RD, Bredeson DE, Davis RL, et al: Herpes virus neurologic diseases associated with AIDS: Recovery of viruses from CNS tissues, peripheral nerve and CSF (Abstract M-82). International Conference on AIDS, Atlanta, 1985
14. Dix RD, Bredesen DE, Davis RL, Mills J: Herpesvirus neurological diseases associated with AIDS: Recovery of viruses from central nervous system (CNS) tissues, peripheral nerve, and cerebrospinal fluid (CSF) (Abstract 43). International Conference on AIDS, Atlanta, 1985

15. Dix RD, Bredesen DE, Erlich KS, et al: Recovery of herpes-viruses from cerebrospinal fluid of immunodeficient homosexual men. Ann Neurol 18:611-614, 1985
16. Dix RD, Waitzman DM, Follansbee S, et al: Herpes simplex virus type 2 encephalitis in two homosexual men with persistent adenopathy. Ann Neurol 17:203-206, 1985
17. Dolin R, Reichman RC, Mazur MH, et al: Herpes zoster and varicella infections in immunosuppressed patients. Ann Intern Med 89:375-388, 1978
18. Douglas JM, Critchlow C, Benedetti J, et al: Double blind study of oral acyclovir for suppression of recurrences of genital herpes simplex virus infection. N Engl J Med 310:1551-1556, 1984
18a. Emanuel D, Cunningham I, Jules-Elysee K, et al: Cytomegalovirus pneumonia after bone-marrow transplantation successfully treated with the combination of ganciclovir and high-dose intravenous immune globulin. Ann Intern Med 109:777-782, 1988
19. Erice A, Chou S, Biron K, Stanat S, Balfour HH Jr, Jordan C: Ganciclovir (GCV) resistant strains of cytomegalovirus (CMV) in GCV-treated patients with AIDS. IV International Conference on AIDS (Abstract 7190), Stockholm, 1988
20. Erlich KS, Mills J, Chatis P, et al: Acyclovir-resistant herpes simplex virus infections in patients with the acquired immunodeficiency syndrome. N Engl J Med 320:293-296, 1989
21. Felsenstein D, D'Amico DJ, Hirsch MS, Neumeyer DA, Cederberg DM, de Miranda P, Schooley RT: Treatment of cytomegalovirus retinitis with 9-[2-hydroxy-1-(hydroxymethyl) ethoxymethyl] guanine. Ann Intern Med 103:377-380, 1985
22. Friedman-Kien AE, Lafleur FL, Gendler E, et al: Herpes zoster: A possible early clinical sign for development of acquired immunodeficiency syndrome in high-risk individuals. J Am Acad Dermatol 14:1023-1028, 1986
23. Goodell SE, Quinn TC, Mkrtichian E, et al: Herpes simplex proctitis in homosexual men: Clinical, sigmoidoscopic, and histopathologic features. N Engl J Med 308:868-871, 1983
24. Hawley DA, Schaefer JF, Schulz DM, Muller J: Cytomegalovirus encephalitis in acquired immunodeficiency syndrome. Am J Clin Pathol 80:874-877, 1983
25. Jacobson MA, Berger TG, Fikrig S, et al: Acyclovir (ACV)-resistant varicella zoster virus (VZV) infection following chronic oral ACV therapy in patients with AIDS. Twenty-Ninth Interscience Conference on Antimicrobial Agents and Chemotherapy (Abstract 63), Houston, 1989
26. Kahlon J, Chatterjee S, Lakeman FD, et al: Detection of antibodies to herpes simplex virus in the cerebrospinal fluid of patients with herpes simplex encephalitis. J Infect Dis 155:38-44, 1987
27. Kinghorn GR, Abeywickreme I, Jeavons M, et al: Efficacy of combined treatment with oral and topical acyclovir in first episode genital herpes. Genitourin Med 62:186-188, 1986
28. Laskin O: Acyclovir: Pharmacology and clinical experience. Arch Intern Med 144:1241-1246, 1984
29. Nahmias AJ, Josey WE: Herpes simplex viruses 1 and 2. In Evans A (ed.): Viral Infections of Humans: Epidemiology and Control, ed. 2. New York, Plenum Press, 1982
30. Nahmias AJ, Whitley RD, Visintine AN, et al: Herpes simplex virus type 2 encephalitis: Laboratory evaluations and their diagnostic significance. J Infect Dis 146:829-836, 1982
31. Nerurkar L, Goedert J, Wallen W, et al: Study of antiviral antibodies in sera of homosexual men. Fed Proc 42:6109, 1983.
32. Nusinoff-Lehrman S, Douglas JM, Corey L, et al: Recurrent genital herpes and suppressive oral acyclovir therapy: Relation between clinical outcome and in-vitro sensitivity. Ann Intern Med 104:786-790, 1986
33. Quinnan GV, Masur H, Rook AH, et al: Herpes simplex infections in the acquired immune deficiency syndrome. JAMA 252:72-77, 1984
33a. Reed EC, Bowden RA, Dandliker PS, et al: Treatment of cytomegalovirus pneumonia with ganciclovir and intravenous cytomegalovirus immunoglobulin in patients with bone marrow transplants. Ann Intern Med 109:783-788, 1988
34. Revision of the CDC Surveillance Case Definition for Acquired Immunodeficiency Syndrome. MMWR 36(Suppl):1S-15S, 1987
35. Rogers MF, Morens DM, Stewart JA, et al: National case control study of Kaposi's sarcoma and *Pneumocystis carinii* pneumonia in homosexual men: Part 2, Laboratory results. Ann Intern Med 99:151-158, 1983

36. Ryder JW, Croen K, Kleinschmidt-DeMasters BK, et al: Progressive encephalitis three months after resolution of cutaneous zoster in a patient with AIDS. Ann Neurol 19:182-188, 1986

37. Sandor E, Croxson TS, Millman A, et al: Herpes zoster ophthalmicus in patients at risk for AIDS. N Engl J Med 310:1118-1119, 1984

38. Shepp DH, Dandliker PS, de Miranda P, et al: Activity of 9-[2-hydroxy-1-(hydroxymethyl) ethoxymethyl] guanine in the treatment of cytomegalovirus pneumonia. Ann Intern Med 103:368-373, 1985

39. Shepp DH, Dandliker PS, Meyers JD: Treatment of varicella zoster virus infection in severely immunocompromised patients. N Engl J Med 314:208-212, 1986

40. Shepp DH, Newton BA, Dandliker PS, et al: Oral acyclovir therapy for mucocutaneous herpes simplex virus infections in immunocompromised marrow transplant recipients. Ann Intern Med 102:783-785, 1985

41. Siegel FP, Lopez C, Hammer BS, et al: Severe acquired immunodeficiency in male homosexuals, manifested by chronic perianal ulcerative herpes simplex lesions. N Engl J Med 305:1439-1444, 1981

42. Skoldenberg B, Alestig K, Burman L, et al: Acyclovir versus vidarabine in herpes simplex encephalitis. Lancet 2:707-711, 1984

43. Spruance Sl, Overall JC, Kern ER, et al: The natural history of recurrent herpes simplex labialis: Implications for antiviral therapy. N Engl J Med 297:68-75, 1977

44. Straus SE, Smith HA, Brickman C, et al: Acyclovir for chronic mucocutaneous herpes simplex virus infection in immunosuppressed patients. Ann Intern Med 96:270-277, 1982

45. Straus SE, Seidlin M, Takiff H, et al: Oral acyclovir to suppress recurring herpes simplex virus infections in immunodeficient patients. Ann Intern Med 100:522-524, 1984

46. Teich S, Orellana J: Retinal lesions in cytomegalovirus infection. Ann Intern Med 104:132, 1986

47. Verroust F, Lemay D, Laurian Y: High frequency of herpes zoster in young hemophiliacs (Letter). N Engl J Med 316:166-167, 1987

48. Wade JC, Newton B, Flournoy N, et al: Oral acyclovir for prevention of herpes simplex virus reactivation after marrow transplantation. Ann Intern Med 100:823-828, 1984

49. Wade JC, Newton B, McLaren C, et al: Intravenous acyclovir to treat mucocutaneous herpes simplex virus infection after marrow transplantation. Ann Intern Med 96:265-269, 1982

50. Weller TH: Varicella and herpes zoster: Changing concepts of the natural history, control, and importance of a not-so-benign virus (parts 1 and 2). N Engl J Med 309:1362-1368, 1434-1440, 1983

51. Whitley RJ, Alford CA, Hirsch MS, et al: Vidarabine versus acyclovir therapy in herpes simplex encephalitis. N Engl J Med 314:144-149, 1986

52. Whitley RJ, Levin M, Barton N, et al: Infections caused by herpes simplex virus in the immunocompromised host: Natural history and topical acyclovir therapy. J Infect Dis 150:323-329, 1984

53. Whitley RJ, Soong SJ, Dolin R, et al: Adenine arabinoside therapy of biopsy proved herpes simplex encephalitis: National Institute of Allergy and Infectious Diseases collaborative antiviral study. N Engl J Med 297:289-294, 1977

22

THE MALIGNANCIES ASSOCIATED WITH AIDS

LAWRENCE D. KAPLAN, MD

Malignancies as a complication of immunodeficiency have been well described in the literature, being recognized long before the advent of the HIV epidemic.[22,37,40] The incidence of both Kaposi's sarcoma and non-Hodgkin's lymphoma are markedly increased in immunosuppressed allograft recipients. It is therefore not surprising that patients with HIV infection, who also have profound defects in cell-mediated immunity, also develop these two malignancies. The marked rise in the incidence of both Kaposi's sarcoma and B-cell lymphoma in populations at risk for HIV infection in the years since 1982 (Table 22–1) strongly suggests a causal relationship between immunodeficiency and the development of these malignancies.[36] As a result of this, these neoplasms are included in the AIDS case definition established by CDC.[8] We can therefore refer to these as "AIDS-defining" malignancies. They are listed in Table 22–2 along with other malignancies that have been reported in HIV-infected individuals but for which no clear causal relationship has been established.

Regardless of the causal relationship between various malignancies and the underlying immunodeficiency state, reports in the literature suggest that the natural history of cancer may be altered in the setting of HIV infection.[19,74,87] Patients tend to present with more advanced disease, which is more rapidly progressive and responds less well to therapy than in the non–HIV-infected population. The shortened survival observed in these patients is best illustrated in a group of HIV-infected Hodgkin's disease patients treated at San Francisco General Hospital.[45] These 14 patients had a median survival of less than 1 year compared with a historical control population of patients treated for Hodgkin's disease in San Francisco prior to 1980, in which the median survival was 12 years.

Management of the HIV-infected patient with a malignancy imposes obstacles rarely encountered in the non–HIV-infected population. Poor

TABLE 22–1. AVERAGE ANNUAL INCIDENCE OF SELECTED MALIGNANCIES PER 100,000 NEVER-MARRIED MEN IN SAN FRANCISCO COUNTY PRIOR TO (1975–1978) AND DURING (1982–1985) THE AIDS EPIDEMIC

MALIGNANCY*	AGE 25–44 Y				AGE 45–54 Y			
	1975–1978		1982–1985		1975–1978		1982–1985	
	RATE	NO.	RATE	NO.	RATE	NO.	RATE	NO.
Kaposi's sarcoma	0.00	0	158.36	477†	0.00	0	151.28	57†
Non-Hodgkin's lymphoma	3.89	8	26.66	81†	21.56	7	34.46	13
Hodgkin's lymphoma								
Mixed cellularity	1.35	3	2.34	7‡	0.00	0	5.27	2‡
Nodular sclerosing	2.40	5	3.80	11‡	9.17	3	5.32	2
Other	1.55	3	1.31	4	0.00	0	8.12	3
Respiratory	7.09	15	7.71	23	162.82	53	126.63	47
Oral squamous	2.89	6	2.64	8	18.15	6	37.64	14‡
Anorectal squamous	1.03	2	0.64	2	2.97	1	13.19	5‡
Skin and lip	10.36	22	7.53	22	15.20	5	29.34	11‡

*International Classification of Diseases for Oncology, (ICD-O)[15] Morphology codes: Kaposi's sarcoma (code 9140); non-Hodgkin's lymphoma (codes 9590-9642, 9690-9701, and 9740-9750); Hodgkin's lymphoma: mixed cellularity (code 9652), nodular sclerosing (codes 9656 and 9657); other (codes 9650, 9651, 9653-9655, and 9658-9662); squamous sites (codes 8070-8076). Topography codes: respiratory (codes 162.0-162.9); oral squamous (codes 141.0-149.9); anorectal squamous (codes 154.0-154.8) skin and lip (codes 173.0-173.9).
†Significance of chi-square trend test on annual incidence for 1980-1985, P <.001.
‡Increase in rates predates 1982 and the AIDS epidemic.
From Harnly ME, et al: Temporal trends in the incidence of non-Hodgkin's lymphoma and selected malignancies in a population with a high incidence of acquired immunodeficiency syndrome (AIDS). Am J Epidemiol 128(2):261-267, 1988.

TABLE 22—2. MALIGNANCIES IN HIV INFECTION

AIDS DEFINING	NON-AIDS DEFINING	REFERENCE
Kaposi's sarcoma	Hodgkin's disease	41,45,80
B-cell lymphoma	Squamous carcinoma	12,19,31,87
	Head and neck	
	Anus	
	Melanoma	86
	Plasmacytoma	87
	Adenocarcinoma colon	7
	Small cell lung carcinoma	31,87
	Germ cell (testicular)	85
	Basal cell	38

bone marrow reserve and the risk of intercurrent opportunistic infections, problems frequently observed in this patient population, may compromise the delivery of adequate dose-intensity. In addition, administration of chemotherapy may lead to further immunosuppression, resulting in a greater likelihood of opportunistic infection. Finally, toxic responses to chemotherapeutic agents, antibiotics, and radiotherapy are excessive and often severe, further impairing the physician's ability to administer adequate therapy.

This chapter will focus on the two AIDS-defining malignancies, Kaposi's sarcoma and non-Hodgkin's lymphoma, from a clinical perspective. The natural history of these malignancies will be presented along with various therapeutic options, followed by a brief discussion of Hodgkin's lymphoma.

KAPOSI'S SARCOMA

Kaposi's sarcoma (KS), once a rarely reported malignancy, is the most common neoplasm affecting HIV-infected individuals. It is seen primarily in homosexual men and has only rarely been reported in intravenous drug users or other risk groups.[63,78] The proportion of AIDS patients with KS as the initial AIDS diagnosis has changed since the first cases were reported in 1981.[13] In New York City, KS was the initial AIDS diagnosis in 50 percent of non–intravenous-drug-using homosexual men diagnosed between 1981 and 1983. Between 1984 and 1987, however, this proportion had fallen to 30 percent. Similar trends have been reported from San Francisco.[77]

The pathogenesis of KS in HIV-infected patients remains uncertain, as do the reasons for its apparent confinement to the homosexual male population. In addition to this unusual epidemiologic pattern, the clinical behavior of KS is unusual; the tumors appear to be multifocal, sites of disease regression can sometimes be observed alongside sites of progression, and the histologic appearance of the tumor may be relatively benign. This has led to the suggestion that KS represents a form of reversible vascular hyperplasia rather than a true malignancy.[5] Laboratory studies implicating retrovirus-induced endothelial growth factors[16,65,79] in the development of KS support this concept. Recently, studies in transgenic mice[89] suggest that one of these presumed endothelial growth factors may, in fact, be the *tat* gene product. The possibility that another sexually transmitted virus may be involved in the pathogenesis of KS has not yet been excluded[15] and may explain the decline in the proportion of AIDS cases presenting as KS. A better understanding of the pathogenesis of the disease may have implications for future therapeutic strategies.

Clinical Presentation and Diagnosis

Unlike the more indolent, endemic form of KS, in the HIV-infected individual the disease tends to be aggressive and unpredictable.[63,78] The skin is most commonly the first site of presentation. Palpable, firm, cutaneous nodules ranging from 0.5 to 2 cm in diameter are frequently observed. However, in early stages, smaller, nonpalpable lesions may be seen. Some early lesions may have the appearance of a small ecchymosis. In more advanced disease, cutaneous lesions may become confluent and form large tumor masses involving extensive cutaneous surfaces. In light-skinned individuals, the lesions are typically violaceous (Color Plate IG), while in dark-skinned individuals, the lesions are a hyperpigmented, brown or even black. Rather than being limited to a single cutaneous site as in endemic KS, in the setting of the HIV infection KS may involve any cutaneous surface. Involvement of the head and neck is frequent, and the appearance of oral KS lesions is often the first sign of disease (Color Plate IH).

The natural history of KS associated with HIV infection closely resembles that observed in immunosuppressed allograft recipients. The disease tends to progress with time and is associated with the appearance of larger, more numerous cutaneous lesions. However, the course of the disease is unpredictable. A patient may present with relatively few lesions which remain stable over time. New cutaneous lesions may not appear for many months but may then be followed by a sudden and rapid increase in disease activity. Visceral involvement is extremely common, and almost any visceral site may be affected. Careful endoscopic examination will reveal gastrointestinal sites of disease in most patients.

Although KS is rarely a direct cause of death in HIV-infected patients, the morbidity associated with more advanced disease can be significant. Bulky cutaneous lesions may become painful and, if large cutaneous surfaces are involved, may restrict movement. Lymphatic obstruction is common and may result in severe edema, most commonly involving the extremities (Color Plate IE) or the face. Visceral spread of KS is rarely symptomatic, particularly when it involves the gastrointestinal tract. However, rare cases of obstruction, perforation, or gastrointestinal bleeding have been reported.[20] In contrast, pulmonary KS may cause cough, bronchospasm, and dyspnea, and death due to respiratory failure is not uncommon.[47,69] Finally, the social problems associated with this disfiguring neoplasm in the setting of an already socially stigmatizing disease cannot be overemphasized.

Careful examination of the skin and oral cavity at each clinic visit is the key to early diagnosis. Once lesions are identified, histologic confirmation should be obtained. For cutaneous lesions, a small punch biopsy is generally used; conventional biopsy techniques may be used at other sites. In patients with suspected pulmonary KS, violaceous endobronchial lesions are typically observed on bronchoscopic examination. Unfortunately, attempts at endobronchial biopsy are frequently unsuccessful due to the submucosal nature of the lesions. However, bronchoscopic visualization of typical lesions is generally accepted for the purpose of diagnosis of pulmonary disease in patients who have KS at other sites.[47]

Except for those patients with pulmonary involvement, most patients do not die as a result of KS. The most common cause of death in this group is opportunistic infection.

Staging

Currently employed staging systems are based primarily on tumor bulk. A modification of the staging system to include the presence or absence of constitutional symptoms is shown in Table 22-3. Unfortunately, these systems have not proven useful because a majority of patients fall into the most advanced stages. In addition, tumor bulk may not be the most important predictor of survival in this group of patients.

Analysis of data from 190 individuals with HIV-associated KS at UCLA Medical Center demonstrated the most important predictor of survival to

TABLE 22–3. MODIFIED STAGING SYSTEM FOR KAPOSI'S SARCOMA

STAGE	CHARACTERISTICS
I	Limited cutaneous (<10 lesions or 1 anatomic area)
II	Disseminated cutaneous (>10 lesions or more than 1 anatomic area)
III	Visceral only (gastrointestinal, lymph node)
IV	Cutaneous and visceral
Subtypes	
A	No systemic signs or symptoms
B	Fevers >37.8° C unrelated to identifiable infection for >2 wk, or weight loss >10% of body weight

From Mitsuyasu RT, Groopman JE: Biology and therapy of Kaposi's sarcoma. Semin Oncol 11:53-59, 1984

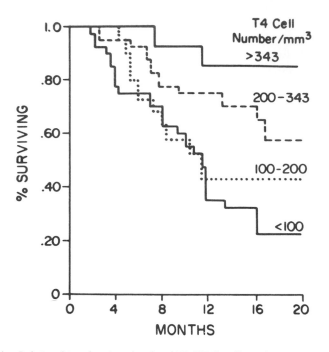

FIGURE 22–1. Relationship of various levels of T4 (CD4) cell numbers to survival in AIDS–Kaposi's sarcoma patients (Kaplan-Meier graph). (From Taylor J, et al.: Prognostically significant classification of immune changes in AIDS with Kaposi's sarcoma. Blood 67:666-671, 1986.)

be the absolute CD4+ lymphocyte count (Fig. 22-1).[84] Only 30% of patients with fewer than 100 CD4 lymphocytes survived for 1 year. Other features associated with a negative impact on survival in various studies have included history of opportunistic infection,[62] presence of bulky tumor[62,64] or constitutional symptoms,[62,64] and initial presentation that involves a mucosal surface or cutaneous sites other than the lower extremities or the lymph nodes.[64]

Based upon these known predictors of survival in AIDS-associated KS, the Oncology Subcommittee of the NIH–sponsored AIDS Clinical Trials Group (ACTG) has proposed a new staging classification (Table 22-4).[54] This system takes into account tumor bulk, immune function, and systemic illness, including history of opportunistic infection and the presence of constitutional symptoms. It will require validation in future prospective clinical trials.

Treatment

Since few patients die as a direct result of KS, it would seem unlikely that therapy directed towards this malignancy would have a significant

**TABLE 22–4.   ACTG PROPOSED STAGING CLASSIFICATION FOR
KAPOSI'S SARCOMA**

	GOOD RISK (0)— ALL OF THE FOLLOWING	POOR RISK (1)— ANY OF THE FOLLOWING
Tumor (T)	Confined to skin, lymph nodes, or minimal oral disease* or any combination of these	Tumor-associated edema or ulceration Extensive oral KS Gastrointestinal KS KS in other nonnodal viscera
Immune System (I)	CD4 cells ≥200/mm³	CD4 cells <200/mm³
Systemic illness	No history or OI or thrush	History of OI and/or thrush
(S)	No "B" symptoms† Karnofsky performance status ≥70	"B" symptoms† present Karnofsky performance status <70 Other HIV-related illness (e.g., neurologic disease, lymphoma)

ACTG: AIDS Clinical Trials Group; OI: opportunistic infection.
*Confined to the palate in nonnodular KS.
†Unexplained fever, night sweats, >10% involuntary weight loss, diarrhea persisting more than 2 weeks.
From Krown SE, Metroka C, Wernz JC: Kaposi's sarcoma in the acquired immunodeficiency syndrome: A proposal for uniform evaluation, response, and staging criteria. J Clin Oncol 7:1201-1207, 1989.

impact on survival. Although the data is retrospective, a review of 194 cases of KS by Volberding et al[91] suggests that this is, in fact, the case. There was no significant difference in median survival between the group of patients treated with chemotherapy (or α-interferon) and those who received no treatment.

Treatment is not appropriate for every patient with KS. Subgroups of patients therefore must be defined in terms of whom treatment will benefit most. Treatment must be optimized for the individual patient so that the best treatment modality will be selected. The primary goals of therapy for KS are palliation of symptoms and cosmesis.

Cosmesis is perhaps the most common indication for therapy of KS and often the most important. Achievement of good cosmetic results may not only improve appearance, but may significantly improve the patient's overall outlook.

There are several situations in which palliative therapy may be indicated:

1.   Painful or uncomfortable intraoral or pharyngeal lesions may cause pain and interfere with eating or swallowing. Bulky KS may even result in airway compromise.

2.   Lymphedema is common in advanced KS. Because of its propensity for infiltrating lymphatics, obstruction and edema formation may occur relatively early. The face and the lower extremities are the sites most com-

TABLE 22–5. THERAPEUTIC OPTIONS FOR KAPOSI'S SARCOMA

Local therapy
Radiation
Cryotherapy
Intralesional chemotherapy
Laser
Systemic therapy
Chemotherapy
α-Interferon

monly affected. Lower extremity edema may be the result of direct lymphatic invasion through bulky cutaneous lesions or from obstruction due to bulky lymphadenopathy in the femoral, inguinal, or iliac regions. Edema may be observed even in the absence of visible KS.

3. Painful or bulky lesions may occur at any site. Lesions involving the plantar surfaces of the feet may be particularly uncomfortable during ambulation.

4. Pulmonary KS is frequently symptomatic and can result in a variety of respiratory symptoms. Disease progression may be rapid, resulting in severe respiratory compromise and death.[24,47]

Another indication for therapy may be rapidly progressive disease. Although it is impossible to prove benefit in the absence of a randomized trial, it is likely that without treatment, such patients will rapidly develop either symptomatic disease requiring palliative therapy or cosmetically problematic disease.

Treatment options include a variety of local and systemic therapies (Table 22-5). Systemic chemotherapy may result in subjective toxicities as well as myelosuppression and immunosuppression, leaving the patient more susceptible to a variety of opportunistic infections.

Local Therapy

Radiotherapy has been the mainstay of local therapy in this disease. A single dose of 800 cGy or the equivalent fractionated dose can be highly effective in achieving local palliation.[10,39]

Radiotherapy is not appropriate for the patient with widespread disease but is best suited for the patient with a single or a few locally symptomatic areas. It often relieves lymphatic obstruction and can be applied to a field encompassing the whole face in patients with facial edema. In addition, smaller facial lesions, conjunctival lesions, or other unsightly cutaneous lesions may be treated with radiotherapy. Intraoral and pharyngeal lesions are frequently treated with radiotherapy. However, a high frequency of severe mucositis has been observed in these patients.[39] As a result, laser surgery has more recently been employed for treatment of some intraoral lesions at our institution.

Intralesional chemotherapy may be utilized for cosmetic purposes in small cutaneous lesions.[68] This is generally accomplished by intralesional injection of 0.01 mg of vinblastine in 0.1 ml of sterile water using a tuberculin syringe. Repeated treatments may be necessary. A hyperpigmented area frequently remains following treatment.

Cryotherapy using liquid nitrogen has been successfully used for the treatment of isolated small KS lesions.[42] Formal clinical trials are currently underway to determine the efficacy of this newer therapeutic modality.

Systemic Therapy

For the patient with more rapidly progressive disease or with advanced, widespread, symptomatic disease, systemic therapy may be most appropriate. Several antineoplastic agents used alone or in combination are active against KS (Table 22-6).

Vincristine[60] and vinblastine[90] have been commonly employed for systemic therapy in AIDS-related KS because each is subjectively well tolerated and the incidence of serious toxicity is low. However, when administered on a weekly basis, vinblastine may cause significant myelosuppression necessitating dose reduction, and vincristine may result in significant peripheral neuropathy. The cumulative toxicities of each of these drugs can be reduced by administering each drug on an alternate-week basis.[44]

Etoposide (VP-16) is also an active agent in KS.[56] However, the frequent occurrence of alopecia in patients treated with etoposide makes it a poor

TABLE 22–6.   CHEMOTHERAPY IN AIDS–KAPOSI'S SARCOMA

Agents	Dose		Reported Response (Percent)	Reference
Vincristine	2 mg/wk		20–59	60
Vinblastine	0.5–1 mg/kg/wk		25–30	90
VP-16	150 mg/m² i.v. q.d. for 3 d. q. 3-4 wk		75	56
Adriamycin	20 mg/m² alternate weeks		53	25
Combination Chemotherapy				
Vincristine	2 mg	Alternate weeks	45	44
Vinblastine	0.1 mg/kg			
Vincristine	2 mg	q. 14 d.	100*	24
Bleomycin	10 mg/m²			
Adriamycin	20 mg/m²			
Bleomycin	10 mg/m²	q. 14 d.	87	25
Vincristine	2 mg			

*Results reported only for patients with pulmonary KS; No. = 3.

choice for patients being treated primarily for cosmetic purposes. In addition, this agent tends to be more highly myelosuppressive than the vinca alkaloids. Clinical trials investigating oral administration of etoposide are currently underway.

Doxorubicin (Adriamycin) may be the most active single agent in AIDS-associated KS[25] and may be useful in the management of patients with more advanced disease or in those in whom prior therapy had failed to produce a response. A recent randomized trial has suggested that the combination regimen of doxorubicin, bleomycin, and vincristine (ABV) is more efficacious against KS than doxorubicin used as a single agent.[25] This regimen has been successfully used in patients with widespread, advanced KS, including those with peripheral edema and pulmonary involvement.[24] It is not unusual to see rapid improvement in peripheral edema or in respiratory symptoms following administration of this combination. The major short-term toxicity associated with doxorubicin is myelosuppression, which may require periodic dose reductions.

The combination of vincristine and bleomycin has significant antitumor activity and may be especially useful for those patients with granulocytopenia, who are likely to be intolerant of more myelosuppressive regimens.[24,27,60]

α-Interferon is an attractive agent for use in the treatment of AIDS-associated KS because it possesses both antiproliferative[53] and apparent anti-HIV activity.[51,55] α-Interferon used as a single agent in the treatment of AIDS-related KS has significant antitumor activity as demonstrated in a large number of clinical trials.[1,25,30] The importance of dose-intensity in the administration of α-interferon is demonstrated in Table 22-7. These data, compiled from several institutions,[30,76] demonstrate that high doses (>20 million units per square meter) of interferon are more effective in inducing antitumor responses than are lower doses. Several studies have demonstrated that patients with better immune function (higher CD4 cell

TABLE 22–7. α-INTERFERON IN AIDS-RELATED KAPOSI'S SARCOMA: EFFICACY OF LOW-DOSE VS. HIGH-DOSE THERAPY

RESPONSE	LOW DOSE < 20,000,000 U/m²	HIGH DOSE ≥ 20,000,000 U/m²
	n = 65	n = 105
Complete	1 (2%)	18 (17%)
Partial	3 (5%)	27 (26%)
Minor or stable	13 (20%)	17 (16%)
Progression	48 (74%)	43 (41%)

Data compiled from published studies at San Francisco General Hospital, the University of California at Los Angeles, Memorial Sloan-Kettering Cancer Center, The M. D. Anderson Hospital and Tumor Institute, and the National Cancer Institute. See text for references.

counts), without a prior history of opportunistic infection, and without "B" symptoms, are more likely to respond to α-interferon than those whose cellular immune function is more compromised and who have had a prior opportunistic infection and are symptomatic.[61,88]

Despite the frequency of objective responses and reports of long disease-free remissions, the use of α-interferon in high doses as a single agent has been limited by its toxicity. While most patients will develop tachyphylaxis to the common flulike symptoms which occur with initiation of therapy, chronic anorexia, fatigue, and weight loss frequently complicate the administration of this agent and limit its usefulness as long-term therapy.

Antiretroviral Agents

Zidovudine (ZDV) is the only currently available antiretroviral agent with proven benefit in patients with HIV infection.[17] However, as a single agent, in our experience, it does not appear to have significant anti-KS activity. Because of the possible occurrence of granulocytopenia in patients treated with ZDV, the concurrent administration of potentially myelosuppressive chemotherapeutic agents is not recommended at this time. Clinical trials are currently underway to evaluate chemotherapy regimens which may be compatible with concurrent administration of ZDV. However, because of its demonstrated efficacy in a variety of stages of HIV infection, ZDV may benefit patients with limited and relatively stable KS who are not candidates for systemic therapy. Zidovudine may be safely administered along with radiotherapy or nonmyelosuppressive chemotherapeutic agents such as vincristine, provided that frequent hematologic evaluation is performed.

Other Treatment Approaches

Clinical trials investigating the concurrent administration of ZDV and low doses of α-interferon are currently in progress. The results of a single trial with this combination were recently reported from the National Cancer Institute.[50] In this trial, ZDV doses ranged from 50 to 250 mg every 4 hours, and α-interferon doses ranged from 0.5 million units per day to more than 25 million units per day. Doses of α-interferon greater than 15 million units per day were not tolerated with ZDV at any dose. However, the lower doses of α-interferon could be safely administered with ZDV. The dose-limiting toxicity was granulocytopenia. Overall, 11 of 26 patients (42 percent) achieved complete or partial tumor response. The majority of these patients were treated with 50 to 100 mg of ZDV every 4 hours and between 0.5 and 15 million units per day of α-interferon. This response rate is significantly higher than that observed in patients treated with these same low doses of α-interferon as a single agent. Since ZDV does not appear

TABLE 22–8. RECOMMENDATIONS FOR TREATMENT FOR KAPOSI'S SARCOMA

Minimal disease	
Stable or slowly progressive	1. Observation only
	2. Investigational agents
	3. Zidovudine $+/-$ α-interferon
Rapidly progressive	1. Vincristine alternating with vinblastine
	2. α-Interferon $+/-$ zidovudine
Widespread, symptomatic	1. Adriamycin
	2. ABV*
Locally symptomatic	1. Radiotherapy
	2. Laser (oral lesions)
Local cosmesis	1. Intralesional chemotherapy
	2. Radiotherapy
	3. Cryotherapy
Cytopenic patients	1. Vincristine
	2. Bleomycin
	3. Vincristine and bleomycin

*ABV: adriamycin, bleomycin, vincristine.

to be particularly effective against KS as a single agent, it would appear that this combination of agents may have synergistic activity in this disease.

Therapeutic Recommendations

Table 22-8 summarizes the recommendations for treatment of patients with AIDS-associated KS. Patients with minimal disease (fewer than 25 cutaneous lesions), unless cosmetically unsightly or painful, are generally not candidates for KS-directed therapy. Those patients may benefit from ZDV or other antiretroviral therapy or from participation in clinical trials of investigational agents. Systemic therapy is recommended for patients with asymptomatic but rapidly progressive disease or for patients with widespread symptomatic disease.

The Adriamycin-containing regimens should generally be reserved for patients with more advanced disease or patients with previously unsuccessful therapy. Vincristine with or without bleomycin may benefit those patients with cytopenias. Locally symptomatic disease can be palliated with localized therapy, generally radiation. Local cosmetic problems may be successfully treated with radiotherapy, intralesional chemotherapy, or possibly cryotherapy. α-Interferon as a single agent may be considered in those patients with more intact immune function (CD4 count $>200/mm^3$). The use of α-interferon and ZDV together or chemotherapy in combination with ZDV may also prove efficacious. However, widespread use of these agents in combination should await the results of large clinical trials currently in progress.

NON-HODGKIN'S LYMPHOMA

The non-Hodgkin's lymphomas (NHL) are a heterogenous group of malignancies. Their biologic behavior ranges from indolent, requiring no therapy, to aggressive malignancies with few long-term survivors. Approximately 70 percent of NHL are of B-cell origin, and another 20 percent are derived from T-cells.

In the most commonly used classification system for the NHLs,[67] these malignancies are divided into three major categories: low grade, intermediate grade, and high grade, according to pathologic characteristics of involved lymph nodes and morphologic criteria of the lymphoma cells.

The first cases of NHL in homosexual men were reported in 1982,[94] and increasing numbers of cases have been reported since that time. The finding of an intermediate or high-grade B-cell NHL in an HIV-infected individual constitutes an AIDS diagnosis as defined by the CDC.[8] Advanced extranodal disease is commonly found at presentation, and median survivals have been short.

Epidemiology

The incidence of NHL is markedly increased in individuals with impaired cell-mediated immunity.[22,40] The best described of these groups are immunosuppressed allograft recipients, a group in which the incidence of NHL is 30 to 50 times that of the general population.[40,70,71] Similarly, Harnly et al[36] have demonstrated a statistically significant increase in the incidence of NHL among never-married men, ages 25 to 44 years, in San Francisco between the years 1980 and 1985. The increase in census tracks with a high incidence of AIDS was greater than the increase in other San Francisco census tracks. In 1985, the incidence of NHL was five times greater than the rate in 1980. However, increases in incidence rates were not observed for other malignancies. Similar trends have been observed for New York City.[52] At San Francisco General Hospital, NHL comprises approximately 2.5 percent of all primary AIDS diagnoses. At this time, it is not known whether the incidence of this malignancy is rising out of proportion to the rising incidence of diagnosed cases of AIDS.

Pathogenesis

The etiology of NHL in patients with HIV infection is not known. In immunosuppressed allograft recipients, molecular data has implicated Epstein-Barr virus (EBV) as a potential etiologic agent in the development of NHL. Several studies have documented the presence of EBV-DNA sequences in the vast majority of B-cell lymphomas from transplant recipicnts.[34,71,81] The majority of lymphomas described in this population have been classified as immunoblastic lymphomas. However, in this patient population, aggressive lymphoproliferative processes have also been described that appear to be polyclonal by both immunologic and morphologic criteria.[21,34,35] In some of these cases, a typical monoclonal lymphoma has subsequently developed.[33]

Although the finding of chromosome t(8;14) translocations, like those seen in Burkitt's lymphoma, and the finding of EBV nuclear antigen in some tumors[4,9,29,72] suggested that EBV might also be implicated in the etiology of HIV-associated lymphomas, more recent observations indicate that EBV-DNA sequences are present in a minority of patients with HIV-associated lymphoma.[46,83] In addition, evaluation of immunoglobulin gene rearrangements using Southern blot hybridization techniques demonstrates that while many of the B-cell tumors observed in this patient population have clonal immunoglobulin gene rearrangements, clonal rearrangements are not observed in other lymphomas.[47a] These tumors may represent "polyclonal" processes, not unlike those observed in allograft recipients.[35] Lymphomagenesis in this population may, in fact, occur by a variety of different pathways. The roles of a variety of potential etiologic agents are currently the subject of extensive laboratory research.

Clinical Characteristics

The vast majority of the NHLs observed in the setting of HIV infection are classified as B-cell malignancies.[57,93] A small number of NHLs of other histologic and immunologic subtypes have been observed, including T-cell lymphoma[46,66,73] and others of uncertain lineage.[49] Of 327 cases reported in the literature from five centers, 73 percent were classified as high-grade, 24 percent as intermediate-grade, and 3 percent as low-grade lymphomas.[3,23,46,48,59,93] The majority of B-cell lymphomas in these individuals are classified as diffuse large-cell tumors of either intermediate-grade type or the high-grade immunoblastic type. In addition, approximately one third of patients present with tumors of the high-grade, small non-cleaved-cell variety.[46]

Widespread disease involving extranodal sites is the hallmark of AIDS-associated lymphoma at the time of diagnosis. Ziegler et al[93] reported that 95 percent of patients had evidence of extranodal disease; 42 percent of patients had central nervous system (CNS) disease, and 33 percent had bone marrow involvement. In a series of 89 patients diagnosed at New York University,[48] 87 percent had extranodal disease at presentation. The most common sites of disease included the gastrointestinal tract, CNS, bone marrow, and liver. At San Francisco General Hospital, two thirds of the patients presented with stage IV disease, and 31 percent presented with extranodal disease alone, with no identifiable site of nodal disease.[46]

As observed in other immunosuppressed patients with NHL, unusual extralymphatic presentations are common. Sites of disease have included the rectum,[6] heart and pericardium,[2,32] and common bile ducts.[43] Gastrointestinal involvement has been reported in up to 27 percent of individuals with lymphoma,[20] and virtually any site in the gastrointestinal tract or hepatobiliary tree can be involved. In the San Francisco General Hospital series,[46] other unusal sites of disease included subcutaneous and soft tissue, epidural space, appendix, gingiva, parotid gland, and paranasal sinus.

Non-Hodgkin's lymphoma confined to the CNS has frequently been reported in association with HIV infection.[18,26,82] The most common presenting symptoms have been confusion, lethargy, and memory loss. Other symptoms have included hemiparesis, aphasia, seizures, cranial nerve palsies, and headache. Single or multiple discreet lesions are the most common findings on computed tomography (CT) or magnetic resonance imaging (MRI) of the brain. The lesions are frequently hypodense and contrast enhancing. Both clinical presentation and CT or MRI findings are frequently indistinguishable from those associated with toxoplasmosis.

Given the similarity in clinical presentation and radiographic findings to other CNS disorders, the diagnosis of primary CNS lymphoma can be difficult to make. Patients presenting with neurologic symptoms should have prompt evaluation with CT or MRI of the brain. Lumbar puncture should be performed if not contraindicated by the CT findings. Patients with focal lesions should have a serum specimen sent for cryptococcal antigen and *Toxoplasma* titers. Since toxoplasmosis is rare in individuals with negative *Toxoplasma* serologies,[28] brain biopsy should be performed in a timely fashion in this group of patients. Individuals with focal intracerebral lesions and positive serologic studies for *Toxoplasma* are typically started on anti-*Toxoplasma* therapy and observed closely for signs of improvement or deterioration.

Treatment and Prognosis

The use of multiagent chemotherapeutic regimens for the treatment of intermediate and high-grade NHL in *non*-HIV-infected individuals has resulted in a dramatic improvement in prognosis for this group.[14] Complete response rates as high as 86 percent[11] and long-term survivals as high as 65 percent[11] have been reported in patients treated for aggressive, large-cell lymphomas.

In HIV-infected individuals, however, the use of similar chemotherapeutic regimens has not resulted in as favorable an outcome (Table 22-9). Complete response rates are lower than the corresponding rates in the non-HIV-infected population, and these responses tend to be of short duration. In the retrospective review by Ziegler et al of patients treated at multiple institutions, 53 percent of 66 evaluable patients achieved complete response

**TABLE 22–9.   RESPONSE TO CHEMOTHERAPY AND SURVIVAL
IN HIV-ASSOCIATED NHL**

INSTITUTION	NO.	TREATMENT REGIMEN	COMPLETE RESPONSE (%)	MEDIAN SURVIVAL (MO.)	REFERENCE
USC	22	m-BACOD	45	NA	23
		& others	32		
NYU	83	various	33	5.0	48
UCSF	65	various	54	5.5	46
MSKCC	30	various	56	6.0	59
Pacific Medical Center	31	CHOP	39	7.0	3
		MACOP-B			
Multicenter	66	various	53	NA	93
ACTG	36	m-BACOD*	42	NA	58
Italian Cooperative Group	72	various	35	4.0	41

USC: University of Southern California; NYU: New York University; UCSF: University of California, San Francisco; MSKCC: Memorial Sloan-Kettering Cancer Institute; Multicenter: UCSF, USC, NY Hospital/Cornell, University of Texas/MD Anderson, NYU/Kaplan Cancer Center, MSKCC; ACTG: AIDS Clinical Trials Group, National Institute of Health; 6 CHOP: Cyclophosphamide, hydroxydaunomide (doxorubicin), oncovin (vincristine), and prednisone.
*Reduced dose.

to combination chemotherapy, but 54 percent of the complete responders subsequently relapsed.[93]

Morphologic subtype appears to predict response to chemotherapy in one series of patients reported from New York University.[48] The best complete response rate was reported for those patients classified as having large non-cleaved-cell lymphoma (52 percent), while those having small non-cleaved-cell and immunoblastic lymphoma had response rates of 26 and 21 percent, respectively. One group[3] has reported a 64 percent complete response rate in a series of 11 patients treated with the MACOP-B regimen (methotrexate, doxurubicin, cyclophosphamide, vincristine, prednisone, bleomycin). However, it cannot be determined from this small number of patients whether this represents significant improvement in the complete response rate over that observed in other series of patients.

Survival times from a number of large series of patients reported in the literature are shown in Table 22-9. Median survivals in these groups range from 4 to 7 months. In the series of 23 patients who received chemotherapy at the Pacific Medical Center[3] the median survival was 20 months in those patients achieving complete response to therapy.

While overall survival times in patients with AIDS-associated NHL are disappointing, subgroups of patients can be identified in which the therapeutic outcome is significantly better than for other groups of patients. Morphologic subtypes predictive of response to therapy in patients treated at New York University[48] were also predictive of survival in this same series. Patients with intermediate-grade large-cell lymphoma had the longest me-

TABLE 22–10. PREDICTORS OF SURVIVAL IN CHEMOTHERAPY-TREATED HIV-ASSOCIATED NON-HODGKIN'S LYMPHOMA (NO. = 65)

CHARACTERISTIC	MEDIAN SURVIVAL (MO)	P VALUE
CD4 count $< 100/\text{mm}^3$	4.1	0.01
CD4 count $> 100/\text{mm}^3$	24	
Prior AIDS: Yes	2.2	0.0001
Prior AIDS: NO	8.3	
KPS $< 70\%$	3.8	0.03
KPS $\geq 70\%$	6.8	
Extranodal disease: Yes	4.2	0.01
Extranodal disease: No	12.2	

KPS: Karnofsky performance score.

dian survival (7.5 months), whereas those with small, non-cleaved-cell lymphoma had a median survival of 5.5 months, and those with immunoblastic lymphoma had a median survival of only 2.0 months.

In the San Francisco General Hospital series,[46] median survival for all 65 patients receiving chemotherapy was only 5.5 months. However, life-table analysis for subgroups within this population illustrates the importance of prognostic features (Table 22-10). Those features identified as being predictive of significantly improved survival included an absolute CD4+ lymphocyte count $>100/\text{mm}^3$, absence of a prior AIDS diagnosis, Karnofsky performance score of 70 percent or more and the absence of an extranodal site of disease. Evaluation of newly diagnosed patients for these prognostic features may help determine how to approach therapy in this disease. The patient without a prior AIDS diagnosis whose immune function is relatively good is a much better candidate for therapy than is a patient whose diagnosis of lymphoma comes after a history of multiple opportunistic infections. Since many patients will fall between these extremes, these prognostic characteristics can only serve as rough guidelines in determining which patients to treat.

What the most appropriate therapeutic regimen will be for a given patient also must be individualized, as there is no known "best" regimen. Poor bone marrow reserve and opportunistic infections often result in dose reductions and delays in therapy. In addition, one must consider the risk of further immunosuppression when treating HIV-infected patients with aggressive combination chemotherapy.

Contrary to the belief that more intensive chemotherapy is associated with improved clinical outcome in non-HIV-associated lymphoma, retrospective data from two centers have suggested that in HIV-infected individuals with NHL, survival may be improved in those treated with less aggressive regimens. Survival data from the San Francisco General Hospital cohort of chemotherapy-treated patients with NHL revealed that patients receiving chemotherapy regimens containing 1 g/m² or more of cyclophosphamide had a median survival of only 4.6 months compared with those treated with regimens containing less than 1 g/m² of cyclophosphamide, who had a median survival of 12.2 months ($P = .02$).[46] Similarly, in a study of nine patients treated with a novel, more aggressive, chemotherapeutic regimen consisting of high-dose cytosine arabinoside, 1-asparaginase, vincristine, prednisone, cyclophosphamide (high-dose), methotrexate, and leucovorin,[23] only three patients achieved complete remission. This intensive regimen was associated with a high risk of mortality due to opportunistic infection. Recently, data was presented from a multicenter clinical trial evaluating the efficacy of a low-dose chemotherapeutic regimen.[58] In this regimen, patients were treated with a *modification* of the standard m-BACOD regimen (methotrextate, bleomycin, doxorubicin, cyclophosphamide, vincristine, and dexamethasone). Instead of administering cyclophosphamide at 600 mg/m², and doxurubicin at 45 mg/m², these two agents were administered at 300 mg/m² and 25 mg/m², respectively. Complete responses were observed in approximately 42 percent of patients (not different from other series of patients reported in the literature treated with standard chemotherapy regimens). There have been several sustained remissions following this therapeutic approach. This indicates that relapse-free survival is possible using reduced doses of chemotherapeutic agents. No direct comparison between this regimen and more standard dose regimens has yet been carried out. Ongoing clinical trials are currently investigating the concurrent administration of growth factors as well as prophylaxis of *Pneumocystis carinii* pneumonia to determine whether these adjunctive therapies will make standard chemotherapy more tolerable in this patient population.

Lymphoma confined to the brain has been particularly difficult to treat. Many cases have been diagnosed at autopsy,[93] and those presenting antemortem often have advanced immunodeficiency and have suffered multiple previous bouts of opportunistic infections.[18,26,82] In a series reported by Formenti et al,[18] 6 of 10 patients with primary CNS lymphoma presented with a prior history of one or more opportunistic infections. In this series, complete responses to cranial irradiation occurred in 6 of the 10 patients. Two of the six died from opportunistic infections, two had recurrent lymphoma, and two were alive at 8 and 14 months after diagnosis. Overall, 50 percent of the patients died of opportunistic infections, and the median survival of the group as a whole was 5.5 months. Others have also reported short survivals despite therapy with whole brain irradiation. Gill et al[26] reported only one of six patients alive at 28 months from diagnosis, and So et al[82] reported a median survival of only 2.7 months in seven patients treated with whole brain irradiation. The most common cause of death in all these series has been opportunistic infection. It would appear, based upon these studies, that pursuing therapy for primary CNS lymphoma is fruitless. However, since the routine use of prophylaxis against *P. carinii* and the use of active antiretroviral agents is now commonplace, the frequency of occurrence of opportunistic infections in these patients may be reduced. Therefore, if effective therapy for the lymphoma can be identified, and if patients are diagnosed early, before severe neurologic compromise has occurred, survivals may be prolonged.

In selecting therapy for HIV-associated NHL, the emphasis should be on individualized treatment. While standard-dose chemotherapy may be appropriate for the patient with good immune function and without a prior opportunistic infection, a lower dose treatment regimen might be selected for the patient with more severe immune compromise, marginal Karnofsky performance score, and history of opportunistic infection. For some patients who are severely ill, a decision may be made to withhold therapy altogether. These decisions must take into account not only the patient's history and present condition, but also the patient's own desires for a given therapeutic approach.

HODGKIN'S DISEASE

As discussed earlier, Hodgkin's disease is not an AIDS-defining illness. The precise relationship of this malignancy to the underlying immunodeficiency state is unclear. Hodgkin's disease has rarely been reported in patients with primary immunodeficiency disorders[22] and has not been reported in immunosuppressed transplant recipients.[40] The observation that the frequency of Hodgkin's disease in the single male population aged 20 to 49 years in San Francisco has not increased in the years since 1979, when HIV seroprevalence markedly increased,[45,52] argues against a direct causal relationship between HIV-related immunodeficiency and the occurrence of Hodgkin's disease in this population. This is in striking contrast to the earlier mentioned sharp rise in the frequency of NHL observed in the same population during the same time period.[34,52]

Clinical observations suggest that Hodgkin's disease in the setting of HIV infection has a different natural history and therapeutic outcome when compared to cases of Hodgkin's disease in the general population. The clinical features and therapeutic outcome in 14 homosexual men with Hodgkin's disease diagnosed at San Francisco General Hospital have been compared with those in a group of 35 single men between the ages of 20 and 49 diagnosed with Hodgkin's disease between the years 1973 and 1979.[45] Mixed cellularity was found to be the most common histologic pattern among the 14 risk-group patients, whereas nodular sclerosis was significantly more common in the control population. All but one of the risk-group patients presented with advanced (stage III or IV) disease. Bone marrow and liver were the most common sites of extranodal disease.

The outcome of therapy in these patients has been disappointing. Of 12 evaluable patients treated at San Francisco General Hospital,[45] there were seven complete responders to either nitrogen mustard, vincristine, pro-carbizine, and prednisone (MOPP) or MOPP with doxurubicin (Adria-mycin), bleomycin, vinblastine, and decarbizine (MOPP-ABVD). Six of these seven complete responders subsequently relapsed. Eight patients (62 percent) developed *P. carinii* pneumonia during treatment. None of these patients are currently living. One half of the patients died with advanced Hodgkin's disease, and the remaining patients died as a result of oppor-tunistic infections. Median survival was less than 1 year in this population, compared with 12 years in the control population. There were no differ-ences in either response or survival between those patients treated with MOPP alone and those treated with MOPP-ABVD.

The mean dose intensity of chemotherapy delivered to our patients was only 41 percent of the planned therapeutic dose. This was a result of the need for frequent dose reductions and delays in chemotherapy because of poor bone marrow reserve and intercurrent opportunistic infections. The very low dose intensity of chemotherapy may account for the high relapse rate observed in complete responders.

The Italian Cooperative Group for AIDS-related tumors recently re-ported 35 cases of Hodgkin's disease occurring in HIV-infected individ-uals.[41] Eighty-nine percent of these patients were intravenous drug abusers, 3 percent were homosexual males, and 9 percent were intravenous drug-using homosexual males. Fifty-three percent of the patients presented with mixed-cellularity histologic type, 31 percent with nodular sclerosis, and 16 percent with lymphocyte depletion. Seventy-eight percent of patients pre-sented with either stage III or IV disease. Seventeen patients were treated with MOPP, ABVD, ABV, or MOPP alternating with ABVD. Only eight patients (30 percent) achieved complete remission. Of 13 patients who died, seven (54 percent) died of opportunistic infections, three died of progres-sion of Hodgkin's disease, and two died of disseminated intravascular co-agulation. In one patient the cause of death could not be determined. The median survival of these patients with Hodgkin's disease was 15 months.

Any illness may be complicated by coexisting HIV infection without a cause and effect relationship. Although frequency data for San Francisco do not support the development of Hodgkin's disease as a direct result of HIV infection, those Hodgkin's disease patients who are HIV-seropositive are more likely to present with advanced stage and poor prognosis histologic pattern. They are more likely to have a poor therapeutic outcome and to develop AIDS-associated opportunistic infections during therapy. These observations suggest that HIV serologic testing can provide important prognostic information in selected patients with Hodgkin's disease.

As is the case for NHLs in HIV-seropositive patients, experience thus far does not suggest that survival with Hodgkin's disease will be improved with more aggressive chemotherapeutic regimens. Poor bone marrow re-serve and opportunistic infections have made it difficult to administer full doses of standard Hodgkin's disease chemotherapy to these patients. The use of less intensive and less myelosuppressive chemotherapeutic regimens is currently being explored as well as the use of more standard chemotherapeutic regimens with hematopoietic growth factors. Since a significant proportion of these patients will die as a result of opportunistic infection, prophylaxis against *P. carinii* pneumonia is strongly encouraged during chemotherapy.

SUMMARY

Patients with HIV infection, like immunosuppressed transplant recipients, are at high risk for the development of both Kaposi's sarcoma and B-cell non-Hodgkin's lymphoma. While other malignancies may be seen in the HIV-infected patient, epidemiologic evidence does not suggest a causal relationship between the underlying immunodeficiency state and the subsequent development of malignancy. Whether causally related or not, however, any malignancy occurring in the setting of HIV infection is likely to have a more aggressive course and to be associated with short survival.

Kaposi's sarcoma is the most common malignancy seen in the setting of HIV infection. The etiology of Kaposi's sarcoma is uncertain, as are the reasons for its nearly exclusive confinement to the homosexual male population with HIV infection. Prognosis is related to the extent of disease, immune function, and the presence of systemic and local symptoms. A variety of local and systemic therapeutic modalities are available including radiotherapy, cryotherapy, chemotherapy, and α-interferon. Which treatment approach is most appropriate for an individual will depend upon the extent of disease, the presence of local symptoms including pain or edema, or the presence of cosmetically unsightly disease. Early studies suggest that the concurrent use of α-interferon and zidovudine may make the use of lower doses of α-interferon possible. The concurrent use of zidovudine with other chemotherapeutic regimens is currently being explored.

Patients with B-cell lymphoma tend to present with advanced extranodal disease, and primary lymphoma of the CNS has frequently been reported as well. Not unlike B-cell lymphoma seen in allograft recipients, lymphoma in the presence of HIV infection appears to arise out of background of polyclonal B-cell activation. Although a viral etiology has been suspected, the cause of lymphoma in these patients remains unknown. Response to therapy in these patients has been disappointing. Response rates to chemotherapy have been lower than those observed in other lymphoma patients, and treatment has been complicated by lack of adequate bone marrow reserve and occurrence of frequent opportunistic infections. While overall survivals have been short, factors predictive of improved survival include better immune function, absence of a prior AIDS diagnosis, good Karnofsky performance score, and absence of an extranodal site of disease. Experience suggests that in some patients, more aggressive chemotherapy may be associated with shortened survival. Current therapeutic modalities being explored include lower dose chemotherapeutic regimens and standard dose chemotherapy with the concurrent use of a hematopoietic growth factor, such as granulocyte–monocyte colony–stimulating factor (GM-CSF).

Treatment of the patient with an HIV-associated malignancy poses challenges which are unique in medicine. It is for this reason that it is especially important that treatment be carefully individualized, with the patient playing an important role in determining which therapeutic alternative is most appropriate.

REFERENCES

1. Abrams DI, Volberding PA: Alpha interferon therapy of AIDS-associated Kaposi's sarcoma. Semin Oncol 14:43-47, 1987
2. Balasubramanyam A, Waxman M, Kazal HL, Lee MH: Malignant lymphoma of the heart in acquired immunodeficiency syndrome. Chest 90:243-246, 1986
3. Bermudez M, Grant K, Rodvien R, Mendes F: Non-Hodgkin's lymphoma in a population with or at risk for acquired immunodeficiency syndrome: Indications for intensive chemotherapy. Am J Med 86:71-76, 1989
4. Bernheim A, Berger R: Cytogenetic studies of Burkitt lymphoma-leukemia in patients with acquired immunodeficiency syndrome. Cancer Genet Cytogenet 32:67-74, 1988
5. Brooks JJ: Kaposi's sarcoma: A reversible hyperplasia. Lancet 2:1309-1311, 1986
6. Burkes RL, Meyer PR, Gill PS, Parker JL, Rasheed S, Levine A: Rectal lymphoma in homosexual men. Arch Intern Med 146:913-915, 1986
7. Cappell MS, Yao F, Cho KC: Colonic adenocarcinoma associated with the acquired immunodeficiency syndrome. Cancer 62:616-619, 1988
8. Centers for Disease Control: Revision of the case definition of acquired immunodeficiency syndrome for national reporting - United States. MMWR 34:373-374, 1985
9. Chaganti R, Jhanwar S, Koziner B, Arlin Z, Mertelsmann R, Clarkson B: Specific translocations characterize Burkitt's-like lymphoma of homosexual men with the acquired immunodeficiency syndrome. Blood 61:1269-1272, 1983
10. Chak LY, Gill PS, Levine AM, et al: Radiation therapy for AIDS-related Kaposi's sarcoma. J Clin Oncol 5:863-867, 1988
11. Connors JM, Klimo P: MACOP-B Chemotherapy for malignant lymphomas and related conditions: 1987 Update and additional observations. Semin Hematol 25(Suppl 2):41-46, 1988
12. Daling JR, Weiss NS, Klopfenstein LL, et al: Correlates of homosexual behavior and the incidence of anal cancer. JAMA 247:1988-1990, 1982
13. Des Jarlais DC, Stoneburner R, Thomas P: Declines in proportion of Kaposi's sarcoma among cases of AIDS in multiple risk groups in New York City. Lancet 2:1024-1025, 1987
14. DeVita VT, Hubbard SM, Young RC, Longo DL: The role of chemotherapy in diffuse aggressive lymphomas. Semin Hematol 25(Suppl 2):2-10, 1988
15. Drew WL, Mills J, Hauer LB, et al: Declining prevalence of Kaposi's sarcoma in homosexual AIDS patients paralleled by fall in cytomegalovirus transmission. Lancet 1:66, 1988
16. Ensoli B, Nakamura S, Salahuddin SZ, et al: AIDS-Kaposi's sarcoma-derived cells express cytokines with autocrine and paracrine growth factors. Science 243:223-226, 1989
17. Fischl MA, Richman DD, Greico MH, et al: The efficacy of azidothymidine (AZT) in the treatment of patients with AIDS and AIDS-related complex. A double-blind, placebo-controlled trial. N Engl J Med 317:185-191, 1987
18. Formenti SC, Gill PS, Rarick M, et al: Primary central nervous system lymphoma in AIDS: Results of radiation therapy. Cancer 63:1101-1107, 1989

19. Frager DH, Wolf EL, Competiello LS, Frager JD, Klein RS, Beneventano TC: Squamous cell carcinoma of the esophagus in patients with acquired immunodeficiency syndrome. Gastrointest Radiol 13:358-360, 1988

20. Friedman SL: Gastrointestinal and hepatobiliary neoplasms in AIDS. Gastroenterol Clin North Am 17:465-486, 1988

21. Frizzera G, Hanto DW, Gajl Peczalkska K, et al: Polymorphic diffuse B-cell hyperplasias and lymphomas in renal transplant recipients. Cancer Res 41:4262-4279, 1981

22. Frizzera G, Rosai J, Dehner LP, Spector BD, Kersey JH: Lymphoreticular disorders in primary immunodeficiencies: New findings based on an up-to-date histologic classification of 35 cases. Cancer 46(4):692-699, 1980

23. Gill P, Levine A, Krailo M, et al: AIDS-related malignant lymphoma: Results of prospective treatment trials. J Clin Oncol 5:1322-1328, 1987

24. Gill PS, Akil B, Colletti P, et al: Pulmonary Kaposi's sarcoma: Clinical findings and results of therapy. Am J Med 87:57-61, 1989

25. Gill PS, Krailo M, Slater L, et al: Randomized trial of ABV (adriamycin, bleomycin and vinblastine) vs A (adriamycin) in advanced Kaposi's sarcoma (KS) (Abstract). Am Soc Clin Oncol, New Orleans, 1988, p 11

26. Gill PS, Levine A, Meyer P, et al: Primary central nervous system lymphoma in homosexual men. Am J Med 78:742-748, 1985

27. Glaspy J, Miles S, McCarthy S: Treatment of advanced stage Kaposi's sarcoma with vincristine and bleomycin (Abstract). Am Soc Clin Oncol, Los Angeles, 1986, p 10

28. Grant I, Gold J, Armstrong D: Risk of CNS Toxoplasmosis in patients with acquired immune deficiency syndrome. Proceedings of Interscientific Conference on Antimicrobial Agents and Chemotherapy (Abstract 441), New Orleans, 1986, p 177

29. Groopman J, Sullivan J, Mulder C, et al: Pathogenesis of B-cell lymphoma in a patient with AIDS. Blood 67:612-615, 1986

30. Groopman JE, Gottlieb MS, Goodman J, et al: Recombinant alpha-2 interferon therapy for Kaposi's sarcoma associated with the acquired immunodeficiency syndrome. Ann Intern Med 100:671-676, 1984

31. Groopman JE, Mayer K, Zipoli T, et al: Unusual neoplasms with HTLV-III infection. Proc Am Soc Clin Oncol 5:14, 1896

32. Guarner J, Brynes RK, Chan WC, Birdsong G, Hertxler G: Primary non-Hodgkin's lymphoma of the heart in two patients with the acquired immunodeficiency syndrome. Arch Pathol Lab Med 111:254-256, 1987

33. Hanto DW, Frizzera G, Gajl-Peczalkska K, et al: Epstein-Barr virus induced B-cell lymphoma after renal transplantation. N Engl J Med 306:913-918, 1982

34. Hanto DW, Frizzera G, Purtilo, et al: Clinical spectrum of lymphoproliferative disorders in renal transplant recipients and evidence for the role of Epstein-Barr virus. Cancer Res 41:4253-4261, 1981

35. Hanto DW, Gajl-Peczalkska KJ, Frizzera G, et al: Epstein-Barr virus induces polyclonal and monoclonal B-cell lymphoproliferative disease occurring after renal transplantation. Ann Surg 198:356-369, 1983

36. Harnly ME, Swan SH, Holly EA, Kelter A, Padian N: Temporal trends in the incidence of non-Hodgkin's lymphoma and selected malignancies in a poplulation with a high incidence of acquired immunodeficiency syndrome (AIDS). Am J Epidemiol 128(2):261-267, 1988

37. Harwood AR, Osoba D, Hofstader SL, et al: Kaposi's sarcoma in recipients of renal transplants. Am J Med 67:759-765, 1979

38. Heyer DM, Desmond S, Volberding P, Kahn J: Changing prevalence of malignancies in men at San Francisco General Hospital during the HIV epidemic. Proc V International Conference on AIDS (Abstract WBO 19), 1989, p 206

39. Hill DR: The role of radiotherapy for epidemic Kaposi's sarcoma. Semin Oncol 14 (Suppl 3):1207, 1987

40. Hoover R, Fraumeni JF: Risk of cancer in renal transplant recipients. Lancet 2:55-57, 1973

41. Italian Cooperative Group for AIDS-related Tumors: Malignant lymphomas in patients with or at risk for AIDS in Italy: Reports. J Natl Cancer Inst 80:855-860, 1988

42. Kahn J: Personal communication.

43. Kaplan L, Kahn J, Jacobson M, Bottles K, Cello J: Primary bile duct lymphoma in the acquired immunodeficiency syndrome (AIDS). Ann Intern Med 110:162, 1989
44. Kaplan LD, Abrams D, Volberding P: Treatment of Kaposi's sarcoma in acquired immunodeficiency syndrome with an alternating vincristine-vinblastine regimen. Cancer Treat Rev 70:1121-1122, 1986
45. Kaplan LD, Abrams DA, Volberding PA: Clinical course and epidemiology of Hodgkin's disease in homosexual men. International Conference on AIDS (Abstract M.11.3.), Washington, DC, June, 1987
46. Kaplan LD, Abrams DI, Feigal E, McGrath M, Kahn J, Neville P, Ziegler J, Volberding P: AIDS-associated non-Hodgkin's lymphoma in San Francisco. JAMA 261:719-724, 1989
47. Kaplan LD, Hopewell PC, Jaffe H, Goodman PC, Bottles K, Volberding PA: Kaposi's sarcoma involving the lung in patients with the acquired immunodeficiency syndrome. J AIDS 1:23-30, 1988
47a. Kaplan LD, Meeker T, Feigal E, et al: Clonality of AIDS-associated non-Hodgkins lymphom predicts survival. Paper presented at American Federation of Clinical Research National Meeting (Abstract). Washington, DC, April 1989, p 467a.
48. Knowles DM, Chamulak G, Subar M, et al: Lymphoid neoplasia associated with the acquired immunodeficiency syndrome (AIDS). Ann Intern Med 108:744-753, 1988
49. Knowles DM, Inghirami G, Ubraico A, Dalla-Favera R: Molecular genetic analysis of three AIDS-associated neoplasms of uncertain lineage demonstrates their B-cell derivation and the possible pathogenic role of Epstein-Barr virus. Blood 73:792-799, 1989
50. Kovacs JA, Deyton L, Davey R, et al: Combined zidovudine and interferon-α therapy in patients with Kaposi's sarcoma and the acquired immunodeficiency syndrome (AIDS). Ann Intern Med 111:280-286, 1989
51. Kovacs JA, Lance HC, Masur H, et al: A phase III, placebo-controlled trial of recombinant alpha interferon in asymptomatic individuals seropositive for the acquired immunodeficiency syndrome. Clin Res 35:479A, 1987
52. Kristal AR, Nasca PC, Burnett WS, Mikl J: Changes in the epidemiology of non-Hodgkin's lymphoma associated with epidemic human immunodeficiency virus (HIV) infection. Am J Epidemiol 128:711-718, 1988
53. Krown SE: The role of interferon in the therapy of epidemic Kaposi's sarcoma. Semin Oncol 14(Suppl 3):27-33, 1987
54. Krown SE, Metroka C, Wernz JC: Kaposi's sarcoma in the acquired immunodeficiency syndrome: A proposal for uniform evaluation, response, and staging criteria. J Clin Oncol 7:1201-1207, 1989
55. Lane HC, Feinberg J, Davery V, et al: Anti-retroviral effects of interferon-alpha in AIDS-associated Kaposi's sarcoma. Lancet 2:1218-1222, 1988
56. Laubenstein LJ, Krigel RL, Odajnyk CM, et al: Treatment of epidemic Kaposi's sarcoma with etoposide or a combination of doxorubicin, bleomycin and vinblastine. J Clin Oncol 2:1115-1120, 1984
57. Levine A, Meyer P, Begandy M, Parker W, et al: Development of B-cell lymphoma in homosexual men. Ann Intern Med 100:7-13, 1984
58. Levine A, Wernz J, Kaplan L, et al: Low dose chemotherapy with CNS prophylaxis and zidovudine (AZT) maintenance for AIDS-related lymphoma: Follow-up data from a multi-institutional trial. American Society of Hematology (Abstract 897), Dec 1989, 239a
59. Lowenthal D, Straus D, Campbell S, et al: AIDS-related lymphoid neoplasia. The Memorial Hospital Experience. Cancer 61:2325-2337, 1988
60. Mintzer DM, Real FX, Jovino L, Krown SE: Treatment of Kaposi's sarcoma and thrombocytopenia with vincristine in patients with the acquired immunodeficiency syndrome. Ann Intern Med 102:200-202, 1985
61. Deleted
62. Mitsuyasu R, Taylor J, Glaspy J, et al: Heterogeneity of epidemic Kaposi's sarcoma. Implications for therapy. Cancer 57:1657-1661, 1986
63. Mitsuyasu RT, Groopman JE: Biology and therapy of Kaposi's sarcoma. Semin Oncol 11:53-59, 1984

64. Myskowski PL, Niedzweicki D, Shurgot BA, et al: AIDS-associated Kaposi's sarcoma: Variable associated with increased survival. J Am Acad Dermatol 18:1299-1306, 1988
65. Nakamura S, Salahuddin SZ, Biberfeld P, et al: Kaposi's sarcoma cells: Long-term culture with growth factor from retrovirus-infected CD4+ T cells. Science 242:426-430, 1988
66. Nasr S, Brynes R, Garrison C, Chan W: Peripheral T-cell lymphoma in a patient with acquired immunodeficiency syndrome. Cancer 61:947-951, 1988
67. National Cancer Institute: NCI-sponsored study of classifications of non-Hodgkin's lymphoma. Summary and description of a working formulation for clinical usage. The Non-Hodgkin's Lymphoma Pathologic Classification Project. Cancer 49:2112-2135, 1982
68. Newman SB: Treatment of epidemic Kaposi's sarcoma (KS) with intralesional vinblastine injection (IL-VLB). Am Soc Clin Oncol (Abstract), New Orleans, 1988, p 5
69. Ognibene FP, Steis RG, Macher AM, et al: Kaposi's sarcoma causing pulmonary infiltrates and respiratory failure in acquired immunodeficiency syndrome. Ann Intern Med 102:471-475, 1985
70. Penn I: The incidence of malignancies in transplant recipients. Transplant Proc 7:323-326, 1975
71. Penn I: Lymphomas complicating organ transplantation. Transplant Proc 15(Suppl 1):2790-2797, 1983
72. Petersen JM, Tubbs RR, Savage RA, et al: Small non-cleaved B-cell Burkitt-like lymphoma with chromosome t(8;14) translocation and Epstein-Barr virus nuclear-associated antigen in a homosexual man with acquired immune deficiency syndrome. Am J Med 78:141-148, 1985
73. Presant CA, Gala K, Wiseman C, et al: Human immunodeficiency virus-associated T-cell lymphoblastic lymphoma in AIDS. Cancer 60:1459-1461, 1987
74. Ravalli S, Chabon AB, Khan AA: Gastrointestinal neoplasia in young HIV-positive patients. Am J Clin Pathol 91:458-461, 1989
75. Real FX, Oettgen HF, Krown SE: Kaposi's sarcoma and the acquired immunodeficiency syndrome: Treatment with high and low doses of leukocyte A interferon. J Clin Oncol 4:544-551, 1986
76. Rios A, Mansell PWA, Newell GA, et al: Treatment of acquired immunodeficiency syndrome-related Kaposi's sarcoma with lymphoblastoid interferon. J Clin Oncol 3:506-512, 1985
77. Rutherford GW, Schwarcz SK, Lemp GF, et al: The epidemiology of AIDS-related Kaposi's sarcoma in San Francisco. J Infect Dis 159:569-572, 1989
78. Safai B: Pathophysiology and epidemiology of epidemic Kaposi's sarcoma. Semin Oncol 2(Suppl 3):7-12, 1987
79. Salahuddin SZ, Nakamura S, Biberfeld P, et al: Angiogenic properties of Kaposi's sarcoma-derived cells after long-term culture *in vitro*. Science 242:430-433, 1988
80. Schoeppel SL, Hoppe RT, Dorfman RF, et al: Hodgkin's disease in homosexual men with generalized lymphadenopathy. Ann Intern Med 102:68-70, 1985
81. Shearer WT, Ritz J, Finego MJ, et al: Epstein-Barr virus-associated B-cell proliferations of diverse clonal origins after bone marrow transplantation in a 12 year-old patient with severe combined immunodeficiency. N Engl J Med 312:1151-1159, 1985
82. So YT, Beckstead J, Davis R: Primary central nervous system lymphoma in acquired immunodeficiency syndrome: A clinical and pathological study. Ann Neurol 20:566-572, 1986
83. Subar M, Neri A, Inghirami G, Knowles DM, Dalla-Favera R: Frequent c-*myc* oncogene activation and infrequent presence of Epstein-Barr virus genome in AIDS-associated lymphoma. Blood 72:667-671, 1988
84. Taylor J, Afrasiabi R, Fahey JL, Korns E, Weaver M, Mitsuyasu R: Prognostically significant classification of immune changes in AIDS with Kaposi's sarcoma. Blood 67:666-671, 1986
85. Tessler AN, Catanese A: AIDS and germ cell tumors of testis. Urology 30:203-204, 1987
86. Tindal B, Finlayson R, Mutimer K, Billson FA, Munro VF, Cooper DA: Malignant melanoma associated with human immunodeficiency virus infection in three homosexual men. J Am Acad Dermatol 20:587-591, 1989
87. Tirelli V, Vaccher E, Sinicco A, Sabbatani S, Giudic MG, Zagni R, Monfardini S: Forty-

nine unusual HIV-related malignant tumors. Proceedings V International Conference on AIDS (Abstract WCP 50), Montreal, 1989, p 600

88. Vadhan-Raj S, Wong G, Gnecco C, et al: Immunological variables as predictors of prognosis in patients with Kaposi's sarcoma and the acquired immunodeficiency syndrome. Cancer 46:417-425, 1986

89. Vogel J, Hinrichs SH, Reynolds RK, et al: The HIV *tat* gene induces dermal lesions resembling Kaposi's sarcoma in transgenic mice. Nature 335:606-611, 1988

90. Volberding PA, Abrams DA, Conant M, Kaslow K, Vranizan K, Ziegler J: Vinblastine therapy for Kaposi's sarcoma in the acquired immunodeficiency syndrome. Ann Intern Med 103:335-338, 1985

91. Volberding PA, Kusick P, Feigal D: Effects of chemotherapy for HIV associated Kaposi's sarcoma on longterm survival (Abstract). Proc Am Soc Clin Oncol 8:12, 1989

92. Volberding PA, Mitsuyasu R: Recombinant interferon alpha in the treatment of acquired immune deficiency syndrome-related Kaposi's sarcoma. Semin Oncol 2(Suppl 5):2-6, 1985

93. Ziegler J, Beckstead J, Volberding P, et al: Non-Hodgkin's lymphoma in 90 homosexual men. Relation to generalized lymphadenopathy and the acquired immunodeficiency syndrome. N Engl J Med 311:565-570, 1984

94. Ziegler JL, Drew WL, Miner RC, et al: Outbreak of Burkitt's-like lymphoma in homosexual men. Lancet 2:631-633, 1982

IV

SPECIAL ASPECTS OF AIDS

23

THE CHEST FILM IN AIDS

PHILIP C. GOODMAN, MD

The variety of opportunistic infections and neoplasms reported in patients with AIDS has changed little since the initial descriptions of this disease in the summer of 1981.[7,8] The chest radiographic features of these entities may overlap, and this has discouraged some from using the chest film as a means of distinguishing between diseases. Nevertheless, some differences in appearance have proven fairly constant and, if recognized, permit an ordering of diagnoses into a most probable sequence.

OPPORTUNISTIC INFECTIONS

Pneumocystis carinii Pneumonia (PCP)

PCP is the most common opportunistic infection seen in patients with AIDS.[27] Chest film abnormalities are frequently present, yet in approximately 5 to 10 percent of cases, the chest radiograph is normal.[16] The diagnosis in this setting is suggested by clinical and laboratory findings such as shortness of breath, lowered PO_2, decreased diffusing capacity, and occasionally an abnormal gallium lung scan. The diagnosis is then confirmed by observing *P. carinii* in induced sputum, bronchoalveolar lavage, or lung biopsy samples (Chapter 15).

In the great majority of patients with PCP, chest films are abnormal and reveal diffuse bilateral and usually fairly symmetric, fine reticular heterogeneous infiltrates (Fig. 23–1).[11,18] Variations in this pattern occur frequently and include unilateral or focal lung infiltrates of the same quality or rarely focal alveolar consolidation (Fig. 23–2).[14] Occasionally the interstitial pattern is medium to coarse, and on rare occasions a miliary pattern is observed (Fig. 23–3). Focal nodules with cavitation have also been attributed to *P. carinii* infection.[2]

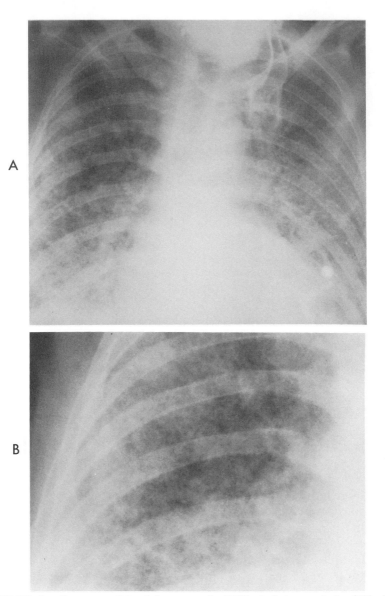

FIGURE 23—1. *Pneumocystis carinii* pneumonia (PCP). *A*, Anteroposterior (AP) chest film demonstrates moderate to severe bilateral reticular heterogeneous densities. *B*, Close-up of the right midlung demonstrates the fine nature of the reticular density seen in PCP. In the peripheral areas of the lung, coalescence of these densities has produced a more homogeneous consolidation as seen in severe episodes of infection.

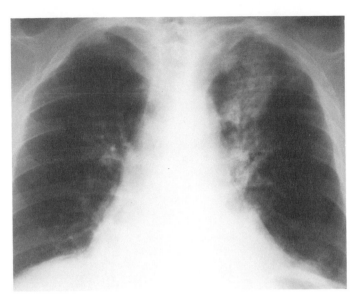

FIGURE 23–2. *Pneumocystis carinii* pneumonia (PCP). Posteroanterior (PA) chest film demonstrates a focal area of fairly homogeneous consolidation in the left upper lobe. Air bronchograms are seen in this region of alveolar density.

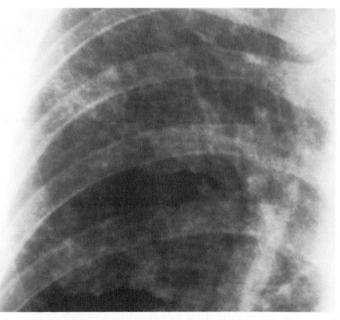

FIGURE 23–3. *Pneumocystis carinii* pneumonia (PCP). Close-up of a PA chest film demonstrates a fine to medium nodular or miliary pattern in the right upper and middle lobes.

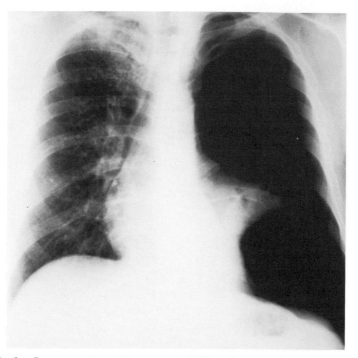

FIGURE 23−4. *Pneumocystis carinii* pneumonia (PCP) and pneumothorax. PA chest film demonstrates large, left-sided tension pneumothorax. The right lung and in particular the right upper lobe demonstrates a medium reticulonodular pattern.

With appropriate therapy, improvement in the radiographic findings is expected within 7 to 10 days. Without therapy, rapid progression to a worsened, diffuse heterogeneous, and in later stages severe bilateral homogeneous, consolidation may occur. Therapy with intravenous trimethoprin-sulfamethoxazole may lead to worsening of the chest film abnormalities within 4 days of the institution of treatment. This is most likely caused by pulmonary edema due to the large amount of fluid required for intravenous therapy with this antibiotic and does not necessarily indicate worsening of pneumonia.[40] If warranted, diuretic therapy will often result in rapid improvement in the patient's radiographic and clinical state. Eventually complete resolution of radiographic abnormalities is expected, although in some instances residual interstitial densities are observed.[32]

A few interesting complications of PCP have been recognized with some frequency in the last 2 to 3 years. Spontaneous pneumothorax has been observed in many patients with PCP (Fig. 23−4).[17] The size of pneumothorax has varied from small to extremely large and may require tube thoracostomy. The timing of the pneumothoraces is not related to treatment but apparently is due to infection with *P. carinii* itself. In some in-

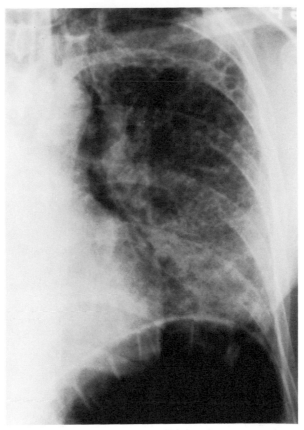

FIGURE 23−5. *Pneumocystis carinii* pneumonia (PCP) and pneumatoceles. Close-up of a PA chest film demonstrates heterogeneous medium interstitial densities in the left lung. In the periphery of the left upper lobe, small thin-walled, air-filled structures representing pneumatoceles are demonstrated. These usually resolve in 3 to 6 months but occasionally lead to pneumothorax.

stances pneumatoceles may precede the appearance of pneumothorax (Fig. 23−5). In one series, 10 percent of patients with PCP were found to have pneumatoceles.[33] These air-containing structures are solitary or multiple and may increase or decrease in size rapidly. Resolution is generally seen in 3 to 6 months. In rare instances, air-fluid levels have been noted within the pneumatoceles. These abnormalities have not been observed in AIDS patients with infections other than PCP. The mechanism for pneumatocele formation in this setting is unclear, and while it may be due to a check valve mechanism, there is little pathologic proof of this occurring in these patients.[29] Other air-filled structures have been described in patients with PCP, including cavitary nodules.[2] These generally have thicker walls and appear in sites where soft-tissue nodules have been previously recognized.

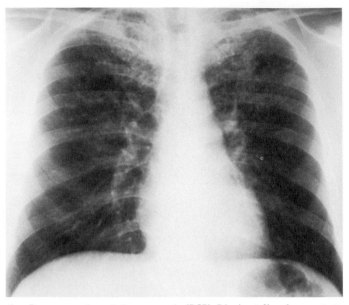

FIGURE 23–6. *Pneumocystis carinii* pneumonia (PCP). PA chest film demonstrates predominantly upper lobe medium reticular densities. This distribution of PCP may be the result of prior prophylactic aerosolized pentamidine therapy and mimics the distribution of reactivation tuberculosis.

Premature formation of bullae as seen on computed tomographic (CT) scan have been described in patients with AIDS.[24]

The distribution of PCP may be altered by prophylactic therapy with pentamidine. In a number of patients who have undergone this therapeutic regimen, new cases of PCP may be preferentially located in the upper lobes (Fig. 23–6).[4,36] The reason for this is thought to be poor coverage of the upper lobes by pentamidine taken in aerosolized form. These unprotected areas are thus more likely to harbor *P. carinii* and to be selectively involved with pneumonia.

Mycobacterial Infections

Various mycobacterial species have been responsible for pulmonary infections in patients with AIDS.[6,18,21] Clearly the majority of infections have been caused by *Mycobacterium tuberculosis* and *Mycobacterium avium* complex (Chapter 19). The radiographic appearance of tuberculosis in this setting depends upon the stage of HIV infection.[20,30] Early in the course of infection, tuberculosis appears, as it does in otherwise non–immune-suppressed individuals. That is, patients with reactivation tuberculosis, thought to be

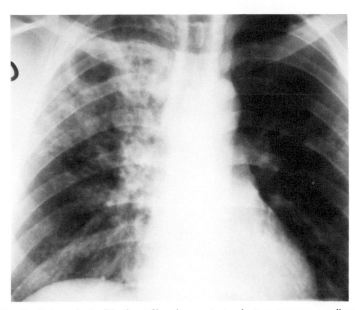

FIGURE 23–7. Tuberculosis. PA chest film demonstrates heterogeneous medium to coarse reticular densities in the right upper lobe. A large cavity is seen in this area. Minimal left upper lobe heterogeneous changes are seen. This pattern is typical of reactivation tuberculosis seen in the early stages of HIV infection.

the most common pathogenesis of tuberculosis in these patients, will present with heterogeneous nodular and cavitary infiltrates in the superior segments of the lower lobes and apical and posterior segments of the upper lobes (Fig. 23–7). These radiographic findings are not seen later in HIV infection, when diffuse and somewhat coarse interstitial densities are observed with or without the presence of hilar or mediastinal adenopathy (Fig. 23–8).[15] Adenopathy itself may be of different frequency within different AIDS risk groups. Thus in patients with intravenous drug abuse backgrounds or patients from Haiti, a higher percentage of individuals with HIV infection and tuberculosis had lymphadenopathy than in HIV-infected homosexual males with tuberculosis.[35] The overall incidence of tuberculosis in AIDS patients has been reported to be as high as 24 percent.[28] Conversely, nearly 30 percent of adult non-Asian patients with tuberculosis had HIV infection.[5] Late in the course of HIV infection, tuberculosis has not resulted in cavitation. Pleural fluid is seen with varying incidence.[15] The presence of adenopathy, pleural fluid, or a coarse bilateral heterogeneous infiltrate is much more typical of tuberculosis than of PCP.

Antituberculosis therapy should result in chest film improvement, paralleling a clinical response by the patient.[35] Within weeks, any of the radiographic abnormalities seen with this infection should begin to resolve.

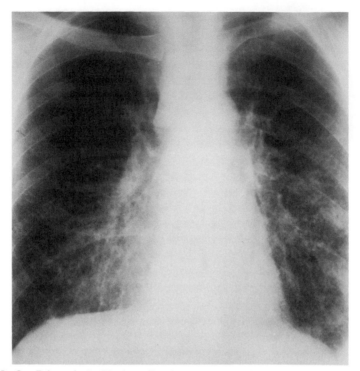

FIGURE 23–8. Tuberculosis. PA chest film demonstrates right paratracheal adenopathy and a diffuse fine to medium reticulonodular infiltrate. This is the pattern seen in patients with late-stage HIV infection and tuberculosis. Since adenopathy is not associated with PCP, it should not be considered a likely cause of disease in this patient.

Worsening of a chest film while a patient is on appropriate medication should prompt a work-up for an alternate infection.

Mycobacterium avium complex is typically seen in lymph nodes, liver, bone marrow, blood, and urine of patients with AIDS. Involvement of pulmonary parenchyma results in diffuse, hetergeneous interstitial patterns with or without lymphadenopathy.[14] No distinguishing features between this species or other species of mycobacterial infection and tuberculosis have been observed on chest films.

FUNGI

A variety of fungal infections have been observed in patients with AIDS. In regions endemic for *Histoplasma capsulatum* and *Coccidioides immitis*, these organisms have been responsible for a number of opportunistic pneumonias in HIV-infected individuals.[1,26] The radiographic appearance of these pneumonias is similar. Commonly, a diffuse, bilateral, poorly defined,

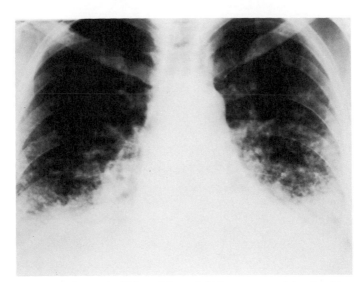

FIGURE 23–9. Histoplasmosis. Diffuse, bilateral, fairly coarse nodular densities are seen in both lungs. This pattern is commonly reported in patients with disseminated histoplasmosis and coccidioidomycosis. Adenopathy is also associated with these diseases in patients with AIDS.

small nodular infiltrate is noted (Fig. 23–9). Lymphadenopathy is reported with variable incidence with both of these fungal infections. Other manifestations, including cavitation and alveolar consolidation, have been reported but are less frequently observed.[1,3]

Cryptococcal infections of AIDS patients generally affect the central nervous system, but some cases of cryptococcal pneumonia have been reported. The radiographic appearance includes single or multiple well-defined nodules with or without cavitation, diffuse reticular interstitial infiltrates, and hilar or mediastinal adenopathy (Fig. 23–10).[38] A miliary pattern may also be seen with this and other fungal infections (Chapter 17).

Cytomegalovirus (CMV)

CMV pneumonia was reported as one of the initial opportunistic infections seen in patients with AIDS. However, our experience suggests that this organism, while frequently observed in patients with AIDS, may not be responsible for pathologic lung changes. Consequently, it is our policy to put less emphasis on this diagnosis compared with the other opportunistic infections. In those patients reported to have CMV pneumonia, a diffuse, fine to medium reticular interstitial pattern has been observed on chest films.[37] However, it is difficult to be certain that the radiographic abnormalities have been caused by this organism since other opportunistic agents

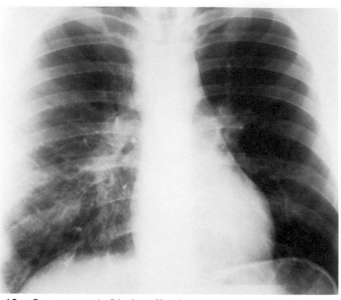

FIGURE 23–10.   Cryptococcosis. PA chest film demonstrates right paratracheal and right hilar adenopathy. Occasionally parenchymal lung nodules and reticular interstitial densities are also seen in patients with intrathoracic cryptococcosis.

frequently coexist. CMV as the sole pathogen responsible for pneumonia is extremely rare[39] (Chapter 21).

PYOGENIC INFECTION

Pneumonias caused by pyogenic organisms such as *Streptococcus pneumoniae* and *Haemophilus influenza* have been reported with increasing frequency in patients with AIDS.[12,31] It has been well established that both T-cell and B-cell immune function is compromised in these patients, thus accounting for the increased frequency of pyogenic infections. The radiographic features are similar to those seen in non-immune-suppressed individuals.[42] Air-space consolidation resulting in homogeneous density in a segment or lobe of lung is frequently observed (Fig. 23–11). Parapneumonic effusions are also seen. Generally patients with pyogenic pneumonia do not have concomitant infection with opportunistic organisms such as *P. carinii*. Response to appropriate antibiotics is similar to that of non-immune-suppressed hosts so that radiographic improvement is seen within 1 to 2 weeks.

Bronchitis caused by pyogenic organisms has also been seen with moderate frequency in patients with AIDS. Radiographically this is manifested by peribronchial thickening and "tram tracking" (Fig. 23–12). The latter

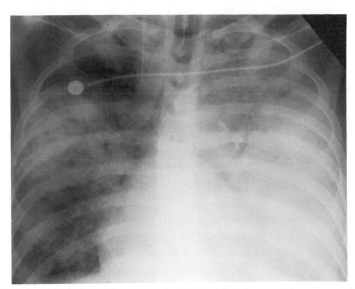

FIGURE 23—11. Pneumococcal pneumonia. AP chest film demonstrates a severe bilateral air-space consolidation, worse on the left than on the right. The findings are typical of severe pyogenic pneumonia.

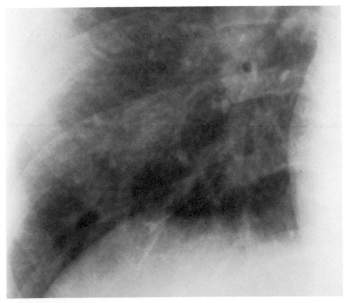

FIGURE 23—12. Bronchitis. Close-up of the right lower lobe demonstrates thin, parallel, linear densities paralleling the course of segmental bronchi. This finding is called "tram tracking" and has been seen in AIDS patients with clinical bronchitis.

finding is caused by bronchial mucosal edema and peribronchial inflammation and is seen as thin, parallel, linear densities following the expected course of bronchi.

NEOPLASMS

Kaposi's Sarcoma

The radiographic features of Kaposi's sarcoma are somewhat distinctive.[16,22,34] Pulmonary parenchymal involvement is manifest by coarse, poorly defined nodular densities scattered throughout the lungs (Fig. 23–13) (Chapter 22). Concommitant coarse, linear densities usually distributed in a perihilar location are also frequent. Pleural fluid is reported in 35 to 50 percent of patients with Kaposi's sarcoma and is probably the result of pleural metastases. Kaposi's nodules generally increase slowly in size over several months. Rapid change in size of a suspected Kaposi's sarcoma pulmonary nodule with progression to lung consolidation should suggest the possibility of hemorrhage in the region of these highly vascular lesions (Fig. 23–14). Hilar and mediastinal adenopathy may be observed but do not occur with the frequency seen in tuberculosis.

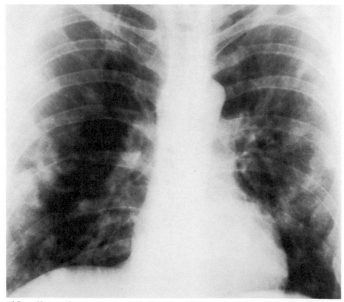

FIGURE 23–13. Kaposi's sarcoma (KS). Scattered, poorly defined nodules are seen in both lungs. This is a classic presentation of pulmonary KS. Other manifestations include pleural fluid and coarse linear interstitial densities.

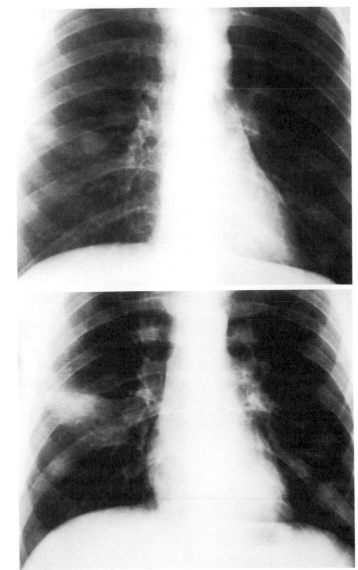

FIGURE 23–14. Kaposi's sarcoma (KS). *A*, PA chest film demonstrates two poorly defined nodules in the right middle lobe and one poorly defined nodule in the left retrocardiac area. These findings are typical of KS. *B*, The same patient 2 weeks later. At this time more homogeneous consolidation is seen in the left lower lobe and right middle lobe. This type of rapid change is most likely due to hemorrhage in the sites of pulmonary KS.

In patients with a background of intravenous drug abuse, differentiating Kaposi's sarcoma nodules from septic emboli may be impossible. However, within a few days, septic emboli will tend to cavitate whereas Kaposi's sarcoma nodules will not.

Non-Hodgkin's Lymphoma

General differences in the lymphomas seen in patients with AIDS as compared to those seen in the general population include a greater stage of involvement at the time of initial discovery, greater aggressiveness of the neoplasm, an almost exclusive tendency for the lymphomas to be non-Hodgkin's variety, and a decreased frequency of intrathoracic involvement.[19] An early study of AIDS patients with non-Hodgkin's lymphoma revealed that only 10 percent of patients had chest manifestations.[43] The radiographic features of non-Hodgkin's lymphoma in this setting include unilateral and bilateral pleural effusions in nearly half the patients. Hilar or mediastinal adenopathy is observed in nearly one fourth of chest films (Fig. 23–15). Pulmonary parenchymal involvement is manifest by reticu-

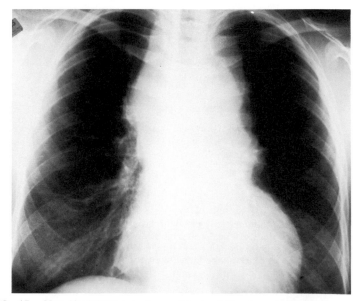

FIGURE 23–15. Non-Hodgkin's lymphoma. PA chest film demonstrates severe mediastinal adenopathy. Intrathoracic involvement in AIDS patients with non-Hodgkin's lymphoma has been observed approximately 10 percent of the time. Adenopathy, pleural fluid, and nodular parenchymal disease have been noted.

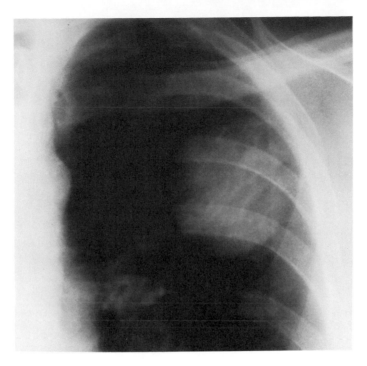

FIGURE 23—16. Non-Hodgkin's lymphoma. This large, well-defined nodule appeared over a period of 6 weeks. A needle biopsy was unrevealing, but an open lung procedure demonstrated a large non-Hodgkin's lymphoma lesion.

lonodular interstitial infiltrates or alveolar consolidation in nearly one quarter of patients. The appearance of well-defined parenchymal nodules remarkable for their rapidity of growth has been noted in rare instances (Fig. 23—16). Cavitation of these nodules may be seen.[19]

MISCELLANEOUS

Lymphocytic Interstitial Pneumonitis (LIP)

LIP has now been recognized as an index diagnosis for AIDS in the pediatric patient. Chest films from these patients are indistinguishable from those of PCP patients, demonstrating diffuse or focal, fine to medium reticular interstitial infiltrates (Fig. 23—17). However, some reports indicate a tendency to small nodular infiltrates correlating well with pathologic findings.[43]

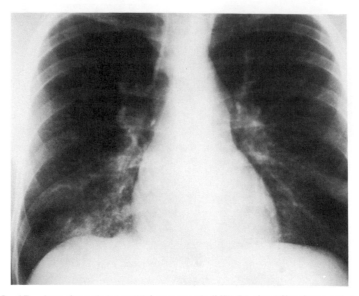

FIGURE 23—17.   Lymphocytic interstitial pneumonia (LIP). PA chest film demonstrates bibasilar fine to medium reticular interstitial densities indistinguishable from PCP. An openlung biopsy revealed LIP.

SUMMARY

The task of interpreting chest radiographs in patients with AIDS will be made easier, it is hoped, through the information contained in this chapter. While the various infections and neoplasms seen with this syndrome occasionally have similar appearances on chest films, some patterns should allow construction of a limited differential diagnosis list. Indeed, there are findings which are nearly specific for certain processes. For example, in this setting, pneumatocele formation is seen exclusively in patients with PCP. The finding of poorly defined nodular densities with associated pleural effusions is almost pathognomonic for Kaposi's sarcoma. On the other hand, some radiographic findings should dissuade one from considering certain diagnoses. For example, pleural fluid and lymphadenopathy are rarely if ever encountered in patients with PCP alone. Other entities such as non-Hodgkin's lymphoma, tuberculosis, or fungal infection should thus be considered. With experience, a more confident interpretation of the chest film will lead to better patient management.

REFERENCES

1. Abrams DI, Robis M, Blumenfeld W, et al: Disseminated coccidioidomycosis in AIDS. N Engl J Med 310:986, 1984
2. Barrio JL, Suarez M, Rodriguez JL, et al: *Pneumocystis carinii* pneumonia presenting as cavitating and non-cavitating solitary pulmonary nodules in patients with the acquired immunodeficiency syndrome. Am Rev Respir Dis 134:1094, 1986
3. Bonner JR, Alexander WJ, Dismukes WE, et al: Disseminated histoplasmosis in patients with the acquired immune deficiency syndrome. Arch Intern Med 144:2178, 1984
4. Case Records of the Massachusetts General Hospital Case 9—1989. N Engl J Med 320:582, 1989
5. Centers for Disease Control: Advisory Committee for Elimination of Tuberculosis. Tuberculosis and human immunodeficiency virus infection. MMWR 38:236, 1989
6. Centers for Disease Control: Diagnosis and management of mycobacterial infection and disease in persons with human immunodeficiency virus infection. Ann Intern Med 106:254, 1987
7. Centers for Disease Control: Kaposi's sarcoma and pneumocystis pneumonia among homosexual men: New York City and California. MMWR 30:305, 1981
8. Centers for Disease Control: Pneumocystis pneumonia—Los Angeles. MMWR 30:250, 1981
9. Chaisson RE, Theuer CP, Schechter GF, et al: HIV infection in patients with tuberculosis. Presented at the 4th International Conference on AIDS (Abstract 7544), Stockholm, June, 1988
10. Davis SD, Henschke CI, Chamides BK, et al: Intrathoracic Kaposi sarcoma in AIDS patients: Radiographic-pathologic correlation. Radiology 163:495, 1987
11. DeLorenzo IJ, Huang CT, Maguire GP, et al: Roentgenographic patterns of *Pneumocystis carinii* pneumonia in 104 patients with AIDS. Chest 91:323, 1987
12. Fimberkoff MS, El Sadr W, Schiffman G, et al: *Streptococcus pneumoniae* infections and bacteremia in patients with acquired immune deficiency syndrome with report of a pneumococcal vaccine failure. Am Rev Respir Dis 130:1174, 1984
13. Garay SM, Belenko M, Fazzini E, et al: Pulmonary manifestations of Kaposi's sarcoma. Chest 91:39, 1987
14. Goodman PC: Pulmonary manifestations of AIDS. Curr Probl Diagn Radiol 17:81, 1988
15. Goodman PC: Pulmonary tuberculosis in patients with the acquired immunodeficiency syndrome. J Thorac Imaging 5:38-45, 1990
16. Goodman PC, Broaddus VC, Hopewell PC: Chest radiographic patterns in the acquired immunodeficiency syndrome. Am Rev Respir Dis 129:26, 1984
17. Goodman PC, Daley C, Minagi H: Spontaneous pneumothorax in AIDS patients with *Pneumocystis carinii* pneumonia. AJR 147:29, 1986
18. Goodman PC, Gamsu G: Radiographic findings in the acquired immunodeficiency syndrome. Postgrad Radiol 7:3, 1987
19. Haskal ZJ, Lindan C, Goodman PC: Lymphoma in the immunocompromised patient. Radiol Clin North Am 28:885-889, 1990
20. Hopewell PC: Tuberculosis and human immunodeficiency virus infection. Semin Respir Infect 4:111, 1989
21. Hopewell PC, Luce JM: Pulmonary manifestations of the acquired immunodeficiency syndrome. Clin Immunol Allergy 6:489, 1986
22. Kaplan L, Hopewell PC, Jaffe H, et al: Kaposi's sarcoma involving the lung in patients with the acquired immunodeficiency syndrome. J AIDS 1:23, 1988
23. Kovacs A, Forthal DN, Kovacs JA, et al: Disseminated coccidioidomycosis in a patient with acquired immune deficiency syndrome. West J Med 140:447, 1984
24. Kuhl JE, Knowles MC, Fishman EK, et al: Premature bullous pulmonary damage in AIDS: CT diagnosis. Radiology 173:23, 1989
25. Lowery S, Fallat R, Fiegal DW, et al: Changing patterns of *Pneumocystis carinii* pneumonia on pentamidine aerosol prophylaxis. Abstracts from the IV International Conference on AIDS 1:419, 1988
26. Mandell W, Goldberg DM, Neu HC: Histoplasmosis in patients with the acquired immune deficiency syndrome. Am J Med 81:974; 1986

27. Murray JF, Garay SM, Hopewell PC, et al: Pulmonary complications of the acquired immunodeficiency syndrome: An update. Am Rev Respir Dis 135:504, 1987
28. Page JW, Liautaud B, Thomas F, et al: Characteristics of the acquired immunodeficiency syndrome (AIDS) in Haiti. N Engl J Med 309:945, 1983
29. Panicek DM: Cystic pulmonary lesions in patients with AIDS. Radiology 173:12, 1989
30. Pitchenik AE, Burr J, Suarez M, et al: Human T-cell lymphotropic virus-III (HTLV-III) seropositivity and related disease among 71 consecutive patients in whom tuberculosis was diagnosed. Am Rev Respir Dis 135:875, 1987
31. Polsky B, Gold JWN, Whimbey E, et al: Bacterial pneumonia in patients with the acquired immunodeficiency syndrome. Ann Inter Med 104:38, 1986
32. Ramaswany G, Jagadha V, Tchnentkoff V: Diffuse alveolar damage and interstitial fibrosis in acquired immunodeficiency syndrome. Patients without concurrent pulmonary infection. Arch Pathol Lab Med 109:408, 1985
33. Sandhu JS, Goodman PC: Pulmonary cysts associated with *Pneumocystis carinii* pneumonia in patients with AIDS. Radiology 173:33, 1989
34. Sivit CJ, Schwartz AM, Rockoff SD: Kaposi's saroma of the lung in AIDS: Radiologic-pathologic analysis. AJR 148:25, 1987
35. Small P, Goodman PC: Utility of serial chest radiographs in the management of tuberculosis in HIV infected patients
36. Small P, Goodman PC, Montgomery AB: Case 9—1989: AIDS and a cavitary pulmonary lesion (Letter). N Engl J Med 321:395, 1989
37. Stover DE, White DA, Romano PA, et al: Spectrum of pulmonary diseases associated with the acquired immune deficiency syndrome. Am J Med 78:429, 1985
38. Suster B, Akerman M, Orenstein M, et al: Pulmonary manifestations of AIDS: Review of 106 episodes. Radiology 161:87, 1986
39. Wallace JM, Hannah J: Cytomegalovirus pneumonitis in patients with AIDS. Chest 92:198, 1987
40. Wharton J, Coleman DL, Wofsy CB, et al: Trimethoprin-sulfamethoxazole or pentamidine for *Pneumocystis carinii* pneumonia in the acquired immunodeficiency syndrome. Ann Intern Med 105:37, 1986
41. Wheat IJ, Slama TG, Zeckel ML: Histoplasmosis in the acquired immune deficiency syndrome. Am J Med 78:203, 1985
42. White S, Tsou E, Waldhorn R, et al: Life threatening bacterial pneumonia in male homosexuals with laboratory features of the acquired immunodeficiency syndrome. Chest 87:486, 1985
43. Zieler JL, Beckstead JA, Volberding PA, et al: Non-Hodgkin's lymphoma in 90 homosexual men. N Engl J Med 311:565, 1984

24

SPECIAL PROBLEMS IN THE CHILD WITH AIDS

MOSES GROSSMAN, MD

AIDS in children presents many special problems for the infected child, for the family, for the physicians involved with the child's care, and for society.

The number of infected children appears small compared with the huge epidemic affecting adults in our country. As of October 1, 1989, some 1860 cases of AIDS had been reported in children (under age 13), representing about 2 percent of all reported cases. The disease has almost certainly been underreported for a variety of reasons,[11] but even at this level of reporting it is already the most common cause of childhood immunodeficiency and one of the 10 leading causes of death in children.[19] Seventy-five to eighty percent of HIV infections are acquired perinatally; that proportion will increase in the future because blood and blood products have been screened since 1985; thus transfusion as a route of infection will be very substantially diminished over the next few years.

The important issue epidemiologically is the number of HIV-infected children (as opposed to children with AIDS) and the number and prevalence of HIV-infected childbearing women. The cord blood studies now being conducted by CDC and others show widely ranging rates in different geographic areas, from a low of 0.03 percent positive antibodies in cord blood (reflecting maternal infection) to a high of 3 to 4 percent in New York City.[1] The majority of births in infected women are in racial minority groups (48 percent in blacks and 22 percent in Hispanics), and they occur predominantly in inner city areas associated with poverty and drug abuse.[8] As the number of affected children increases, more physicians will find themselves confronted with HIV-infected children as patients. Thus it is

385

important for all physicians treating children to be acquainted with the diagnosis and principles of management of this infection.

PERINATAL HIV INFECTION—APPROACH AND DIAGNOSIS

The key to prevention of HIV infection and AIDS in children is the prevention of infection in childbearing women. Thus, we need a vigorous and continued educational effort among that population group. Minority women residing in inner urban areas and drug users in particular are at the highest risk of infection. Programs which will effectively reach these women need the highest priority. Women at risk need to be taught how to protect themselves against infection and encouraged to test their own HIV antibody status prior to considering a pregnancy.

It is currently customary to recommend testing the HIV antibody status only in pregnant women who find themselves in one of the so-called high-risk categories.[27] This should be done as early as feasible so that the HIV-antibody–positive mother could be counselled and an informed decision made about continuing or interrupting the pregnancy. There is a serious debate at present about whether HIV antibody testing should be restricted to women in the high-risk categories or whether all pregnant women should be offered the HIV antibody test routinely.[4] The hepatitis B experience during the perinatal period has shown that 40 percent of women who are surface antigen–positive and thus capable of transmitting infection to their infants are missed when testing is restricted to high-risk categories. As a result, the current CDC recommendation is that *all* pregnant women be tested for hepatitis B surface antigen.[22] While the epidemiology of HIV infection is similar to that of hepatitis B, it is not identical; the prevalence of HIV infection is less than that of hepatitis B at present, but certain similarities can nevertheless be drawn between the two. Another argument for routine testing of all pregnant women is that such a policy would diminish the stigma of performing the test (suggesting that the patient is at increased risk of HIV infection and possibly jeopardizing health or life insurance). On the other side of the argument, routine testing will increase the cost of pregnancy and the current national prevalence of HIV infection may not justify this increased cost.

A serious unresolved problem is when during pregnancy the infection actually occurs. It is known that HIV infection can occur as early as 20 weeks of gestation.[11] What proportion of infections occurs transplacentally as opposed to intrapartum is not known. It is also known that infection can be transmitted through breast milk.[18]

The delivery of an HIV-positive mother needs to be approached with full attention to body substance precautions, as should every delivery. Once the baby has had the first bath and maternal blood and secretions are washed off, the baby does not require any precautions other than when handling blood.

At the time of birth it is impossible to tell clinically which babies will be infected. Some studies state that 20 to 50 percent of infants born to infected mothers will themselves be infected (30 to 35 percent is the most likely current estimate).[6,28] Serologic diagnosis, which is the mainstay of diagnosis in adults, is fraught with problems in infancy.[11,19] Initially all babies will reflect the presence of maternal IgG and will be antibody-positive whether they are infected or not. The majority of infants will begin to synthesize their own IgG and will remain antibody-positive after the maternal IgG dissipates (around a year of age). However, some 10 percent of infected infants are unable to synthesize IgG by the age of 1 year, and these will become HIV antibody–negative.[12,30] Infected babies do not uniformly synthesize anti-HIV IgM; thus this test which is so useful in many vertically transmitted perinatal infections is not reliable or usable in HIV infection.[19] Because p24 antigen is not uniformly present in infected neonates,[16] a positive p24 test is meaningful, but a negative test does not rule out infection. Culture for the presence of HIV virus is the gold standard at present but not generally available to the practicing physician.

Polymerase chain reaction (pcr), a method that amplifies the small amount of viral DNA which may be present, is a promising new method just now becoming commercially available.[24] However, the method is not yet standardized and is flawed by false-positive reactions; even a minute amount of maternal blood contaminating a cord blood specimen will produce a false positive test.

It is clear that for early laboratory diagnosis of HIV infection in young infants more sensitive and more specific laboratory assays must be developed. In the meantime, the responsible physician must use whatever laboratory tests are available in the community, interpret results as best he or she can, and use clinical information as well to come to a conclusion about the presence or absence of infection. As we approach the era when we might be treating asymptomatic HIV-infected infants, early diagnosis becomes even more important (Table 24-1).

TABLE 24–1. DIAGNOSTIC TESTS AVAILABLE FOR DETERMINING INFANT INFECTION

HIV viral culture	Gold standard Specific, not 100% sensitive
Anti-HIV IgG (ELISA, Western blot, or immunoassay)	Positive result indicates *maternal* antibody in the first 9 months of life. After 1 year is specific but only 90% sensitive
Anti-HIV IgM	Specific, only 65% sensitive
p24 antigen	Specific, only 65% sensitive
Polymerase chain reaction (pcr)	Very sensitive; promising test Specificity can be a problem; not entirely standardized

In the vast majority of instances, infants declare themselves infected through a combination of repeated clinical and laboratory observations by 9 to 12 months of age. Negative serology in the presence of a *totally healthy* infant by 15 to 18 months of age can be taken as firm evidence of lack of HIV infection.

SIGNS AND SYMPTOMS OF AIDS

The first signs and symptoms of vertically transmitted HIV infection usually appear in the second half of the first year, although some infants develop opportunistic infections as early as the first month of life. Half of the infected children will qualify for a diagnosis of AIDS by a year of age, 80 percent by 3 years of age[11]; a few children, however, may have a quiescent period of infection for as long as 7 years.

The principal signs and symptoms of pediatric HIV infection are listed in Table 24-2.[16] It is obvious that many of them are nonspecific. Lymphadenopathy, hepatosplenomegaly, and failure to thrive are frequent manifestations of HIV infection, but they are nonspecific. Repeated common infections in young infants (for example, invasive *Haemophilus influenzae* infections) might arouse one's suspicion of underlying HIV infection.[26] Thrush or candidal dermatitis are common in HIV-infected children, but so they are in many normal children. In a child whose background puts him or her at risk for AIDS (for example, baby of an intravenous drug user), these nonspecific signs and symptoms should lead to early suspicion of HIV disease and to laboratory investigation.

Some manifestations are very suggestive of HIV infections.

TABLE 24–2.   PRINCIPAL SIGNS AND SYMPTOMS OF PEDIATRIC AIDS

Failure to thrive
Diarrhea
Frequent otitis media
Frequent other common pediatric infections
Invasive or disseminated infections
Thrush
Opportunistic infections
Lymphocytic interstitial pneumonia
Skin diseases (candidiasis and seborrhea)
Parotid swellings
Neurologic involvement
   Developmental delay
   Loss of attained milestones
   Dementia
   Encephalopathy

among these is lymphocytic interstitial pneumonia (LIP) which occurs in 35 to 40 percent of children with AIDS.[26] Children develop nodular peri-bronchial lymphoid infiltrates, often with hilar adenopathy. The definitive diagnosis of LIP is histologic; experienced radiologists can make an accurate radiologic diagnosis of the condition, but in diagnosing LIP it is important to exlude other forms of lung disease. LIP causes ventilatory compromise, and clubbing may occur.

Salivary gland enlargement (particularly of the parotid glands) is a unique manifestation in childhood. All body organs are subject to HIV infection, which may become clinically manifest—cardiomyopathy, hepatitis, pancreatitis, thrombocytopenia, and hemolytic anemia have all been described.

Neurologic disease, namely, encephalopathy, is a common and devastating clinical finding in most HIV-infected children (Chapter 12).[5] Classically, it causes developmental delay as well as the loss of developmental milestones which have already been acquired. Progression may be slow, rapid, or intermittent. Acquired microcephaly is common. Computed tomographic scans and magnetic resonance imaging show brain atrophy, ventricular enlargement, attenuation of white matter, and calcification of basal ganglia.

Opportunistic infections occur in children as they do in adults. *Pneumocystis carinii* pneumonia is the most common of these, occurring in some 50 percent of children with AIDS. Most other opportunistic infections have been described in children, notably *Mycobacterium avium-intracellulare* infections, candidal infections, and many others.[11]

Children with vertically transmitted HIV infection have a very poor prognosis. The median survival after the diagnosis of AIDS is made using CDC criteria is 9 months.[25] Children diagnosed in the first year of life have an even shorter survival time.

CDC has defined AIDS in the pediatric population, a definition with which physicians seeing children should be familiar.[23] CDC also has a classification system for HIV-infected children, briefly summarized in Table 24-3.[9]

TABLE 24–3.   CDC CLASSIFICATION FOR HIV-INFECTED CHILDREN*

P-0	Indeterminate infection in perinatally exposed children younger than 15 mo
P-1	Asymptomatic infection
P-2	Symptomatic infection (causes other than HIV excluded)
	A Nonspecific findings
	B Progressive neurologic disease
	C Lymphocytic interstitial pneumonia
	D Secondary infectious diseases

*Abbreviated from Centers for Disease Control MMWR 36:225-236, 1987.

**TABLE 24–4.   PRINCIPAL LABORATORY FINDINGS IN PEDIATRIC
HIV INFECTION**

Presence of anti-HIV antibody (confirmed by Western blot or
   radioimmunoassay)
Isolation of HIV virus
Polymerase chain reaction (not yet standardized)
Polyclonal hypergammaglobulinemia
Reverse CD4/CD8 ratio
Loss of cell-mediated immunity (anergy)
Poor antibody response to antigen challenge
Positive CSF findings (pleocytosis, elevated protein)

LABORATORY FEATURES

The diagnosis of AIDS can be made clinically, but it depends heavily on
laboratory confirmation. The diagnosis of HIV infection is based on laboratory findings. The principal laboratory findings are listed in Table
24-4. HIV-infected children have early and major B-cell involvement; this
manifests itself as polyclonal hypergammaglobulinemia and poor antibody
response to specific antigens.[11,26] Hypergammaglobulinemia is common in
HIV-infected children and thus a useful laboratory screening tool for suspected HIV infections. The use of the other tests, particularly during the
perinatal period, has already been described.

ADOLESCENT HIV INFECTIONS

Adolescents (age 13 to 18 years) present special problems and special
concerns within the spectrum of pediatric HIV disease.[14] The number of
actual reported cases of AIDS in this group is small (about 1 percent of all
reported cases). There are no meaningful studies about the prevalence of
HIV infections in this population. There is a high probability that young
adults presenting with clinical AIDS in their early twenties have in fact
acquired the infection as teenagers. There is currently a surge in the incidence of other sexually transmitted diseases among teens, which may be
an ominous sign for HIV infections. It is urgent and imperative that all
teenagers be exposed to intensive, culture- and age-appropriate education
about HIV infection and its prevention. Centers for counselling and testing
of adolescents who wish to be tested must be organized; adult test centers
often lack the experience and orientation for counselling adolescents.

The legal and ethical issues concerning consent by teenagers need clarification. Adolescents may legally give consent in all issues involving sexually
transmitted diseases. HIV is sexually transmitted, but consent here involves
far weightier issues than consent for the treatment of gonorrhea. Can an

adolescent refuse the physician permission to disclose the diagnosis of HIV infection to the parents? Is such a refusal legally binding? Can the adolescent consent to be treated with an experimental highly toxic drug? Finally, most current HIV treatment protocols are for individuals over the age of 18 or for young children. Adolescents have been excluded in part because there are not enough of them in any one location to make a valid series and in part because of the issues mentioned above and the resultant increased liability for these decisions. It is urgent that we address these issues involving adolescents in our country and in our communities.

MANAGEMENT

The principal management issues are listed in Table 24-5. Management must be interdisciplinary; these children have social and emotional problems of extraordinary complexity in addition to their medical problems. Many have mothers who are dead, ill, or unable to function by virtue of disease or drug addiction. Many need foster care; thus they are involved with the social service as well as with the juvenile justice system.

Physicians cannot and should not try to manage these children without an appropriate team. Many of these children are poor, and access to care is a problem. California has made an enlightened decision: all babies of HIV-positive mothers are eligible to be paid for by California Children Services. This ensures that in the difficult early period when it is not clear whether the infant is infected, financing and case management will be paid for, as well as the care of the symptomatic child with AIDS. These children may receive their care from physicians around the State but must be seen in consultation in approved pediatric centers capable of dealing with this infection. This scheme will also insure that children have access to treatment protocols as they develop.

HIV-infected children need diligent primary care. Minor symptoms may be signs of severe, even life-threatening infections. Febrile episodes need to be taken seriously. Cough may be the first manifestation of serious

TABLE 24-5.   MANAGEMENT OF AN HIV-INFECTED CHILD

Access to care
Continued health supervision
Vigorous therapy of common pediatric infections
Aggressive and early therapy of opportunistic infection
Immunization
Attention to caloric intake
Provision of an opportunity for social and emotional development
Prevention of *Pneumocystis carinii* infection (prophylactic therapy)
Prevention of common infections (IV immunoglobulin)
Antiretroviral therapy

TABLE 24–6.   RECOMMENDATIONS FOR ROUTINE IMMUNIZATION OF HIV-INFECTED CHILDREN*

VACCINE	AGE
Diphtheria pertussis tetanus (DPT)	Routine schedule
Inactivated polio vaccine (IPV)	Routine schedule
Measles, mumps, rubella, live attenuated (MMR)	15 mo
Conjugated *H. influenzae* (PRP-D)	18 mo
Pneumococcal polysaccharide vaccine	24 mo
Influenza vaccine	12 mo

*Adapted from American Academy of Pediatrics Report of Committee on Infectious Diseases.

pulmonary disease. Nutrition is important—every effort must be made to supply adequate calories and protein. Timely immunization is also important. Current recommendations call for the use of the normal immunization schedule (DPT, MMR, PRP-D) with the single exception that killed polio vaccine (Salk) is recommended instead of the live attenuated product (Sabin).[2,15] The recipient as well as other family members might be immunocompromised by virtue of their HIV infections and thus susceptible to paralysis by the attenuated vaccine strain. For the same reason the other children in the household should also not receive live attenuated polio vaccine. These children should certainly receive conjugated *H. influenzae* vaccine; unfortunately at present this product is not recommended for children younger than 15 months; it will be of much greater benefit when a conjugated vaccine is approved for use in infancy. Immunizations with pneumococcal polysaccharide vaccine should also be considered, but unfortunately this also is not presently possible before the age of 18 months. Finally, children over a year of age should be immunized with the appropriate influenza vaccine. These recommendations are summarized in Table 24-6. Thus it is clear that children who are known or suspected of being HIV-infected need to have a supportive and knowledgeable primary care physician in addition to close supervision at a recognized pediatric HIV center.

MANAGEMENT OF BACTERIAL INFECTIONS

Unlike adults, HIV-infected children are subject to frequent and serious bacterial infections (encapsulated bacteria and *Salmonella* are particularly common), usually involving common microbial pathogens. These infections often occur before the first opportunistic infection and may be the early manifestation of clinical AIDS.

Such bacterial infections need to be treated promptly, preferably using bactericidal antimicrobials and ensuring compliance in taking oral medications. In an attempt to prevent such bacterial infections, a number of investigators and clinicians have administered monthly intravenous immunoglobulin,[11,17] 200 to 400 mg/kg. There are no controlled randomized studies to test the efficacy of this preventive measure. Some experienced clinicians are convinced of its efficacy, but a controlled multicenter study has been under way for only a few months. For that reason it is also not clear when the regimen should be started. Some investigators recommend beginning such therapy based on clinical history of infection; others base it on laboratory evaluation of B-cell function. The final resolution of this issue will be further complicated by the fact that antiretroviral drugs such as azidothymidine (AZT) may also affect B-cell function and thus the possible need for immunoglobulin therapy.[19]

MANAGEMENT OF OPPORTUNISTIC INFECTIONS

The two principal opportunistic infections affecting children are *P. carinii* pneumonia (PCP) and candidal infections. The entire spectrum of such infections affecting adults (discussed in detail elsewhere in this volume) has also been seen in children. The medications and approaches to therapy in children are similar to those used in adults.[11] The most common clinical problem is the presentation of a child with pulmonary infiltrates.[11] This clinical situation presents the physician with a broad differential—PCP, LIP, bacterial or viral or mycobacterial infection. Radiologic appearance of the lungs is often helpful but not foolproof. Rapid clinical onset with cough and rapidly developing hypoxia suggest PCP; specific diagnosis and early therapy for this infection are urgent because of its rapid progression. Bronchoscopy and bronchoalveolar lavage with examination of the stained specimens is usually the best approach. Therapy includes the use of trimethoprim-sulfamethoxazole 20 mg (TMP)-100 mg (SMX)/kg/d divided into four doses, orally or intravenously, whichever is appropriate, for 14 to 21 days; or pentamidine isethionate, base 4 mg/kg/d intramuscularly or intravenously for 14 days (Chapter 15).

Prevention of *Pneumocystis* infection is of particular concern and is addressed elsewhere in this volume. Children often tolerate trimethoprim-sulfamethoxazole better than adult patients, but toxic reactions are frequent and need to be monitored. The use of aerosolized pentamidine is promising, but there is little published experience with children.[13]

The most common fungal infection is candidiasis, oral or esophageal. Nystatin (4 to 6 mg, 100,000 U/ml q.6h.), clotrimazole troches, or ketoconazole (5 to 10 mg/kg/d once or twice daily) usually provide adequate therapy, thus avoiding amphotericin (Chapter 10).

Antiviral and antimycobacterial agents are described elsewhere in this volume.

LIP need not be treated unless it interferes with ventilation and oxygenation. In this event it is important to first exclude other causes of pulmonary disease. The current therapy for LIP is glucocorticoids[26]; unfortunately, there are no controlled treatment trials to guide us as to optimal dose or duration of therapy.

ANTIRETROVIRAL THERAPY

Azidothymidine (AZT, zidovudine, marketed as Retrovir) was released by the U.S. Food and Drug Administration for use in adult patients in 1987 and is in widespread use today. It is discussed in Chapter 8. Experimental use of AZT in children lags far behind that in adults. This has been the traditional approach in introducing new drugs, particularly when dealing with toxic agents; however, the rapid progression of HIV infection combined with early death requires a more vigorous application of evolving new therapies to children. Finally, preliminary phase I studies have been completed in different pediatric age groups, and phase II studies based on protocols have been initiated through the NIH AIDS Clinical Treatment Group pediatric centers.[11,19] In October 1989, AZT was approved for the treatment of children outside of research protocols. Some clinicians have already been using this drug in children outside of research protocols, but the results of their work cannot be evaluated. The preliminary results of organized protocol studies in children show that, as in adults, AZT prolongs life but is not curative.[11,21]

Pizzo, at the National Cancer Institute, performed a particularly interesting study.[21] He treated a group of children with a constant intravenous infusion of AZT (0.9 to 1.4 mg/kg/h). The analysis of the study showed that the patients had a significant and occasionally sustained improvement in their encephalopathy. Many of these children showed significant improvement in their IQ scores. The continuous intravenous route is not convenient, and studies using the oral route are in progress. There is no recommended or accepted pediatric dose for AZT. Oral doses of 180 mg/m² every 6 hours by mouth appear reasonable based on current information.

There is also no unequivocal recommendation about the optimal timing of AZT therapy. It is not clear that the absolute number of 200 CD4 cells or less used in adult guidelines for initiating therapy applies to children of different ages. Protocols attempting to treat infected pregnant mothers in order to prevent vertical transmission are being developed as are protocols calling for the treatment of newborn babies starting at birth (before it is known that the infant is infected). It is hoped that the next few years will clarify some of these issues.

AZT may turn out to be only one of several drugs suitable for children. As new drugs become available, they are tried singly or in combination for their effectiveness and toxicity in children. The use of 2'3'-dideoxycytidine (ddc)[20] and dideoxyinosine (ddI)[7] has been reported in a very preliminary way.

Another newcomer to a possible list of useful agents is recombinant CD4 (rCD4). This agent has a different mechanism of action and might find a significant role in the future.

The number of children available for these studies is limited; thus it is particularly important to have well thought out collaborative protocols so that we may reach statistically significant answers in the near future. Our one recommendation with respect to antiretroviral treatment is to enroll each HIV-infected child into the most suitable and most promising research protocol.

SOCIAL-SOCIETAL ISSUES

We have already emphasized the importance of general supportive care for the HIV-infected child. Such support systems need to be extended beyond strict health matters. Access to health care, financially and geographically, has been mentioned. Many infected children require foster care because of parental inability to provide the needed care. Arrangements for foster care normally are left to Departments of Social Services. However, in the case of HIV-infected children, teamwork is needed between the health and social services components. Prospective foster parents need to be recruited, trained with continued in-service training, and supported by a health professional and must receive high compensation and a smaller number of children to care for than foster parents normally receive. For testing and for experimental drug regimens, permissions must be obtained from juvenile courts.[27] Foster parents and social service professionals need help with these issues as well.

Many infected children would benefit from the infant stimulation they are likely to receive in a day care center. The concern about placing these children in day care is their overexposure to many infections, gastrointestinal and respiratory, that tend to spread when children in diapers are commingled.[3] There is no concern about spreading HIV infection since horizontal spread by casual contact has not been demonstrated.[29] Thus the decision about day care should be made about each child individually, balancing the gain of infant stimulation against the risk of acquired nosocomial infection.

Early in the epidemic the CDC stated[10] that children with AIDS would benefit by normal classroom schooling and that they did not pose a hazard to their classmates. Although initially controversial, this position has been widely accepted. The reality is that few children with vertically transmitted infection will live long enough to go to school; those whose infection was transmitted through blood products encompass youngsters of all ages, but they will be an ever diminishing number.

At very high risk for acquiring HIV infection are runaway adolescents who live on the street and often subsist by engaging in prostitution. These teenagers have few support systems. They are usually school dropouts and have severed their family connections. We need to plan the care of this group of youngsters, some of whom will inevitably develop AIDS.

The key to preventing further spread of HIV transmission is education. Education is discussed elsewhere in this volume; however, in addressing the issues of children it is only right to stress that education needs to begin during childhood. Age- and culture-appropriate curricula have now been designed and are in use in many communities. It is our obligation to see to it that our own communities, where we live and practice, have incorporated the education of youth into their community AIDS planning.

REFERENCES

1. AIDS and human immunodeficiency virus in the United States: A review of current knowledge. MMWR 38(Suppl):1-14, 1989
2. American Academy of Pediatrics Report of Committee on Infectious Disease. Elk Grove Village, Ill, 1988
3. American Academy of Pediatrics Committee on Infectious Disease Health Guidelines for the Attendance in Day Care and Foster Care Settings of Children Infected with Human Immunodeficiency Virus. Pediatrics 79:466-471, 1987
4. Barbacci M, Quinn T, Kline R, et al: Failure of targeted screening to identify pregnant women. Johns Hopkins University. V International Conference on AIDS (Abstract MBP5), Montreal, 1989, P222
5. Belman Al, Diamond G, Dickson D, et al: Pediatric acquired immunodeficiency syndrome: Neurologic syndrome. Am J Dis Child 142:29-35, 1988
6. Blanche S, Ramzioux C, Muscato M-LG, et al: A prospective study of infants born to women seropositive for human immunodeficiency virus type 1. N Engl J Med 320:1643-1648, 1989
7. Butler K, Eddy J, Einloth M, et al: Dideoxyinosine (ddI) in children with symptomatic HIV infection. Interscientific Conference on Antimicrobial Agents and Chemotherapy, 1989
8. Centers for Disease Control. AIDS surveillance report. June 1989
9. Classification system for human immunodeficiency virus (HIV) infection in children under 13 years of age. MMWR 36:225-236, 1987
10. Education and foster care of children infected with human T lymphotropic virus type III. MMWR 34:521, 1985
11. Falloon J, Eddy T, Wiener L, Pizzo P: Human immunodeficiency virus infection in children. J Pediatr 114:1-30, 1989
12. Goetz DW, Hall SE, Harbinson RW, Reid MJ: Pediatric acquired immunodeficiency syndrome with negative human immunodeficiency virus antibody response by enzyme-linked immunosorbent assay and Western blot. Pediatrics 81:356-359, 1988
13. Guidelines for prophylaxis against Pneumocystis carinii pneumonia for persons infected with human immunodeficiency virus. MMWR 38:51-58, 1989
14. Hein K: Commentary on adolescent acquired immunodeficiency syndrome: The next wave of the HIV epidemic. J Pediatr 114:144-149, 1989
15. Immunization of children infected with human immunodeficiency virus: Supplementary ACTP statement. MMWR 37:181-183, 1988
16. Johnson JP, Nair P, Hines SE, et al: Natural history and serologic diagnosis of infants born to HIV infected women. Am J Dis Child 143:1147-1153, 1989

17. Ochs HD: Intravenous immunoglobulin in the treatment and prevention of acute infections in pediatric AIDS patients. Pediatr Infect Dis J 6:509-511, 1987
18. Oxtoby MJ: Human immunodeficiency virus and other viruses in human milk: Placing the issue in broader perspective. Pediatr Infect Dis J 7:825-835, 1988
19. Pizzo PA: Pediatric AIDS: Problems within problems. J Infect Dis 161:316-325, 1990
20. Pizzo PA, Einloth M, Butler K, et al: A Phase I-II study of dideoxycitidine (ddc) alone and on an alternating schedule with AZT in children with symptomatic infection. Interscientific Conference on Antimicrobial Agents and Chemotherapy, 1989
21. Pizzo PA, Eddy J, Falloon J, et al: Effect of continuous intravenous infusion of zidovudine (AZT) in children with symptomatic HIV infection. N Engl J Med 319:889-896, 1988
22. Prevention of perinatal transmission of hepatitis B virus: Prenatal screening of all pregnant women for hepatitis B surface antigen. MMWR 37:341-346, 1988
23. Revision of the CDC surveillance case definition for acquired immunodeficiency syndrome. MMWR 36:15-155, 1987
24. Rogers MF, Ou C-Y, Rayfield M, et al: Use of polymerase chain reaction for early detection of proviral sequences of HIV in infants born to seropositive mothers. N Engl J Med 320:1649-1654, 1989
25. Rogers MF, Thomas PA, Starcher ET, et al: Acquired immunodeficiency in children: Report of the Centers for Disease Control National Surveillance 1982 to 1985. Pediatrics 79:1008-1014, 1987
26. Rubinstein A: Pediatric AIDS. Curr Probl Pediatr 16:361-409, 1986
27. Rutherford GW, Oliva GE, Grossman M, et al: Guidelines for the control of perinatally transmitted HIV infection and care of infected mothers, infants and children. West J Med 147:104, 1987
28. Ryder RW, Nsa W, Hassig SE: Perinatal transmission of the human immunodeficiency virus type I to infants of seropositive mothers in Zaire. N Engl J Med 320:1637-1642, 1989
29. Sande MA: Transmission of AIDS: The case against casual contagion. N Engl J Med 314:380-382, 1986
30. Senturia YD, Peckham CS, Ades AE: Seronegativity and Paediatric AIDS. Lancet 1:1151-1152, 1987

25

CLINICAL CARE OF PATIENTS WITH AIDS:
Developing a System

PAUL A. VOLBERDING, MD

Physicians caring for patients with AIDS appreciate that the epidemic has thrust them into the middle of an intense public debate. Much more than just a medical problem, the AIDS epidemic poses important political and social dilemmas. For the medical profession and especially for the hospital involved in the care of patients with AIDS, the disease forces a reexamination of care structures and calls for new approaches to the many difficulties in the care of AIDS patients.

In this chapter some implications of AIDS care are addressed by first considering briefly the experience at San Francisco General Hospital and by then attempting to make generalizations from this experience to providers and medical centers at an earlier stage in their involvement with this epidemic. Limitations in generalizing from the local situation are pointed out.

AIDS IMPACT AT SAN FRANCISCO GENERAL HOSPITAL

The history of AIDS at San Francisco General Hospital began with early and unrecognized cases of opportunistic infections in 1980 and early 1981. The first patient with Kaposi's sarcoma was admitted to the hospital in June 1981, and with the first report of epidemic Kaposi's sarcoma and *Pneumocystis carinii* pneumonia came the awareness that the hospital was already seeing patients with this new epidemic disease.

The clinical experience with AIDS patients at San Francisco General Hospital increased, and in early 1983 patient volume warranted establishment of an outpatient clinic dedicated to the care of these individuals. By the middle of 1983 the hospital averaged eight to 10 inpatients with AIDS. Because of this and problems in appropriately educating hospital personnel in all areas of the hospital, San Francisco General Hospital established the world's first inpatient unit, which opened in June 1983.[13] An academic division of AIDS care and research was formed in the department of medicine in 1984 to help coordinate the growing volume of patients and clinical studies.

Demographic characteristics of AIDS patients at San Francisco General Hospital were an important factor in determining the overall structure and success of our program. In contrast to AIDS patients in many other parts of the country and in particular on the Eastern Seaboard, AIDS patients at San Francisco General Hospital have been predominantly homosexuals rather than users of intravenous drugs and have usually not been from racial or ethnic minority groups. As determined from San Francisco Department of Public Health reports of AIDS cases from July 1981 to November 1989, more than 90 percent of our AIDS patients have been homosexual and 85 percent have been white. Inpatients in most cases have CDC-defined AIDS, either known at the time of admission or established during their stay. Outpatients in the AIDS clinic also usually have CDC-defined AIDS, although one third of the clinic census is composed of patients with severe ARC. This relatively homogeneous background of patients and the visible nature of the gay community in San Francisco have made it relatively easy for San Francisco General Hospital to work with community organizations representing the bulk of the AIDS patient burden. However, this relative homogeneity is changing. The number of patients with HIV infection acquired parenterally through the use of intravenous drugs is increasing.

The volume of AIDS care at San Francisco General Hospital has expanded continually with the epidemic. When the AIDS inpatient unit was formed in mid-1983, the average inpatient census was approximately eight patients and the outpatient unit was handling approximately 100 to 120 appointments per month. By the end of 1989 there was an average of 30 to 35 inpatients and 1800 outpatient visits in the AIDS clinic each month. In mid-1989 the inpatient AIDS census on some days was greater than 50 percent of patients on a medical-surgical service of fewer than 200 beds.

BASIC COMPONENTS OF AIDS CARE

The structure of the care of AIDS patients at San Francisco General Hospital has already been mentioned. This structure can be seen as a triangle, the points of which are the dedicated AIDS outpatient clinic, the AIDS inpatient unit, and community-based organizations with hospital-focused services. For reasons detailed later in the chapter, the care of the

AIDS patients at San Francisco General Hospital has involved many medical and surgical subspecialties and a wide array of psychosocial services.

Psychosocial services are provided by a variety of individuals and organizations. The Shanti Project, a largely volunteer organization, provides extensive nonprofessional counseling and social services to AIDS patients in all parts of San Francisco. At San Francisco General Hospital full-time employees of the Shanti Project work in the inpatient unit and outpatient clinic to permit referral to this important organization with no delay or duplication of patient encounters. Another important organization, the AIDS Health Project, provides professional counseling for patients with AIDS, and employees of this organization are also included in the AIDS clinic at San Francisco General Hospital. Finally, professional counseling and psychiatric care are provided in both inpatient and outpatient settings by full-time faculty and staff.

COMPLEXITIES OF AIDS CARE

A central challenge facing medical institutions in the care of patients with AIDS- and HIV-associated illnesses derives from the enormous medical complexity of these diseases. Manifestations of HIV infection can affect any organ system in the body, and the patients commonly have several critical illnesses at the same time. In treating these illnesses, physicians more frequently encounter the toxic effects of drugs than when the same drugs are used in the care of non-AIDS patients,[5,7,9] and the toxicity of one required drug may overlap with the toxicity of a second drug also required for the care of that patient. Some common HIV-associated illnesses, such as cryptosporidiosis, have no effective treatment, and many drugs required in the care of patients with HIV-associated illnesses are difficult to obtain or cumbersome to administer. This is especially obvious with drugs still considered experimental, which is true of more drugs used in the care of AIDS patients than in other complex diseases. This problem is well known to AIDS medical care providers. For example, until several years into the AIDS epidemic, pentamidine required individual applications for drug release on a compassionate basis from the CDC, and foscarnet, a drug useful in the care of sight-threatening cytomegalovirus (CMV) retinitis, must now also be obtained on an individual, case by case, basis.[2]

In addition to being cumbersome, the use of experimental or nonapproved drugs in AIDS may pose administrative difficulties. Although these drugs can be obtained from the manufacturer, hospitals or practitioners must provide the clerical and administrative staff to maintain records of the drug use, and reimbursement for the drug's use or even for the hospital admission required for drug administration may be difficult or impossible to obtain. In our experience, insurance sources, Medicaid in particular, routinely disallow the costs of entire hospital stays if any experimental agent is administered. Recent changes, in place or proposed, may alter this situation. Various new mechanisms—the "treatment IND (investigational new drug) and parallel track"— have been established to broaden the distribution of new drugs for AIDS prior to the completion of formal clinical trials. Yet even here, the administrative requirements for drug prescription may be daunting.

A final complexity in the case of AIDS patients arises from the poor prognosis of the underlying disease. Patients with advanced HIV illnesses may express a desire for less intense care or less aggressive diagnostic procedures. Physicians may likewise elect to limit therapy because of an underlying poor prognosis. Although in many situations this is an appropriate response to severe underlying disease, this limitation in care frequently poses ethical dilemmas for AIDS care providers.

The medical complexities of the diseases caused by HIV infection are reflected in the administrative burden of coordinating the involvement of relevant health professionals. At San Francisco General Hospital, for example, AIDS clinical research is being conducted by at least seven divisions within the department of internal medicine (oncology, AIDS, infectious disease, gastroenterology, nephrology, endocrine, pulmonary), as well as many other departments, including psychiatry, pediatrics, obstetrics and gynecology, epidemiology and international health, surgery, microbiology, and biochemistry. Although such involvement is understandable and encouraging from the perspective of our understanding this disease, it does require that hospitals and medical centers develop some means of coordinating care and clinical research.

It has seemed important to us at San Francisco General Hospital to deliver care to the fullest possible spectrum of HIV exposure backgrounds and to patients with all stages of HIV disease. To these ends, novel changes are being initiated. For example, the AIDS clinic staff is providing care for HIV-infected clients in the methadone maintenance clinic. Also, because patients with early HIV disease (those still asymptomatic) are still employed, we are opening evening clinic hours. In these and similar ways we seek to keep AIDS clinic providers most current in the aspects of the epidemic that are changing most rapidly.[3,10,14]

PSYCHOSOCIAL NEEDS IN AIDS

In addition to the medical and administrative complexities in AIDS care as discussed, patients have clear and often nearly overwhelming psychosocial needs. Patients with AIDS and HIV infection are commonly young and have limited experience in dealing with medical insurance policies. In fact, many HIV-infected persons, because of their recent entrance into the labor force, are employed by small companies with limited health care benefits or none at all. Thus financial assistance in the form of reviewing insurance status and processing applications for additional coverage are often paramount early in the patient's disease course. With advancing disease, issues of housing and personal assistance may become at least as large a source of concern to the patient as the medical problems. Patients with AIDS are often evicted from housing or forced by reasons of economy or convenience to change their residence during their illness. Patients with AIDS, facing the loss of intellectual capacity and mobility caused by HIV-associated illnesses, may require assistance in such activities as housecleaning and shopping to remain in a community-based environment.

COUNSELING SERVICES

Counseling is also important for patients with HIV infection.[1] Although such patients may require a variety of counseling services during the course of their illness, the most important points are services required at the time of diagnosis and those required as patients enter the terminal phase. Early in the disease course, nonprofessional counseling is often most effective and appropriate. In many cases this remains true as the disease accelerates, although more intensive and individualized approaches may also be required, as may prescription of psychotropic medications. For these reasons we have found it important to have a support staff that can assess the need for and provide aid ranging from the concrete to psychiatric and both nonprofessional and professional psychotherapeutic assistance.

STRESS IN AIDS CARE PROVIDERS

Health professionals who care for AIDS patients experience enormous personal stress. This stress arises from a number of sources, including the medical complexity of the disease, the stigma of AIDS, and AIDS risk behaviors. Other factors contributing to the stress are that AIDS patients are often disfigured by the disease, that they are young, and that death from AIDS often appears inevitable to both the patient and the physician. In many organizations those who provide AIDS care are relatively isolated from their colleagues and peers and receive little external recognition for their efforts.

Several approaches to reducing the stress in AIDS care providers can be considered. Organizations should consider providing staffing levels for AIDS adequate to the acuity level as well as to the patient volume. Health professionals, including physicians, nurses, and others, may require more flexible schedules or a smaller proportion of time involved in the direct provision of AIDS care to reduce accumulated AIDS stress. In addition, physicians and other health professionals should be encouraged to discuss issues of grief and loss in a safe environment. At San Francisco General

Hospital we have begun small meetings of AIDS clinic personnel in a group therapy format to approach some of these issues and have found the experience to be extremely rewarding.

Even after administrative and organizational attempts to reduce stress are made, stress should be expected to continue. Organizations should anticipate a higher than average staff turnover. This should, in general, not be considered to represent administrative weakness but rather to reflect unavoidable and chronic stress. In addition to the concerns of direct providers of AIDS care, concern can be anticipated from other hospital staff. Often this concern is stated in the general question "Why are we getting involved in AIDS?" This concern, often an expression of fear, can be controlled by an aggressive program of education. All staff members should be included in a regular program of education conducted on a repeating basis to reinforce the information and to update it as understanding of the HIV infection changes. Because much of the fear is of occupational transmission, surgeons and nurses, the professionals most likely to receive occupational injuries, should be invited to participate at all levels of the development of educational programs and infection control policies. Hospitals must develop a comprehensive and clearly stated set of policies regarding AIDS, which include infection control aspects, the ethical response and professional responsibility to care for AIDS patients, and guidelines for testing in the hospital setting. These guidelines developed in conjunction with input from surgery and nursing staff members should be widely communicated in writing to minimize the frequent misconception that fear of occupational infection with HIV has not been addressed at the administrative level.

Fear from non-AIDS patients in the hospital must also be considered, as they recognize that AIDS patients are in the hospital and may also be concerned that this will put them at risk for infection with HIV or associated infections.[4] The lack of risk to other patients must be stressed along with a clear statement that AIDS patients are in need of medical care and that policies ensuring the safety of other patients have been addressed and enforced. This education of non-AIDS patients should also stress the positive advantages of newer methods of infection control that help protect them from non-AIDS-related nosocomial infections at least as much as from HIV-associated problems (see Chapter 4).

STRATEGIES FOR ORGANIZING AIDS CARE

AIDS presents a unique set of problems that require a fresh look at the organization of medical services. Most AIDS patients require the services of many medical subspecialties, especially infectious disease, oncology, and pulmonary medicine, at some point in their disease course. If the case volume warrants it, a hospital may benefit from bringing these subspecialties together in a dedicated AIDS outpatient facility. If the volume or the medical structure does not permit this, another approach is to formalize a network of relevant disciplines to minimize miscommunication and duplication of clinic visits and laboratory testing.

Along with subspecialists, generalists in both internal medicine and family practice can be effectively used in the care of patients with AIDS. The medical problems of AIDS patients, although complex, are somewhat predictable. Between acute episodes, when medical subspecialists may be required, the bulk of AIDS care can, and perhaps should, be delivered by a physician with a more general orientation. To be most effective, these generalists must be given additional training and clinical experience with AIDS and recognition of the importance of their role by the hospital or medical center.

A system of AIDS care must also include social services, both counseling and financial assistance, for the reasons described. The precise nature of these services and background of the disciplines involved (clinical psychology, psychiatry, or social work) may vary considerably from hospital to hospital. These staff members, in addition to providing the aforementioned services, should be prepared to work with the physicians to minimize the problems of obtaining experimental drugs and reimbursement for their use.

A final important component for the organization of AIDS care concerns the many ethical dilemmas that can be anticipated. Issues of patients' competency to consent to medical care, given HIV dementia, and the extent to which care should be continued in the face of terminal disease make the establishment and active use of a medical ethics committee essential. This committee should be invited to participate actively in regular conferences regarding patient care and to assist in evaluation in specific cases. It should be urged to provide a practical response to ethical problems in the hope that the AIDS provider staff members will gradually become more skilled in addressing these often uncomfortable situations and preventing them from developing.

CONTROLLING THE COST OF AIDS CARE

AIDS patients require the complete set of services anticipated for any patient group with a difficult, progressive, and ultimately fatal disease. This includes treatment in a hospital's acute care unit and outpatient facilities, community-based services, and some acute and extended care. The cost of AIDS care has been estimated to be $50,000 to $150,000 from diagnosis to death.[6,11,12] Most estimates are still crude and may vary considerably among regions and patient groups. Our experience in San Francisco suggests that a well-conceived system of medical care for AIDS, with a focus as described on community-based services, can reduce these costs. At San

Francisco General Hospital, we have, for example, found that our lifetime medical cost for AIDS patients is approximately $50,000.[11] We have achieved this by intentionally reducing the average length of stay for AIDS patients and by assembling community-based services that can deliver comprehensive yet cost-effective care, which, moreover, our patients prefer over hospitalization for acute care.

One way that AIDS costs have been unexpectedly reduced at San Francisco General Hospital concerns the use of intensive care facilities. Although we have never explicitly attempted to limit the use of intensive care for patients with AIDS, we have found that a more aggressive program of education about the outcome of ventilator support has caused fewer patients to request this form of treatment. A survey of our experience showed that only 10 to 15 percent of patients given ventilator support survived that hospitalization. When our patients were informed of this, the majority declined this intervention, and despite an increasing census in the hospital, we have seen a decrease in intensive care admissions.[15] The wisdom at this approach is underscored by reports that more selective initiation of ventilator support increases survival rates in intensive care units.[8]

Reducing the rate and duration of hospitalization is the principal means of controlling AIDS cost. To do this, we must closely examine outpatient services and facilities. Outpatient transfusions, antibiotics, and chemotherpeutic infusions are obvious ways to reduce hospitalizations; more aggressive outpatient management of *Pneumocystis carinii* pneumonia, the most common opportunistic infection in AIDS, also is critical. Outpatient therapy for *P. carinii* pneumonia has been more possible since the development of regimens of oral trimethoprim-sulfamethoxasole and of a combination of dapsone and trimethoprim. Many investigators are exploring the use of aerosolized pentamidine for the outpatient management of acute *P. carinii* pneumonia. Similar attempts in outpatient therapy for cryptococcal meningitis with amphotericin B or fluconazole, and for cytomegalovirus-associated retinitis with ganciclovir and foscarnet are also worth considering.

In summary, several steps can be used to control the cost of AIDS. Hospitals and medical centers can develop systems that concentrate service as the volume of AIDS patients allows and that focus on outpatient and community-based care. Hospitals should closely monitor the use of intensive care and educate patients and staff to reduce this expensive and frequently unneeded medical treatment. Hospitals can maximize their use of community-based care by explicitly inviting community organizations to participate in the establishment of AIDS care systems, in some cases as full-time staff members within the hospital. Finally, as the medical center is able to shift more care to the outpatient setting, it must seek reimbursement for these services, which may require staff members specifically devoted to this activity.

The impact of AIDS can be further limited by public and private hospitals working together to ensure that the burden of AIDS care is well distributed rather than being unfairly concentrated at one or a small number of facilities. In all facilities, criteria of effectiveness, such as average length of stay and use of intensive care, should be monitored and reported regularly to hospital administrators. Finally, the increased use of physician extenders, such as nurse practitioners and physician's assistants, may prove valuable in controlling the impact of AIDS on the physician and community.

THE POSITIVE SIDE OF AIDS CARE

AIDS patients are often young, well educated about their disease, and extremely compliant with their medical care. Furthermore, they are often extremely appreciative of expert care that is both comprehensive and socially sensitive. AIDS is at the cutting edge of many issues central to medicine and society, and working directly with AIDS patients allows the medical system to participate in a vital debate, which may well change the face of American medicine for decades to come. The final and most obvious reason for physicians and medical systems to become more involved in AIDS care is the clear need of all HIV-infected patients for expert, comprehensive, and efficient care. Given the long tradition of response to these issues in the setting of other diseases, a similar response from the medical system to this epidemic is expected.

REFERENCES

1. Abrams DI, Dilley WJ, Maxey LM, et al: Routine care and psychosocial support of the patient with acquired immunodeficiency syndrome. Med Clin North Am 70:707-720, 1986
2. Felsenstein D, D'Amico DJ, Hirsch MS, et al: Treatment of cytomegalovirus retinitus with 9-[2-hydroxy-1-(hydroxy-methyl) ethoxymethyl] guanine. Ann Intern Med 103:377-380,1985
3. Francis DP, Anderson RE, Gorman ME, et al: Targeting AIDS prevention and treatment toward HIV-1-infected persons: The concept of early intervention. (Special Communication.) JAMA 262:2572-2576, 1989
4. Gerbert B, Maguire BT, Hulley SB, et al: Physicians and acquired immunodeficiency syndrome: What patients think about human immunodeficiency virus in medical practice. JAMA 262:1969-1972, 1989
5. Gordin FM, Simon GL, Wofsy CB, et al: Adverse reactions to trimethoprim-sulfamethoxazole in patients with the acquired immunodeficiency syndrome. Ann Intern Med 100:495-499, 1984
6. Hardy A, Rausch K, Echenberg DF, et al: The economic impact of the first 10,000 cases of AIDS in the United States. JAMA 225:209-211, 1986
7. Jaffe HS, Abrams DI, Ammann AJ, et al: Complications of co-trimoxazole in treatment of AIDS-associated *Pneumocystis carinii* pneumonia in homosexual men. Lancet 2:1109, 1983
8. Luce JM, Wachter RM: Intensive care for patients with the acquired immune deficiency syndrome. Intensive Care Med 15:481-482, 1989
9. Mitsuyasu R, Groopman J, Volberding P: Cutaneous reaction to trimethoprim-sulfa-

methoxazole in patients with AIDS and Kaposi's sarcoma. (Letter.) N Engl J Med 308:1535-1536, 1983

10. Rhame F, Maki D: The case for wider use of testing for HIV infection. N Engl J Med 11:1248-1254, 1989

11. Scitovsky AA, Rice DP, Showstack J, et al: Estimating the direct and indirect economic costs of the acquired immunodeficiency syndrome 1985, 1986 and 1990. Task order 282-85-0061, No 2, 1986. Atlanta, Centers for Disease Control

12. Seidman RL, Williams SJ, Mortensen LM: Assessing the economic impact of AIDS in local communities: Current and projected costs for San Diego County. West J Med 151:467-471, 1989

13. Steinbrook R, Lo B, Tirpack J, et al: Ethical dilemmas in caring for patients with the acquired immunodeficiency syndrome. Ann Intern Med 103:787-790, 1985

14. Volberding PA: HIV infection as a disease: The medical indications for early diagnosis. (Editorial.) J AIDS 2:421-425, 1989

15. Wachter RM, Luce J, Lo B, et al: Life-sustaining treatment for patients with AIDS. Chest 95:647-652, 1989

26

LEGAL RAMIFICATIONS FROM AIDS*

PAULA JESSON, JD

This chapter follows a physician—let's call him Dr. Good—through several incidents that illustrate the need for physicians to be aware of the laws relating to HIV testing, the disclosure of test results, and other HIV-and AIDS-related issues. The discussion of these incidents is based on California law as of December 1989.

Dr. Good's practice has been confined to a geographical area that has no special laws relating to AIDS or HIV. He has moved to California and has heard people refer to the state's various laws regarding AIDS and HIV. He is sure that he can learn these laws quickly. He feels confident that they are based on common sense and a reasoned balance among the needs of physician, patient, and society. If he needs assistance, he plans to rely on the instruction and advice of his sister Ms. Cautious, who is a lawyer. She has promised to be available by phone if questions arise.

DISCLOSURE TO SEXUAL AND NEEDLE-SHARING PARTNERS; INFORMED CONSENT TO TEST

Dr. Good's first patient is a young bisexual man who is worried that he may be infected with HIV. He informs Dr. Good that he has a sexual relationship with Ms. X. The patient tells Dr. Good that if he is infected, he does not want Ms. X to know. The patient reveals that Ms. X is unaware of the high-risk sexual encounters he has with others.

In Dr. Good's opinion this patient should be tested so that his medical status can be accurately evaluated and monitored. Dr. Good is also con-

---

*This chapter does not present legal advice in regard to particular situations. For advice about specific circumstances, a lawyer should be consulted.

cerned that Ms. X be made aware of her risk of infection from her relationship with the patient. He would like to know whether he can tell Ms. X about the patient's HIV status. He is also concerned that he understand what information should be conveyed to the patient to ensure that any consent for the test is "informed." Dr. Good excuses himself in the midst of this visit and makes a quick phone call to his sister.

Ms. Cautious tells Dr. Good that a physician may disclose HIV test result information to a spouse and to sex and needle-sharing partners if the physician complies with these requirements:

1. The patient is under the physician's care.

2. The physician has a confirmed positive test.

3. The third party is reasonably believed to be a spouse or sexual or needle-sharing partner.

4. The disclosure is made for the purpose of interrupting the chain of transmission or for diagnosis, care, and treatment of the third party.

5. Before disclosing the results, the physician
    a. Discusses the test results with the patient
    b. Offers appropriate educational and psychological counseling (including ways to avoid infecting others)
    c. Attempts to get the patient to consent voluntarily to the disclosure
    d. Notifies the patient before he or she makes the disclosure
    e. Does not disclose identifying information regarding the patient
    f. Sees that the third party is provided with appropriate care, counseling, and follow-up

The physician may, rather than disclosing the information directly, notify the county health officer, who can make the disclosure. The county health officer is not permitted to identify the physician who reported the information.

Dr. Good wonders whether he should inform the patient before obtaining his consent to the test that the results may be subject to disclosure to Ms. X. If the patient knows that the test results can be disclosed to Ms. X, he is likely not to have the test or simply to go elsewhere for it and not disclose his relationship to Ms. X.

Ms. Cautious informs Dr. Good that patients considering the HIV test generally should be provided with both medical and nonmedical information that may affect their decision. For example, the physician should warn that a potential for discrimination by employers and insurers exists if they discover the results of a positive test.

Ms. Cautious believes that since this patient has revealed to Dr. Good his concern that Ms. X not be informed of his test results, Dr. Good should disclose that she might be told of the results. If Dr. Good has the test done on the patient without telling him of the possibility of such disclosure and thereafter discloses the information to Ms. X over the patient's objection, the physician could be subject to a claim that he tested the patient without obtaining fully informed consent or a claim of misrepresentation based on his failure to disclose an obviously material fact of which the patient was unaware.

What if the patient had had the test done at an anonymous test site and reported to Dr. Good the fact that he was HIV positive? Could Dr. Good disclose this information to Ms. X? No. The statute requires a confirmed positive test before a physician may disclose the results to a third party. The physician should receive confirmation of the test results and not rely on the patient's own reporting.

What if Ms. X was aware that Dr. Good was her partner's regular physician? Remember that the physician who makes the disclosure may not disclose identifying information regarding the patient. In this situation Ms. X might know that Dr. Good is talking about her partner when he warns of her risk of infection simply because he is her partner's physician. In this situation Dr. Good should inform the county health officer so that someone else can make the disclosure.

Is Dr. Good obligated to disclose the test results to Ms. X if they are positive? No. The law protects a physician from civil or criminal liability if he or she chooses to disclose the information but does not impose a duty to disclose.

Dr. Good returns to the patient and fully discusses with him the advantages and disadvantages of taking the HIV test, as well as the dangers of infecting others. The patient decides to think about it some more.

TESTING AFTER POSSIBLE INFECTION OF A HEALTH WORKER; RECORDING RESULTS IN MEDICAL RECORD; PENALTIES FOR PROHIBITED DISCLOSURE

Dr. Good is now ready to see his second patient. Unfortunately, during this visit Dr. Good suffers a needlestick injury with a needle that has just been used on the patient. He is alarmed at the thought that he may have just been infected. He would like to have the patient's blood tested. He already has two blood samples that could be used for this purpose. Nervously, he calls his sister for advice.

As he feared, Ms. Cautious reminds him that he cannot test the patient's blood without the patient's informed consent. Does he need to get written consent? Since California's law was changed in 1988, a physician treating a patient does not need to obtain written consent to the HIV test. However, the physician still must obtain informed consent. Getting it in writing is good protection against a later claim that the patient did not consent, particularly in this instance in which the test is being done for physician's benefit. Dr. Good fully explains the situation and his concerns to the patient, who willingly consents.

Dr. Good later receives the good news that test results are negative. He assumes that the results of the test should be placed in the patient's medical record. In fact, it is inconceivable to him that they would not be included in the record. However, to be on the safe side, he consults his sister.

Ms. Cautious tells him that before 1988 there was some concern that the inclusion of HIV test results in the medical record could be considered an unauthorized disclosure. This is because the statute prohibited disclosure "to any third party" without defining who "third parties" were. Some worried that a nurse or even another consulting physician might be considered a "third party" and that disclosing the test results to them could be considered unlawful.

The law was changed in 1988 to specify that the placing of the test results in the medical record by the physician who ordered the test is not a prohibited "disclosure." Other changes at the same time made clear that the results could be shared with other physicians and health care workers directly involved in the patient's care.

Notwithstanding this welcome clarification, a danger remains regarding placement of the test results in the patient's record. HIV test results may not be released without written authorization meeting certain requirements, including a separate authorization for each disclosure. If the patient requests the release of general medical information but does not provide authorization for release of the HIV results meeting these requirements, there is a risk that the protected information will mistakenly be copied and sent along with the rest of the medical record. One solution to this problem is to place the results in a separate part of the medical record. This enables medical records personnel to be sure that the results are not unintentionally copied when the record is disclosed pursuant to routine requests for medical information by third parties, such as insurance companies.

Other questions arise regarding references to HIV status in the medical record. What happens if the patient himself tells the physician that he is infected? May the physician record this information in the medical record? What about a reference to the fact that the physician intends to order the test for the patient?

California law protects the "*results* of a blood test to detect antibodies to the probable causative agent of acquired immune deficiency syndrome." This language is probably broad enough to cover a patient's statement to the effect that he has had the test and it is positive or negative. The reference to the test being performed is a harder question. It does not fall within the language of the statute. The statute protects the *results* of the test only. However, the information is still sensitive enough that the safest course of action is to treat it in the same manner as the test results.

What are the penalties if the HIV test results are disclosed without authorization? The penalties for the *negligent* disclosure of test results include a civil penalty (paid to the patient) of up to $1000 plus court costs. In addition, if the patient claims economic, bodily, or psychological harm, the physician may be liable for these damages and may be guilty of a misdemeanor (imprisonment for up to 1 year or a fine not to exceed $10,000 or both). *Intentional* disclosures carry the same penalties, except that the civil penalty may be up to $5000 instead of $1000.

TESTING OF INCOMPETENT PATIENTS

Dr. Good's third patient is a married woman who has been in a coma for 6 months. Dr. Good believes that she may have been at risk of infection before she went into the coma and that knowing her HIV status would be helpful in deciding her course of treatment. Dr. Good knows that he must obtain informed consent to test her but is uncertain who may consent on behalf of this patient. Her husband's whereabouts are unknown. Her mother has been actively involved in her care and says that the patient and her husband had an off-again on-again relationship before she became unconscious, and it is unclear when he is likely to appear on the scene again. The mother is fully agreeable to consenting to the test if that will help. Dr. Good puts in a call to his sister.

Ms. Cautious tells her brother that California law concerning incompetent patients provides that "written consent for the test may be obtained from the [patient's] parents, guardians, conservators, or other person lawfully authorized to make health care decisions for the subject." Is the mother a "parent" within the meaning of this section? Or does "parent" here mean the parent of a minor? The law is not entirely clear. Comparison with other laws on parental consent supports the argument that parents of both adults and minors may consent. However, in light of the uncertainty, the safer interpretation is that it permits parental consent for minors only, not adults.

Is the mother a person "lawfully authorized to make health care decisions for the subject?" Again, it is not entirely clear. She has no specific statutory authorization to make health care decisions on behalf of her adult child. However, court decisions have recognized the right of the immediate family to make health care decisions for incompetent patients under certain circumstances. Arguably, these decisions provide "lawful authorization" for the mother to act as surrogate decision maker. Dr. Good recognizes the uncertainty of the situation but decides that he is willing to take the risk so the patient will receive proper treatment.

Surprisingly, Dr. Good's fourth patient is also an adult, married, comatose woman whose mother is the only member of the family available to make health care decisions for the patient. However, knowing the HIV status of this patient will not affect Dr. Good's care of her. The question of testing arises when a nurse providing care for the patient comes into contact with the patient's blood through a needlestick injury. She is distraught and asks Dr. Good whether he can obtain the mother's consent to test the patient. The mother has indicated that she will consent to the test on her daughter's behalf. Dr. Good checks with Ms. Cautious.

Ms. Cautious informs her brother that there is a serious question whether anyone may consent to the HIV test for an incompetent person when the test is not done to provide care and treatment for the patient. The law states that consent for the testing of incompetent persons can be provided only "when necessary to render appropriate care or to practice preventative measures."

Yes, Dr. Good argues, but what about preventive measures on the nurse's behalf? If the patient is infected, the nurse may decide to take zidovudine. She may also take greater precautions in her intimate relationships to prevent the spread of the infection to others. Ms. Cautious agrees that these arguments can be made. However, it is simply not clear that the relevant language would be construed broadly enough to allow testing for protection of parties other than the patient. Dr. Good decides that the risk is too great and informs the nurse.

TESTING OF CRIMINAL DEFENDANTS: PROPOSITION 96

Dr. Good's final patient is a young woman who has had a work-related injury. She is a deputy sheriff working as a juvenile court bailiff during custody proceedings. A woman who had been attending a hearing regarding her child became upset and disruptive. After escorting the woman from the courtroom, the deputy had to restrain her physically and in doing so suffered a deep bite on her arm. Dr. Good's patient is worried that she may have been infected with HIV by the bite.

She informs Dr. Good that she may be able to obtain a court order compelling the biter to submit to a blood test for HIV but that she needs Dr. Good's help in the court proceeding. The voters adopted a new law, she tells him, that permits a court-ordered test of a criminal defendant if the defendant transmits a body fluid in the course of an assault that constitutes interference with the official duties of a peace officer. Her attorney has told her, however, that she needs expert medical testimony establishing that knowledge of the biter's HIV status will provide useful information to the deputy and her physician in assessing her chance of contracting HIV infection. The court in particular will want to know whether medical evidence exists that a bite can transmit HIV if only saliva and not blood was transmitted.

This last, rather lengthy example is included because it is currently the subject of a lawsuit. The injury occurred in January 1989 in a San Francisco courtroom. The trial court ordered the blood test, and the Court of Appeal considered the question of the order's constitutionality. This case, like the situations described previously, provides a good example of the difficulties involved in balancing the right of citizens to be free from compelled intrusion into a most personal area of their lives with the right of others, such as health care workers or peace officers, to ascertain the HIV status of those who may have been a source of HIV infection.

The following paragraphs briefly summarize some of the arguments raised on behalf of the biter and the victim in this case. A central issue, of course, was whether HIV can be transmitted by saliva. The medical experts agreed on certain facts: that HIV had been found in saliva in low concentrations and that therefore a theoretical risk of transmission existed. They also agreed that no cases of transmission of HIV through saliva had been documented.

The experts disagreed, however, whether the theoretical risk could be considered a realistic possibility. In testimony submitted on behalf of the biter in opposition to the compelled testing, Dr. Paul Volberding stated, after noting studies on saliva transmission, that "there is no reason to think HIV is transmitted by biting." Dr. Marcus Conant stated that he did not consider the possibility of transmission "in any way real or significant."

In contrast, in testimony submitted by the City of San Francisco on behalf of the deputy, both Dr. Merle Sande and Dr. Julie Gerberding distinguished between the transfer of saliva on intact skin and the transfer via a transcutaneous bite. Dr. Sande said that, "If saliva containing lymphocytes infected by HIV is injected into a puncture wound and comes into contact with the lymphocytes of the victim, it is theoretically possible that the victim could get infected with HIV." He called the possibility of such transmission "highly remote" but noted that "it cannot be said, based on currently available information, that HIV could not be transmitted through a bite." Similarly, Dr. Gerberding stated that, although the risk of such transmission is "clearly low, there is insufficient information to determine precisely how low."

The woman who bit the deputy sheriff argued that she has the right to be free from unreasonable invasions into her privacy and unreasonable searches and seizures. She said that compelled testing is unreasonable because the harm to her would be great and no benefit would accrue to the deputy. With respect to the harm to herself, she argued that the physical intrusion of a blood test is a serious invasion of personal privacy. She said that if the results are positive, and that information is disclosed to others, she may suffer substantial discrimination. Moreover, she has the right to refuse medical care and therefore the right *not* to know her HIV status, particularly since learning that one is positive is like receiving a "death sentence."

She also offered several arguments in support of her contention that testing the biter would not benefit the injured deputy. First, there is no realistic possibility of transmission of HIV by the bite; therefore the deputy has no realistic cause for concern. Second, the test provides, at best, inaccurate information and, at worst, misleading information. If the biter has a negative test, that does not necessarily mean that the victim was not infected at the time of the bite. If the test is positive, the victim still does not know whether the bite transmitted the infection. Nor can compelled testing be justified on the grounds that it alleviates the victim's anxiety — a negative test does not establish that she was not infected and therefore should not alleviate her anxiety.

Moreover, the deputy herself has the means of obtaining accurate information. She could have herself tested. It is true that she will not know her HIV status for up to 6 months, but when that time has passed, a test of her own blood will provide accurate information.

In response, the city argued that it had a compelling interest in providing its public safety officers with all available information to assist them and their physicians in ascertaining their medical status and in making life-style decisions relating to their health and that of those close to them. There is debate in the medical community over the risk of infection from saliva by a bite. In light of that debate, the voters may err on the side of caution and adapt a law that provides the injured peace officer with information regarding the potential source of infection. The fact that the test results may be negative even though the biter was infected at the time of the bite does not mean that the information is not useful. Hospitals themselves recognize the value of source testing, albeit on a voluntary basis, to alleviate the anxiety of injured health care workers and to assess the risk to the health care worker and whether azidothymidine or other treatment is appropriate.

This was the first case in the California appellate courts regarding compelled HIV testing. The California Court of Appeal has rendered a decision upholding the validity of Proposition 96 and permitting the compelled testing of the biter of the injured deputy sheriff. At the time this book is going to press, that decision is not yet final and may be appealed.

Proposition 96 is an example of the easing of restrictions on HIV testing and reporting since the California Legislature's adoption of stringent laws in 1985. Laws allowing compelled testing and disclosure have arisen particularly in the context of the criminal justice system. Many concern prisoners, persons convicted of certain crimes such as sex crimes, and even persons accused but not yet convicted.

We have also seen an easing or clarifying of restrictions in the health care setting. The examples considered earlier regarding partner notification and the testing of incompetent patients are laws added in 1987. The partner notification law, which initially allowed disclosure to spouses only, was amended again in 1988 to allow disclosure to sex and needle-sharing partners.

Evidence of the legislative turmoil in this area can be found in the long list of proposed amendments currently under consideration relating to

AIDS, as well as the number of amendments finally enacted, all within the relatively brief period since 1985. In California, which has seen an explosion of the use of the initiative process in the last decade, the legislative dialog occurs at the ballot box as well as in the legislative chambers.

More changes in the law will undoubtedly occur as society continues to assess how best to balance the sometimes competing concerns of those who are infected (or fear infection) and those involved in preventing the spread of infection, and as the medical community's work in understanding the disease continues to advance.

BIBLIOGRAPHY

Arras JD: The fragile web of responsibility: AIDS and the duty to treat. Hastings Center Rep, April/May 1988, pp 10-19

Brennan TA: The acquired immunodeficiency syndrome (AIDS) as an occupational disease. Ann Intern Med 107:581-583, 1987

Goldblum P, Moulton J: AIDS-related suicide: A dilemma for health care providers. Focus 2:1-4, 1986

Greene WH, Gerberding JL, Sande MA: Infection-control policies and AIDS. N Engl J Med 316:1479-1480, 1987

Klein RS, Phelan JA, Freeman K, et al: Low occupational risk of human immunodeficiency virus infection among dental professionals. N Engl J Med 318:86-90, 1988

Lo B, Steinbrook R, Cooke M, et al: Voluntary screening for HIV infection. Ann Intern Med 110:727-733, 1989

Matthews GW, Neslund VS: The initial impact of AIDS on public health law in the United States — 1986. JAMA 257:344-352, 1987

Miller PJ, O'Connell J, Leipold A, et al: Potential liability for transfusion-associated AIDS. JAMA 253:3419-3424, 1985

Mills M, Wofsy CB, Mills J: Special report: The acquired immunodeficiency syndrome; Infection control and public health law. N Engl J Med 314:931-936, 1986

Tashjian VK: The rights of the mentally retarded and mandatory screening for the AIDS virus. JAMA 257:1327-1328, 1987

Turnock BJ, Kelley CJ: Mandatory premarital testing for human immunodeficiency virus: The Illinois experience. JAMA 261:3415-3418, 1989

Wolchok CL: AIDS at the frontier: United States immigration policy. J Legal Med 10:127-142, 1989

Zuger A: Professional responsibilities in the AIDS generation: AIDS on the ward; A residency in medical ethics. Hastings Center Rep 17:16-20, 1987

INDEX

Note: Page numbers in *italics* refer to a figure; page numbers followed by the letter t indicate a table.